A SHORT HISTORY OF OBSTETRICS AND GYNECOLOGY

A SHORT HISTORY OF OBSTETRICS AND GYNECOLOGY

By

THEODORE CIANFRANI, M.D.

Associate Professor of Obstetrics and Gynecology at the Graduate School of Medicine, University of Pennsylvania, Philadelphia, Pennsylvania

CHARLES C THOMAS • PUBLISHER

Springfield • Illinois • U.S.A.

CHARLES C THOMAS • PUBLISHER
BANNERSTONE HOUSE
301-327 East Lawrence Avenue, Springfield, Illinois, U.S.A.

Published simultaneously in the British Commonwealth of Nations by
BLACKWELL SCIENTIFIC PUBLICATIONS, LTD., OXFORD, ENGLAND

Published simultaneously in Canada by
THE RYERSON PRESS, TORONTO

Library of Congress Catalog Card Number: 59-14190

With THOMAS BOOKS careful attention is given to all details of manufacturing and design. It is the Publisher's desire to present books that are satisfactory as to their physical qualities and artistic possibilities and appropriate for their particular use. THOMAS BOOKS will be true to those laws of quality that assure a good name and good will.

Printed in the United States of America

PREFACE

THE NAMES of people who created medicine will be afforded due and proper space in this book, according to their accomplishments. However, we believe that there are other factors necessary for a proper perspective of the history of gynecology and obstetrics, such as a knowledge of social and economic conditions, the geography and the time in which the men lived who made history; in short, the civilization of the period under discussion must be considered in addition to the life of any particular individual. Further, the history of obstetrics and gynecology cannot be divorced from the history of general medicine; therefore, a certain amount of general medical history must be covered, and to this we must add scientific and technical advances such as the discovery of anesthesia, radium and x-ray. They have no direct bearing on our specialty, but are, nevertheless, just as responsible for the progress of obstetrics and gynecology.

Obstetrics, as practiced by physicians rather than midwives, is a young specialty; it is only in recent times that men have taken over the practice of midwifery, in fact the men who pioneered in this field were often subjected to all sorts of embarrassment. Gynecology also is a very young specialty; when it was endeavoring to become a special branch of medicine, many general surgeons ridiculed and abused these efforts. Even to this day he accepts the gynecologist in particular, with reservations. In 1867, Samuel D. Gross wrote, ". . . diseases of the uterus are the fashionable disorders. Not to have an ulcer upon the womb is to be beyond the pale . . . doctors and patients alike have womb on the brain." Again in 1883, at a meeting of the American Gynecological Society, he said, "after six years (the society started its existence in 1876) the gynecological society must certainly have exhausted the field by now. Such a body," he continued, "like all specialties, must work continually in a circle."

There is a graph, in the beginning of this book, from which the progress of obstetrics and gynecology can be followed very simply. From the beginning of recorded history to A.D. 1800, progress is represented by a line that is almost horizontal; actually this line rises almost imperceptibly from its beginning many thousands of years ago to the year A.D. 1800, so minimal was progress in all these years; shortly after the beginning of the 19th Century, 1809, the curve takes an abrupt upward trend, noted in the graph as a forty-five degree upsweep, continuing this course until the middle of the 19th Century. This rise was due to the initiation of gynecological surgery that began with McDowell's performance of ovariotomy. From the middle of the 19th Century to the present time, the line in the graph goes up almost perpendicularly. It will be noted that the greatest advance has come in the years since 1900, shown by a line which is truly perpendicular from 1900 to 1920. This progress is based on the discoveries of anesthesia, bacteriology and pathology in the middle of the 19th Century. For a few years after 1920, we witness a brief lull, then a rise again occurs due to the overenthusiastic use of endocrines, antibiotics and parenteral therapy. Gynecological surgery eased off somewhat; however, some surgery, particularly in malignancies, still received its share of attention. At any rate, obstetrics and gynecology have, at long last, attained their place among the great specialties of medicine.

Some histories are unnecessarily elongated by their anecdotal character, and by too many unauthenticated, bizarre, human interest stories; others are the antithesis of this, that is too concise and factual and therefore difficult to hold the reader's interest. A moderate amount of the unusual component of medical behavior peculiar to the past should be sufficient to support one's interest. It is with this latter point of view in mind that we have proceeded to write "a short history of obstetrics and gynecology."

This book is not a research project; on the contrary, it is, as the name implies, a short history of the subject. It does contain all the important factual data and pertinent information desirable to the average reader, even though the details will be less comprehensive than might be found in a work of reference. The main objective of this presentation is to convey a panoramic view of obstetrics and gynecology, from its inception to the present time, and it is hoped that the brevity of the material will, in some measure, be compensated by the numerous illustrations.

Graph Showing Progress Of Obstetrics And Gynecology

a speculum
b first cesarean
c sounds
d microscope
e forceps
f ovariotomy
g ovum
h lull in progress
i anesthesia
j bacteriology
k vesico-vaginal fistula
l cellular pathology
m mid-19th century (i, j, k, l)
n radiotherapy
o greatest advance
p some endocrines
q menstrual cycle
r lull in advance
s endocrines and antibiotics
t mass literature

(details on following pages)

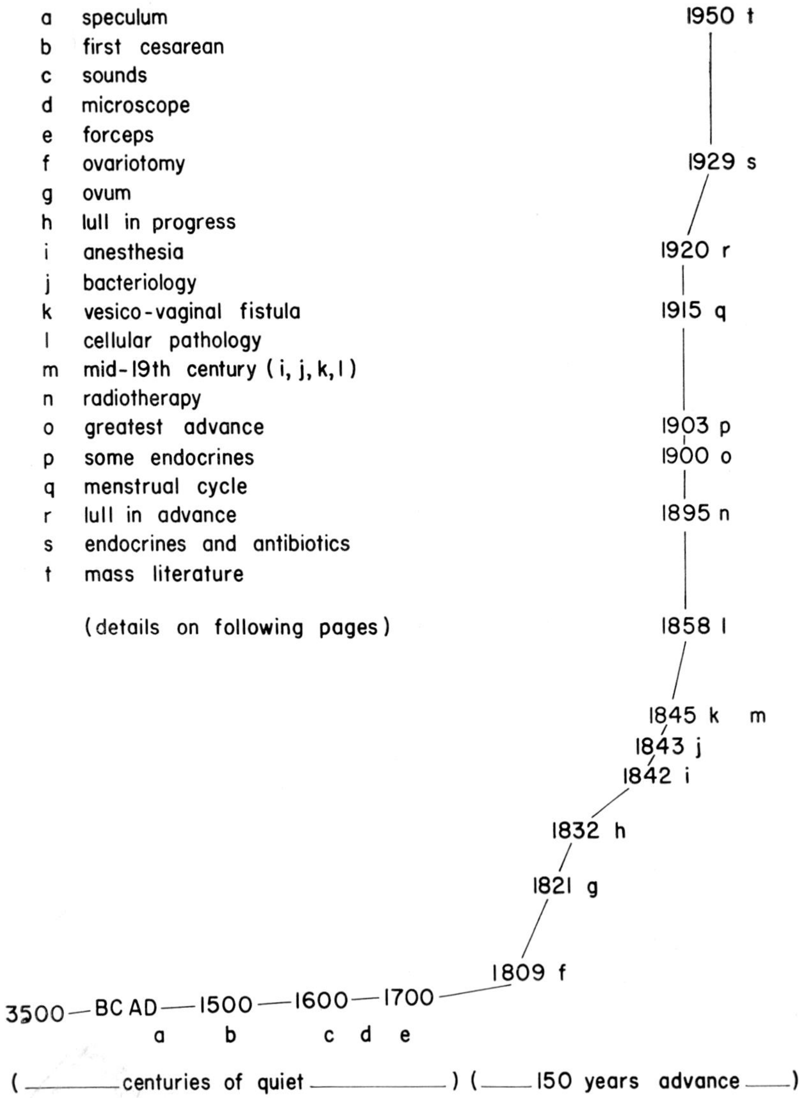

DETAILS OF PROGRESS

a. Speculum	Hebrews, definite record of its use, 2nd Century. Ancients (some Egyptians to Hippocrates), 1500 B.C. to A.D. 500. Sims, 1845.
b. First Cesarean	Jacob Nufer, A.D. 1500, on wife. Christofer Bain, A.D. 1540, in Italy. Trautmann, A.D. 1610, Wittenberg, the first such operation actually recorded. John L. Richmond, A.D. 1827, America.
c. Sounds	Wierus, 1657, for exploration, as our modern sounds. Ancients (Egyptians), 3500 B.C. to A.D. 500 for medication and probing. Simpson, 1843.
d. Microscope	Leeuwenhoek, 16th to 17th Century. Beginning of real great change in medicine. Believed in spontaneous generation. Studied the sperm, said father alone begot child, uterus only an incubator. Started cult of spermatacists.
e. Forceps	Chamberlen, Peter I, invented the forceps circa 1598. Chapman in 1733 divulged the "secret" of the forceps.
f. Ovariotomy	McDowell, 1809, first (with European confreres), abdominal approach to gynecology.

g. Ovum	William Bayer, Leipsic, 1821, or thereabouts. First to report seeing a human ovum.
h. Lull in Progress	1832-1842 quiet. Flush of advance due to abdominal approach reached its peak in 1832, then followed a period of quiet until 1842 when advance began anew as a result of discoveries of the mid-19th Century.
i. Anesthesia	Long, 1842, ether, Georgia. Morton, 1846, (dentist), ether, Massachusetts General Hospital. Simpson, 1847, chloroform, England. (Sir Humphry Davy, 1800, discovered nitrous oxide. Faraday, 1818, worked on inhalation of ether—same effects as nitrous oxide. Horace Wells, 1844, tooth extracted under nitrous oxide.)
j. Bacteriology	Pasteur, 1860, streptococcus (worked 1843 to 1867). Lister, 1867, antisepsis in surgery, based on Pasteur. (Both Pasteur and Lister had scientific basis; streptococcus). Holmes, 1843, and later. Childbed fever. Contagion. Semmelweis, 1860, published *Aetiologie*, began in 1847. (Both Holmes and Semmelweis used clinical approach; they deduced that infected material was the cause.)
k. Vesico-vaginal Fistula	Sims, 1845.
l. Cellular Pathology	Virchow, 1858.
m. Mid-19th Century	Newest and greatest discoveries (i, j, k, l). Transition period from blind empiricism to scientific knowledge of pathologic processes.

n. Radiotherapy	Roentgen, 1895, discovered x-rays. The Curies, 1898, discovered radium. (Pusey and Pfahler, Philadelphia, were the first to apply x-ray treatment to cancer of uterus.)
o. Greatest Advance	1900, the result of discoveries of the 19th Century.
p. Some Endocrines	Fraenkel, 1903, beginning of endocrine consciousness.
q. Menstrual Cycle	Schroeder, 1915, new concepts of shedding of mucous membrane and the menstrual cycle.
r. Lull in Advance	1920 to 1929 quiet. The surgical age, the era of greatest expansion subsided by 1920. Technical processes firmly established and standardized. Indications for major surgery denounced. Gynecology seemed to have reached a static phase—continuing thusly until 1929.
s. Endocrines and Antibiotics	1929, sudden burst of endocrines and, later, antibiotics. Result was another resurgence of gynecology, which continues to this day.
t. Mass Literature	1950, age of mass literature, which is concerned mainly with improvements and refinements in techniques—results of blood, antibiotics, endocrines, x-rays and radium and all other basic discoveries of the recent past.

CONTENTS

A SHORT HISTORY OF OBSTETRICS AND GYNECOLOGY

Chapter I

PRIMITIVE

A. OBSTETRICS AND GYNECOLOGY OF ABORIGINAL PEOPLE

PRIMITIVE MEDICINE undoubtedly was born of instinct. In the beginning man found food instinctively, and most likely found drugs in the same way. Just as the body craves food, it craves drugs which, at first, may be food, but, when overeaten, become a drug, such as the fruit of the fig tree. Even in this day some pregnant women have been seen eating whitewash from walls, because the body craves calcium especially during pregnancy. So it can be said that dietetic and pharmacological therapy was born of instinct; eventually man became conscious of his knowledge of foods and drugs, extended it and passed it on from father to son, or mother to daughter. They added hygiene, because, like animals, it was instinctive to wash or bathe in rivers or lakes to fight against parasites. Surgery, too, started instinctively, such as the removal of a thorn. Self-help came first, then mutual aid followed; even animals delouse one another instinctively.[1]

The practices of primitive peoples have changed little during their entire existence. Apparently the primitive mind is of a fairly uniform character, the customs, folklore and folk medicine and other aspects of culture, which are remarkably alike under various conditions of time and place, are related directly to fundamental instincts. The primitive mind is so basic that it is fair to assume that the behavior of prehistoric man was not too different from the behavior of primitive tribes today.[2] So, in a sense, primitive medicine is a key

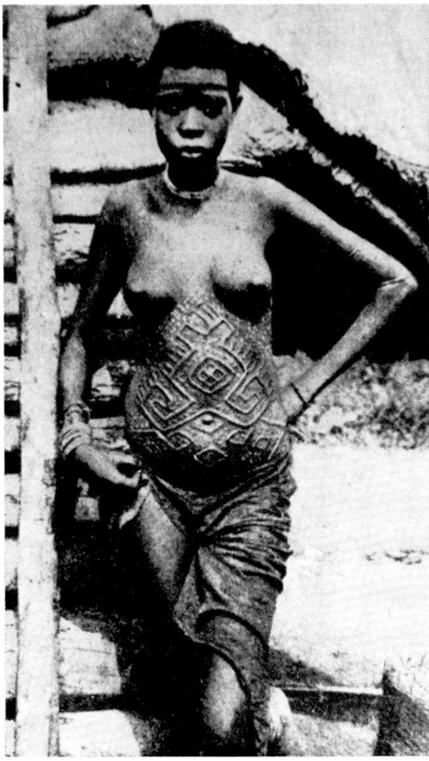

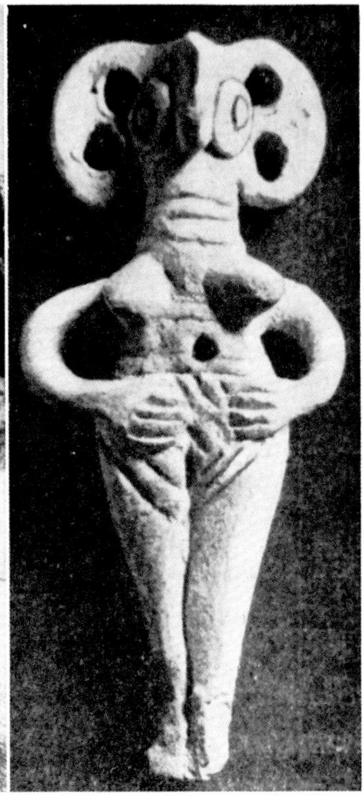

Fig. 1. Native of French Congo with "scarifications sexuelles." (Chauvet, Stephen: *Les Peuples Primitifs* [Prehistoriques et contemporanis]. Paris, Librairie Maloine, 1936.)

Fig. 2. Statuette found about 2000 B.C. "scarifications sexuelles." (Chauvet, Stephen: *Les Peuples Primitifs* [Prehistoriques et contemporanis]. Paris, Librairie Maloine, 1936.)

to our knowledge of prehistoric medicine. This similarity can be noted in the parallel of the "Congo Woman" and the Egyptian "Statuette with Striae."

The picture of the Congo native girl taken in recent times and the statuette made long before 2000 B.C. both show striae of the abdomen (a design of stripes) which in some way is related to the sex life of these individuals. This excellent analogy also shows the fundamental instincts of man regardless of time or race. A number of other such instances have been reported.[3]

The philosophy of primitive medicine is well expressed by Harley in his studies of African tribes, and the Mano people in particular.

He says that primitive man believes that everything animate or inanimate has a sort of spirit power within it; man, beast, tree, stone and even lightning and other natural phenomena are personified in a vague way. To him the struggle for existence between all creatures, including plants and even stones, is a very real struggle, each individual holding its place by some innate strength of personality.

Any substance whose power is under control or known to be controllable is called medicine ("nye" by the African natives). Any method of controlling that power is spoken of as "making medicine." The majority of medicines are directed toward the cure and prevention of disease. To the primitive mind disease is caused by external forces, which are considered unnatural and abnormal and not understood. Also, illness may be the result of an act of malignity produced by the use of "nye" (actual drugs or magic), and, if ordinary and understood, they do not consider it due to witchcraft, but the rare and stubborn cases are explained by the old theory of witchcraft. In fact, anything they cannot explain, they look for in the unknown, what we would call the supernatural. An interesting practice among the GIO people (East Africa) is a direct appeal to the spirits for aid at childbirth. The spirit mask of a late midwife is prayed to, then placed at the foot of the bed of the expectant mother, washed with herbal waters which are afterward rubbed on the woman's abdomen, and finally "thanked" with a suitable sacrifice for a favorable outcome.

To them, death, if it follows upon sickness, is the result of another and separate act not necessarily emanating from the same source. In other words, death is not the natural termination of sickness that preceded it. As an example of death caused by the direct result of some evil power exerted by human or divine agency we have the traditions, as to the origin of death, of the Wachagga, a tribe of the Kilimanjaro district of Africa. They believe mortality is the result of, and the punishment for, the disobedience of man in eating the fruit of a certain tree that the supreme god had forbidden. While the deity had given mankind the liberty to enjoy the fruits of all other kinds, disobedience to divine commands resulted in the offenders and their descendants being doomed to die.

Because they believed that illness resulted from some hidden force (supernatural power) invoked by someone who had made medicine ("nye") against him, successful therapy depended on placation of their gods, by sorcery and witchcraft, diviners, by fetishes and taboos and any other means to influence the supernatural powers.

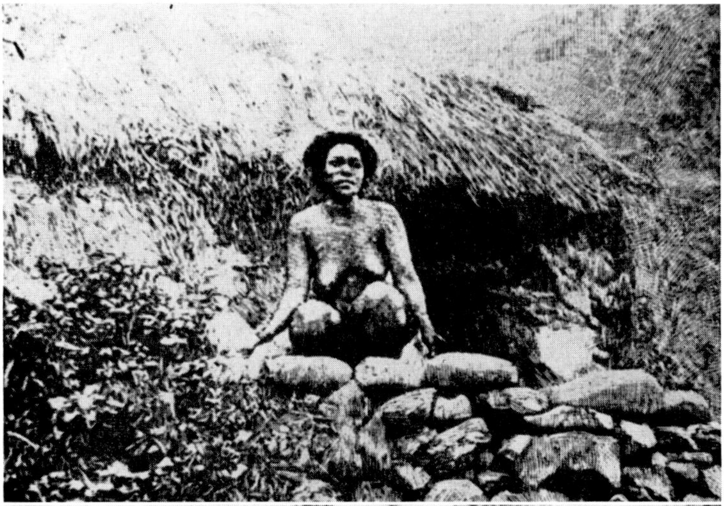

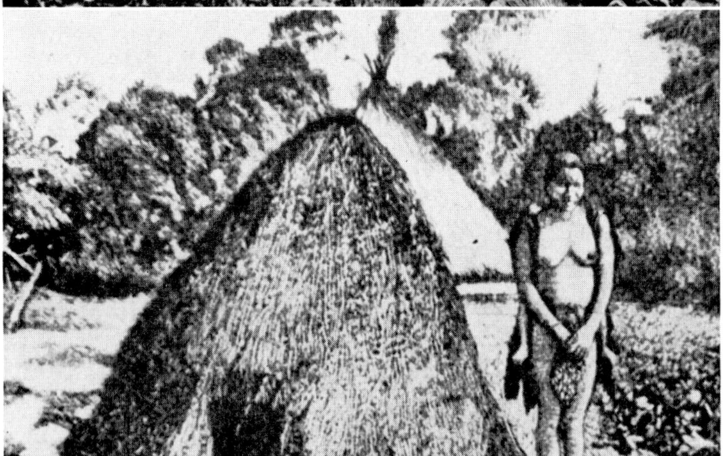

Fig. 3. Young unmarried girl in the Philippine Islands, isolated during her menstrual period. ([Ploss-Bartels] Neufeld and Henius.)

Fig. 4. Birth hut in Ukinga on Lake Nyassa, Africa. ([Ploss-Bartels] Neufeld and Henius.)

One of the taboos of interest is that broken sex taboos are particularly liable to be blamed for illness. If a baby cries a great deal without any demonstrable cause, it is believed that the parents may have had intercourse after pregnancy had been established, which is always taboo. To remove the effects of such an accident, the midwife, "zo," takes a few leaves of an orchid (*Eulophia barteri*), rubs them between her hands, adds a little water, and squeezes the juice into the baby's eyes.

Another taboo was menstruation, an act that purified their bodies of poisonous substances. So menstruating women were confined to special houses and were temporarily taboo. They would remain in a detached hut apart from the family and were carefully screened from roving bands. Menstrual blood was considered poisonous and vile and the cause of numerous disasters, therefore associated with many taboos. An Australian blackfellow discovered that his wife had lain on his blanket while menstruating; he killed her and with justification. To this day the women of certain Australian tribes are forbidden, on pain of death, to touch anything belonging to men. Girls of the Tinneh or Dene tribes, who are nearing their period of maturity, are not permitted to eat from dishes used by anyone else, and when their period appears they are fed by their mothers or near kinsmen. They are not permitted to touch food with their own hands; they may not touch their own heads. Sticks are provided with which they may scratch their backs. They are forbidden to touch venison or any animal lest the hunters fail in the chase. For the very reason that menstrual blood was considered poisonous and vile, the most disgusting remedies were considered the most efficacious to drive out the devils of disease. A similar practice may be noted among the people of the Dark Ages; they considered menstrual blood in the same manner and the most disgusting remedies were thought to be the most efficacious to drive out the spirits of disease, so menstrual blood was prescribed for many diseases, and maidens used it as a love philtre (potion).[5]

As early as Aurignacean times, 25,000 B.C., blood (not menstrual blood) was regarded as the vital fluid which was essential to active existence; this was probably the result of blood loss involved in violent death. This belief explains why blood plays such an important part in the rites of primitive people, and why red objects have ever been associated with blood and with death. The life giving attributes of blood are evident in many customs; thus, among certain Australian tribes, in cases of severe illness, human blood is swallowed as a medicine to impart renewed vitality to the patient. A paste of fat and red clay is rubbed on their bodies by Kaffir women as a "purification" after childbirth. This has also been noted in Tasmania and East Africa.

The practice of medicine by the Manos in Africa illustrates the best of primitive medicine. Each adult Mano native knows at least a few simple remedies which he uses upon himself and his friends. It is the women who know most of the remedies, and the older women act as midwives and carry on the bulk of medical practices. Certain of the men are professional leeches or physicians and they are more likely to know about special treatments. The good remedies are passed on from one generation to another; neighborly interchange of help is customary. A small fee must ensue, lest the medicine be insulted for it's the medicine and not the doctor that counts. They have medicines for genito-urinary diseases, such as urethral discharges and stricture and hematuria, inguinal adenitis and they prescribe aphrodisiacs, e.g. the bark of *neubouldia laevis* rubbed up with white clay and red pepper. The resulting mess is licked by the patient. For dysmenorrhea two large handsful of leaves of *vanilla crenulata* are put into a pot, and brought to a boil. A mat is placed on the floor, covered with a layer of the steaming leaves, and another mat is put down. The patient is made to lie face down on the moist warmth of the mat. Young shoots and fruits of "gnai gba" (*solanum aculeatissimum*) are roasted over the fire in a pouch of leaves. The resulting hot pulp is applied to the woman's abdomen as a poultice. For a powerful diuretic, a quantity of the bark of "bo" (*mitragyna stipulosa*) is beaten, dried and beaten again. The fine powder is sifted through a piece of cloth, and a large spoonful of it taken in water or palm wine. They treat habitual abortion by using an infusion of "longo la" (*ethulia conyzoides*). If the doctor is too far off to give the infusion, the patient herself cooks the leaves and makes the concoction. If the woman already has one child and loses all subsequent pregnancies, she is told to add two buds of "gei yidi" (*erythrina altissima*) to the above. This is probably magical.

Abortifacients are very generally used with apparent safety to the mother, but natives realize that after three months one is no longer entirely free from danger. The root of the cotton yue is used, more often the shrub called "corset leaf" or "wana" (*mareya spica-*

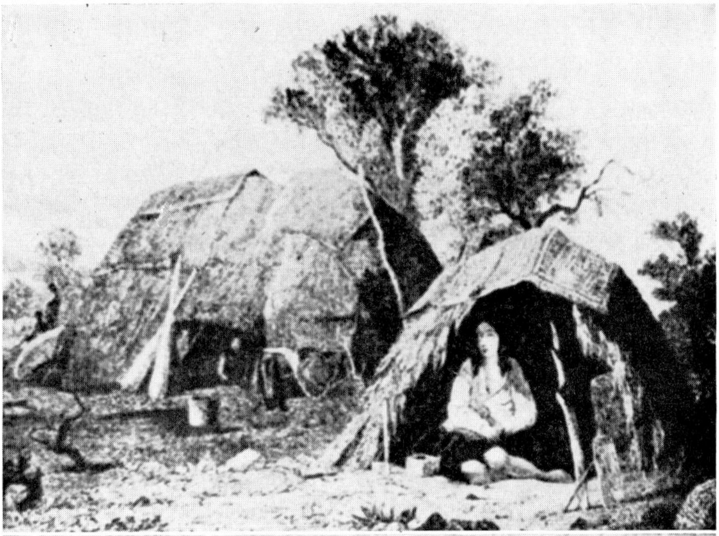

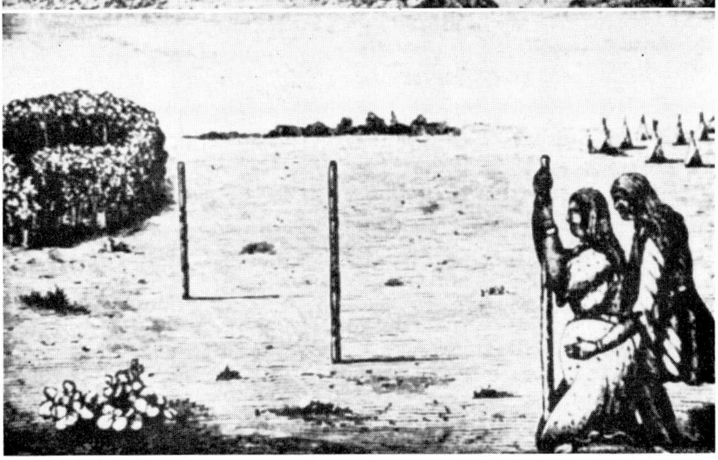

Fig. 5. North American Indian woman in birth hut. ([Ploss-Bartels] Schoolcraft.)

Fig. 6. Birth hut of the Comanche Indians. "The woman grasps the poles as the pains come on, in her journey to the hut." ([Englemann] J. H. Chambers and Co., St. Louis.)

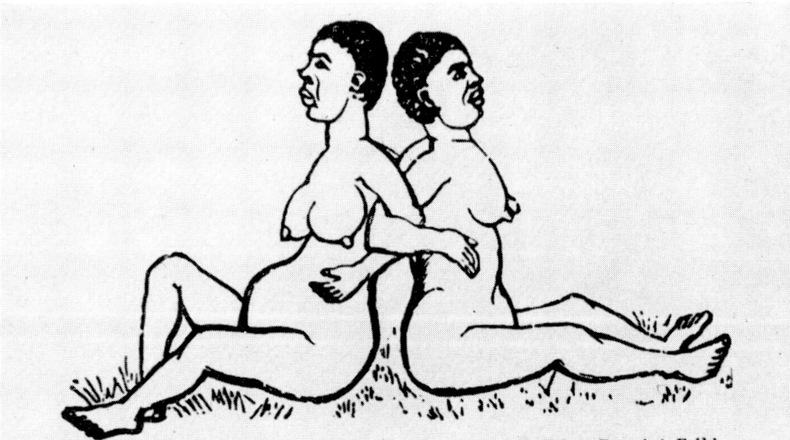

Fig. 7. A Madi Negress of Central Africa supported by another woman while delivering. ([Ploss-Bartels] Felkin.)

ta). The pot used in preparing it is thrown away in order to prevent accidental abortion; even the fumes are dangerous. A pregnant woman will not eat with her neighbors for fear of a jealous wife dropping one of the leaves into her food. The infusion from these leaves acts within a day. It is used for removing the afterbirth and during the postpartum period.

Confinement is usually in the wife's mother's house, rather in the space behind the house. The father sees the baby the next day after the midwife is through and brings her a present. Routine treatment of a woman in labor is remarkably benign in a normal case. In many aboriginal tribes the woman is placed in a hut or cave by herself, and usually assumes the squatting position during her pains and does not cry out for fear of being heard by prowling animals.

In some tribes the lying-in woman is alone in the hut until she is ready to deliver, at which time a big audience presents itself to cheer her up. The Mandingo midwives seem to have a good idea of what not to do. They encourage the patient in labor; if she is having difficulty, the midwife squats before the patient and makes compression and violent motions with her hands on the abdomen, approaching the pubic area from the patient's armpits. If nothing happens a whiff of snuff is used, and this is generally effective. The midwife will try to help the patient by taking her on her back, and walking around with her, shaking her and rolling her around. As the patient is belly down across the back of the other woman, the weight pushing on the uterus is considerable. The cord is tied and cut three inches from the navel. Great care is given to it; it is anointed with some kind of fat.

Usually there is no surgery, only pressure exerted on her abdomen by assistants. Many women kill their offspring by pressing on them or even sitting on them to even grudges they may have against their husbands. If the paternity is doubtful, a midwife often

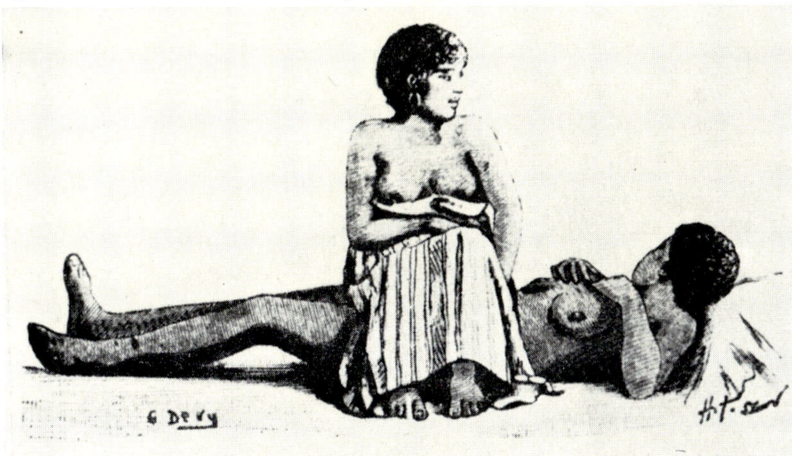

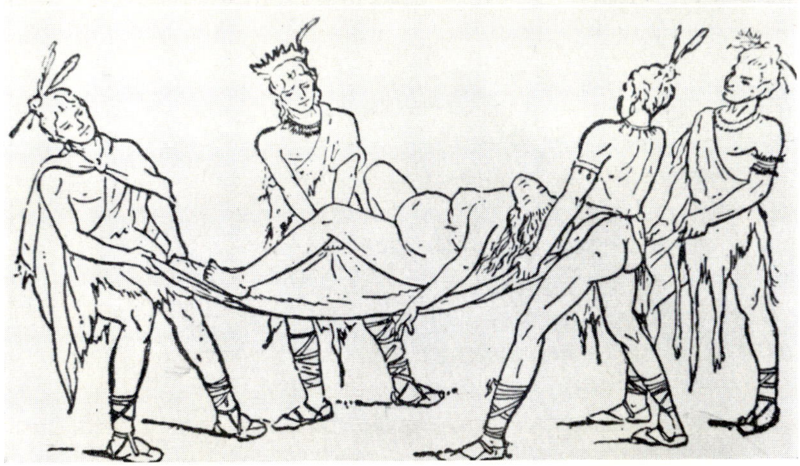

Fig. 8. A difficult delivery in Senegal. ([Witkowski] G. Steinheil, Paris.)
Fig. 9. Western Indians tossing squaw in a blanket to shake baby out. ([Witkowski] G. Steinheil, Paris.)

strangles the baby. Head presentation is the only form of birth liked. Foot presentation is a bad omen, and will cause the parents to die. When this takes place, any people who are in the house, are sent out, a food basket is brought in, the bottom of it cut out, and the child is passed through this, head first, to reverse the order of birth and avert any evil. Offerings are also made to the gods and ghosts to prevent evil results. Version and dismembering procedures have been used in some tribes by one expert in the practices. The performance of cesarean section is not omitted from the literature of the primitive people. In 1879, a Dr. Felkin witnessed a cesarean operation performed by a native specialist in Uganda, in which banana wine was used to disinfect the hands of the operator and as an anesthetic. Following an incision through the abdominal wall and uterus, the child and placenta were removed, the uterus massaged but not sutured, the escaped fluids removed by elevating the patient, the abdominal incision closed by means of pins and figure of eight sutures and the wound covered with a paste of crushed herbs. The patient made an uneventful recovery. Emil Novak suggests that such a well-developed technic must have been under development for a long time, that possibly primitive races had performed the operation for centuries.

That natives were able to appreciate neurotic and hysterical manifestations is indeed interesting; the following incident occurred in one of the tribes discussed by Harley. A frightened woman claimed she was in labor three days; it was believed to be false, hysterical labor. The midwife took a small vine which produces violent itching and rubbed it on the woman's body (Tragia *ep.*). The patient forgot all about being in labor when she found it was so necessary to scratch. Later she was delivered of a baby normally.

During the postpartum period the patient may go and come as she pleases; she has sexual restrictions until the baby is weaned. She does no work for three days, gets applications of hot canna leaves (*canna bidentata*) twice daily on the abdomen, and she drinks one dram of "kpwi" (*waltheria americana*). A small dose of "wana" (*mareya spicata*) is used to bring out the afterbirth. It is also given two to three weeks after the delivery to mark the end of the puerperium, and is supposed to contract the uterus and settle everything in its proper place.

From a medical standpoint they have no knowledge of anatomy, pathology and especially physiology. They know where certain organs are and they recognize some gross lesions, much more so than is credited to primitive people. They learn from animals and sometimes from humans (cannibals). Some, as in the Mano tribes, perform autopsies. The leech opens the cadaver and removes a diseased organ, especially if this organ was the seat of a tumor recognizable before death and supposed to be witch substance. It is removed and burned separately from the rest of the body so that the spirit of the deceased will not pass the disease to some other member of the family. They use a definite part of the forest for this, and no doubt have prevented epidemics by so doing. In Cambodia, because of a belief in the danger of the dead to the living, the dead are car-

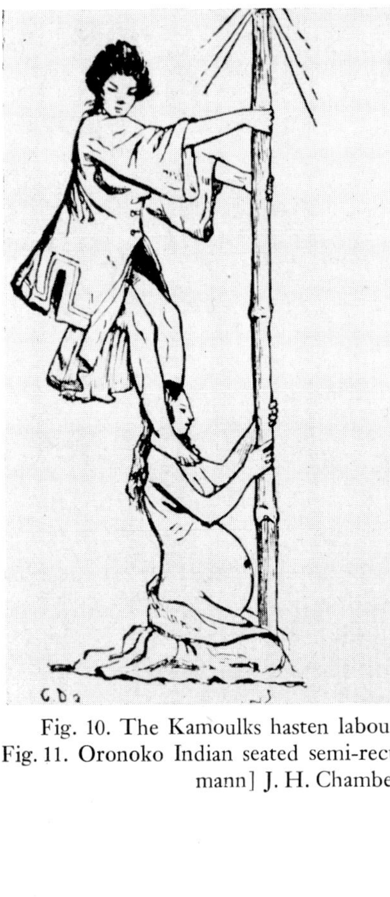

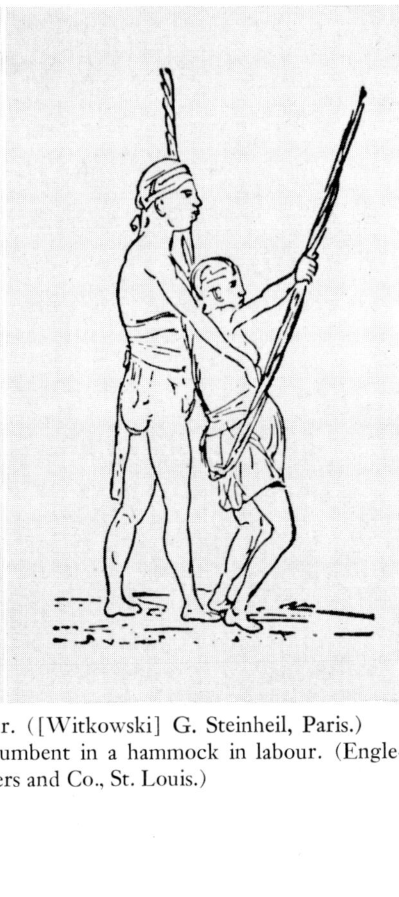

Fig. 10. The Kamoulks hasten labour. ([Witkowski] G. Steinheil, Paris.)
Fig. 11. Oronoko Indian seated semi-recumbent in a hammock in labour. (Englemann] J. H. Chambers and Co., St. Louis.)

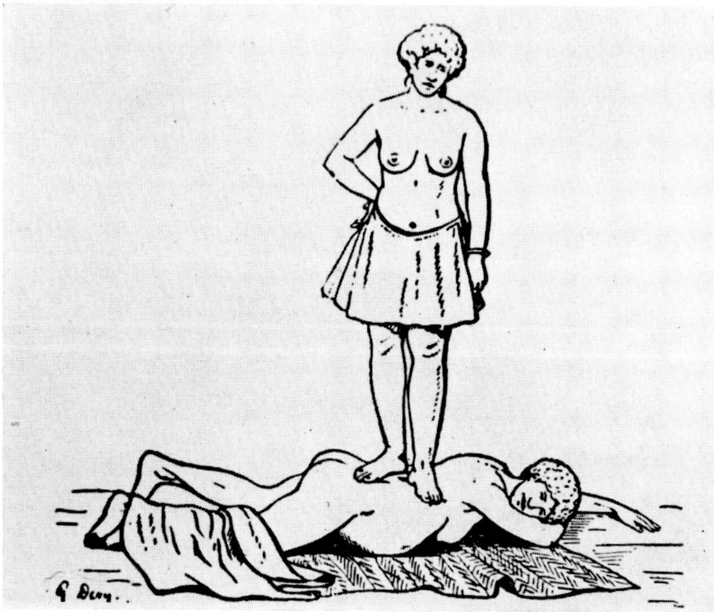

Fig. 12. Labour in Loango. (Witkowski.)

ried out feet first so that the dead man may not see the house, in which event sickness would visit the survivors. Fires are lighted around a house in which a dead body lies in order to keep out evil spirits which are attracted by the corpse and would bring sickness among the living. Similar customs imply a belief in something very like contagion from the dead, and, to protect himself against such risks, the ingenuity of man has devised many measures. The Navajos, when burying their dead, smear their bodies with tar in order to protect themselves from evil influences. This contagion is a spiritual and not a physical one. There is no fear of physical morbid infection by touching the dead body of a person who died of disease. The real fear is that the evil spirits residing in the corpse could transfer themselves or their influence to the living by mere contact. Persons whose duties bring them in contact with the dead are avoided for the same reasons.

We must credit these aborigines with a modicum of rational therapy. For puerperal infection *Harungana madagascariensis, euphorbia hirta* and *bidens bipinnata* are used in the diet; also *scleria Barteri.* Malformations are destroyed at birth and never seen.

Some primitive people attribute conception to the conspiracy of spirits that reside in the woman's food, water or in the air. The span of nine months is never related in any way to the pregnancy.

The practice of circumcision of females was a common one and varied in different countries. Usually the skin fold of the clitoris and nymphae are excised. As an anesthetic in the Mano tribes "Yei pulu" (*Tragia sp.*) is rubbed on the area to be cut. This causes violent itching so that the cutting is welcome rather than painful. To control the hemorrhage the vine "sa kpan" (*Tiliacora Dinklagei*) is used. Other remedies used are "fla la" (*alchornia cordifolia*), and "lolo" (*Harungana madagascariensis*). *Pergularia extensa* is said to be particularly effective. Dried foreskins from boys and some dried clitoris and labia minora were always held in readiness by a midwife and by a "property" man. On the third day after the operation, the dried skins from the boys were cut up fine and cooked in a soup called "teni" and eaten to promote healing of the wounds. Circumcisions were often a preliminary to the scarification of tribal marks. Although performed ceremonially, it is supposed to prevent masturbation.[6]

In ancient Abyssinia, female infibulation was done by sewing the lips of the vulva together, only allowing for the passage of excretions, then, at the time of marriage, the sutured parts were separated with a bistoury. For purposes of preserving chastity, infibulation was also regularly practiced by the ancient natives in the Sudan and also among the Nubians, usually when the girl was about eight years old. Often these Nubians also excised the clitoris and nymphae and scraped the walls of the outer lips of the vulva, thus inducing a very successful infibulation. On the bridal night, if the spouse was unable to rupture the scar tissue from the infibulation, an incision was made, probably with a piece of sharpened flint.[7–9]

Primitive superstitions relative to sexual intercourse are interesting and numerous. Warriors deemed chastity a necessity in order to be strong. In Madagascar the native who goes on a fishing trip will avoid his wife and remain chaste for a month prior to the trip to be sure his arm is strong and his aim accurate. That chastity was held in high esteem by some primitive tribes can be cited by the cessation of sexual intercourse between married couples during the construction of a new village, otherwise the chief would die and the new

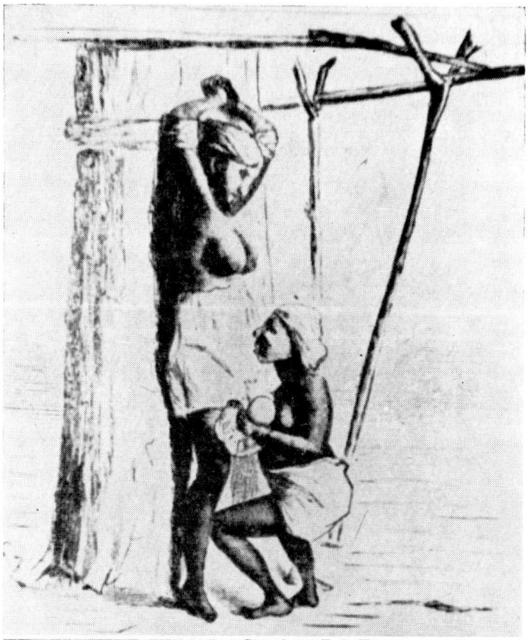

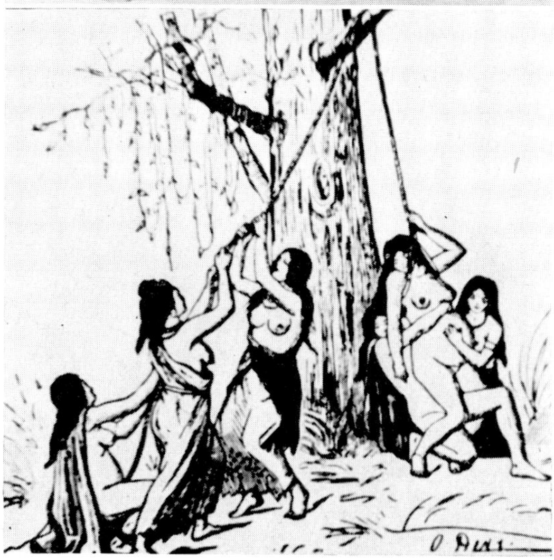

Fig. 13. Native of the Serang Islands delivering in erect position. ([Englemann] J. H. Chambers and Co., St. Louis.)

Fig. 14. A difficult delivery among the Apache Indians. ([Witkowski] G. Steinheil, Paris.)

village would always be unlucky. A native of Indochina could divorce his wife on his return from an elephant hunt if one of his elephants got away, the presumption being that his wife was unfaithful to him during his absence.

The folklore of fertility is well established. Worshipped for their fertility, savage women are considered by their mates not only as the givers of children, but also possessing the power to give or to withhold fertility to the fields and woods, and to all animal life. To insure good crops and a plentiful supply of cattle, women were put to work in the fields. Apparently to insure greater fertility to their fields, savages indulged in intercourse at the time seed was being sown (among the Pipiles of Central America), or at the time that the broom appears upon the rice in Java. According to Sir James Frazer, even in Europe in ancient times, fertility of soil was celebrated by bouts of sexual congress. Even today, or at least in recent times, in the Russian Ukraine, on the 23rd of April of each year, the newly sprouting crops are blessed by the priest in full regalia, after which the young married people lie down in couples on the sown fields and roll several times over on them in the belief that this will promote the growth of the crops.

The practice of contraception has been found among the more ancient tribes. A type of female condom used by a tribe in South America, consisted of one end of a vegetable pod, not unlike our milkweed pod. The end of the pod was snipped off, and inserted into the vagina. Foreign bodies inserted into the vagina were used as contraceptives, and operations on the vagina, or on the male sex organ to prevent insemination were other methods used to prevent conception."

Primitive peoples practiced many cruel abortifacient procedures, and often controlled childbirth by abortion or infanticide. For many centuries people have remained in ignorance of the most elemental concepts of human creation. More than 4000 years ago a mere suggestion of such things as fertility and childbirth may be found in the papyrus of Kahun. It was not until Empedocles (Circa 504-443 B.C.) the theory was advanced that the embryo was created through the union of the male and female semens. He held that the fetus began to take form 36 days after conception and attained its full development on the forty-ninth day.

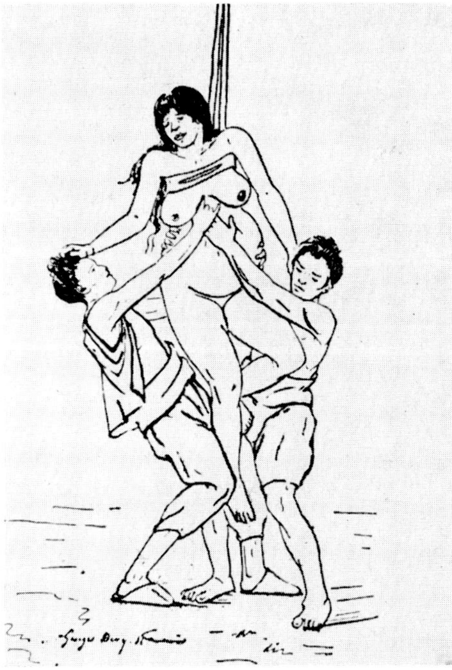

Fig. 15. Delivery of a Siamese native. ([Witkowski] G. Steinheil, Paris.)

As long as babies were born, a certain amount of midwifery must have been employed. In complicated labors, the only recourse was the crude manipulations and incantations of the medicine man. Postnatal complications of the pregnant woman received some sort of primitive gynecological therapy. To the primitive midwife, therefore, goes the honor of being the first medical practitioner.

First Occurrences and Outstanding Events

For the first time, in 25,000 B.C. (Aurignacian Period), blood was regarded as the vital fluid which was essential to active existence.

Menstrual blood was considered poisonous and vile and the cause of numerous disasters.

Abortifacients are commonly used by primitive people.

In 1879, a Dr. Felkin witnessed a cesarean operation performed by a native specialist in Uganda.

Circumcision, and infibulation of females was very common among aboriginal people. These, perhaps, were the first gynecological operations.

The first practitioner of medicine was the primitive midwife.

References

1. Sigerist, H. E.: *A History of Medicine: Primitive and Archaic Medicine*, Vol. 1. London, Oxford, 1951.
2. Findley, P.: *Priests of Lucina.* Boston, Little, 1939, p. 5.
3. Chauvet, S.: *La médecine chez les peuple primitifs* (préhistoriques et contemporanis). Paris, Librairie Maloine, 1936.
4. Harley, G. W.: *Native African Medicine.* Boston, Harvard, 1941.
5. Leonardo, R. A.: *History of Gynecology.* New York, Froben, 1944, p. 5.
6. Harley, G. W.: *Native African Medicine*, Boston, Harvard, 1941.
7. Burckhardt, J. L.: *Travels in Nubbia.* London, J. Murray, 1819.
8. Daniel, W. F.: *Sketches of the Medical Topography and Native Diseases of the Gulf of Guinea.* London, Highley, 1849.
9. Schaefer, G.: Female circumcision. *Obst. & Gynec.*, *6*:235-238, 1955.
10. Langdon-Davies, J.: (Fertility) *A Short History of Women.* New York, Viking, 1927.
11. Hammerton, J. A.: (Contraceptives) *Manners and Customs of Mankind.* New York, Wise, 1937, n.d. p. 139.

B. PREHISTORIC (500,000-6000 B. C.)

The prehistoric age which may be dated from 500,000 to 3500 B.C. gives us very little gynecology and obstetrics, yet there are a few pregnant bits of information that fit into our story, without which a beginning could not be made. Our information on prehistoric medicine comes mainly from two sources. From the study of primitive medicine, briefly covered in the preceding chapter, we can postulate prehistoric medicine inasmuch as the customs of both differed so little since they are so basic. Also we are able to obtain knowledge from the science of Prehistoric Archeology, which may be defined as "the science of antiquities antecedent to the most ancient historical documents." Its methods differ from those of later archeology in that, instead of being based on history, it draws exclusively from the natural sciences of geology, paleontology, ethnology and anthropology. This early period is divided into two ages:

1. Paleolithic age (flaked or chipped stone).
2. Neolithic age (polished stone).

Each of these are subdivided, e.g., under Paleolithic, the first of six subdivisions is the Chellean epoch, 100,000 B.C. The name of the locality where the chief finds were made is applied to the epoch, so this epoch was called Chellean because the finds were made at Chelles; the Aurignacean epoch, 4th subdivision, 25,000 B.C., is so called because the finds were in Aurignac.[1]

Whereas skeletal remains may date as far back as the Chellean era, evidence in the form of statuettes is commonly designated in the

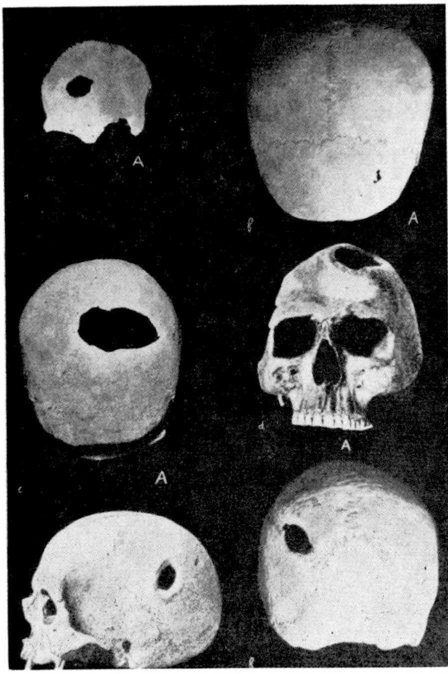

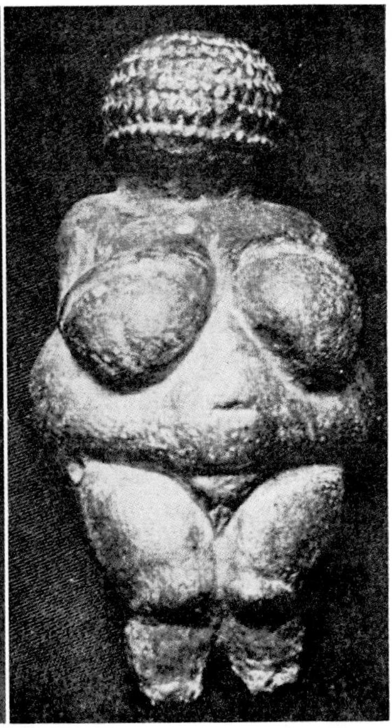

Fig. 16. Trephined skulls found in the ruins of the Swiss lake dwellers. (Chauvet, Stephen: *Les Peuples Primitifs* [Prehistoriques et contemporanis]. Paris, Librairie Maloine, 1936.)

Fig. 17. Venus of Willendorf, a limestone statuette unearthed in the valley of the Danube about 25,000 B.C. (Chauvet, Stephen: *Les Peuples Primitifs* [Prehistoriques et contemporanis]. Paris, Librairie Maloine, 1936.)

Aurignacean period because the first direct manifestation of an art appears in this period, representing realistic figures, or animals such as horses and reindeer. It was in this epoch that evidence was found from which we obtain information applicable to our subject of gynecology and obstetrics.[2]

The skeletal remains of the Chellean era give evidence of fractures with callous formation, of rachitis and arthritis deformans, conditions that we believed to be due to our modern civilization.[3] Trephined skulls, several hundreds of them, have been found in the ruins of the Swiss lake dwellers; perhaps trephining was done to allow the escape of the evil spirits, the spirits of disease, of epilepsy, a most ancient affliction. Poppy seed cakes were found in the same ruins and we have wondered if the poppy seed cakes did not initiate the use of opium.

It is in the Aurignacean period, 25,000 B.C., that we have some finds that bear a modicum of relation to obstetrics and gynecology. Deep in the Danube Valley a limestone statuette of a woman has been unearthed. It is less than five inches high, but her bowed head, her massive breasts and her squat torso suggest in eloquent fashion the obstetrical difficulties that have beset our prehistoric mothers. The date of this statuette, which is called the "Venus of Willendorf," is estimated to be long before 25,000 B.C. If the carving of this misshapen figure is at all typical of the prehistoric women, one is led at once to speculate upon the possible incidence of skeletal deformities and their effect on childbearing.[4]

Victor Robinson describes prehistoric women thusly:

> The Venus of Willendorf should be compared with the living Hottentot Venus of today, since both illustrate the primitive man's penchant for fleshiness in his females. Primitive man himself is depicted as straight and slender, but he liked his women round, and thus the pendulous breasts and overdevelopment of the buttocks were due not only to too much cave life and to too much meat but to selection.[5]

Since gynecological maladies, of certain types at least, follow childbirth, we can assume their presence during the prehistoric age. In fact we possess more tangible evidence of their presence; statuettes have been unearthed, traced to the Aurignacean Period, 25,000 B.C. which contained the structural properties described by Robinson. These statuettes present indubitable evidence of glandular dystrophies that existed even as far back as the prehistoric period. When we compare one of these statuettes with a photograph of a female of today, we may note the similarity.

We must conclude that our knowledge of prehistoric obstetrics and gynecology is indeed meager, but there is sufficient evidence that it did exist. Though minimal in quantity, it is certainly of his-

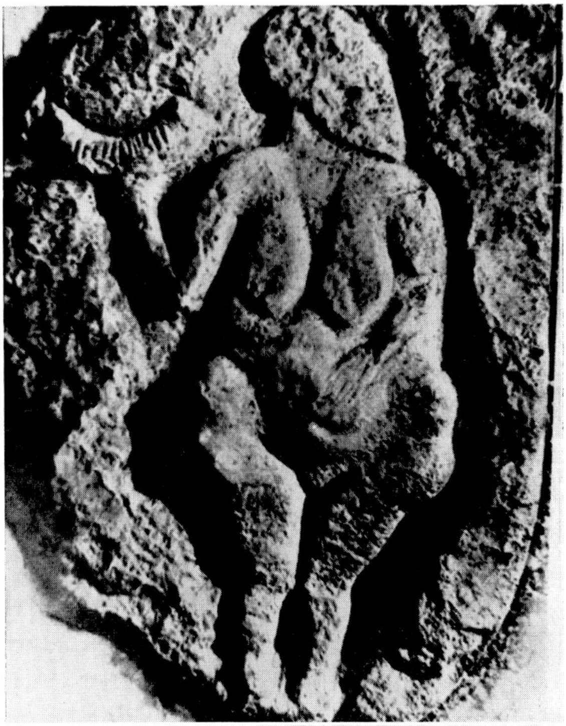

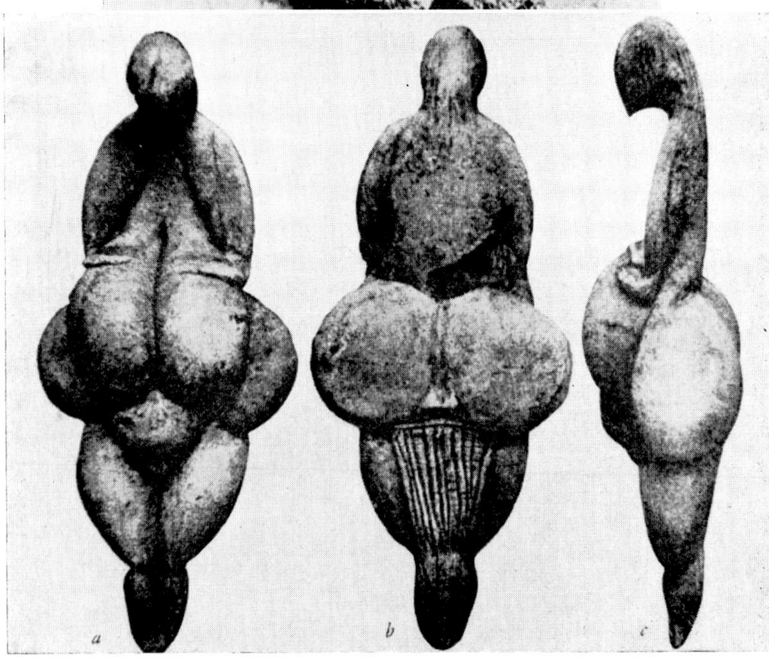

Fig. 18. Relief found in a cave at Laussel, France. (*MD Medical News* Magazine, Mar. 1958. New York, MD Publications, Inc.)

Fig. 19. Statuette of Aurignacean Period shows a glandular dystrophy. (Chauvet, Stephen: *Les Peuples Primitifs* [Prehistoriques et contemporanis]. Paris, Librairie Maloine, 1936.)

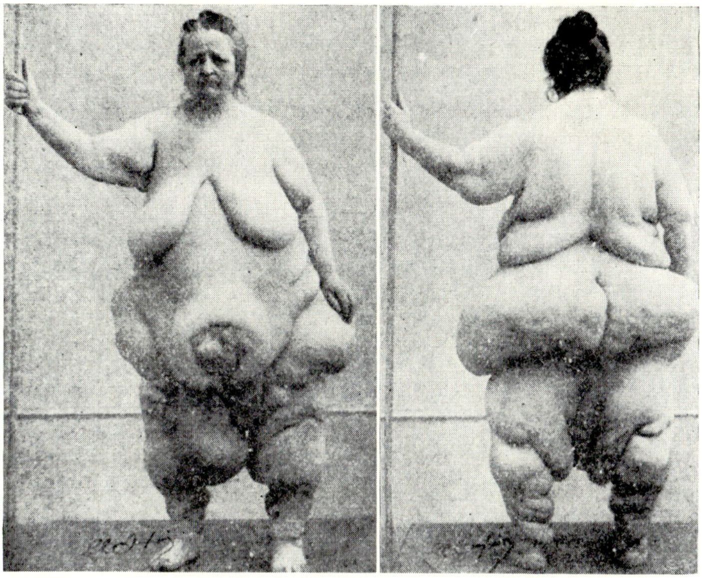

Fig. 20. Woman with evidence of glandular dystrophy taken in recent times. (Chauvet, Stephen: *Les Peuples Primitifs* [Prehistoriques et contemporanis.] Paris, Librairie Maloine, 1936.)

torical importance since it is the point from which our story is developed and our progress in obstetrics and gynecology is measured.

First Occurrences and Outstanding Events

First evidence of obstetrics and gynecology occurred in this period.
Glandular dystrophies were known to have existed in this age.

References

1. Blum and Tatlock: *A Short History of Art*. London, B. T. Batsford, 1926.
2. Leonardo, Richard A.: *History of Gynecology*. New York, Froben, 1944, p. 3.
3. Sudhoff, Karl: *Essays in the History of Medicine*. New York, Medical Life Press, 1926, p. 9.
4. Findley, Palmer: *Priests of Lucina*. Boston, Little, 1939, p. 3.
5. Robinson, Victor: *The Story of Medicine*. New York, Tudor Pub. Co., 1931.

Chapter II

EGYPTIAN (6000-1200 B.C.)

THE EARLIEST CULTURE, of which we have a written record, began in the valley of Egypt, about 6000 B.C. The earliest definitive evidence of the existence of medicine in Egypt came 2000 years later, although medicine in a much more primitive state existed long before this time.

Medicine in Egypt developed on the empirical and rational side early in its history. It remained static because of the conservative character of the Egyptians who believed no improvement was possible since their precepts reflected the wisdom of the gods and the physicians divinely inspired.

Egypt has left us a rich legacy of historical information, from which we are able to deduce quite accurately their culture and medical accomplishments.

The principal source of our knowledge of Egyptian medicine comes from a series of papyri, all of which are anonymous. The longest and most famous of these is the *Ebers Papyrus*, found together with the *Edwin Smith Papyrus* about 1862. The *Ebers Papyrus* was written about 1500 B.C., but some of its passages date back to 3400 B.C. and contain 877 prescriptions and sections. The *Kahun Medical Papyrus*, discovered in 1889, was written during the 12th and 13th Dynasties, circa 2000-1800 B.C. It deals with gynecology only, and contains thirty-four sections. Other sources of our medical information of Egypt are the sculptures, tombs, religious texts and the antiquities preserved in various museums. To this may be added mummification and embalming.

While ailments due to obvious mundane causes were treated on a rational basis, diseases of unknown origin were regarded as visitations from and inflictions of the gods and consequently were treated in the main, by magical and religious appeal. For this they depended

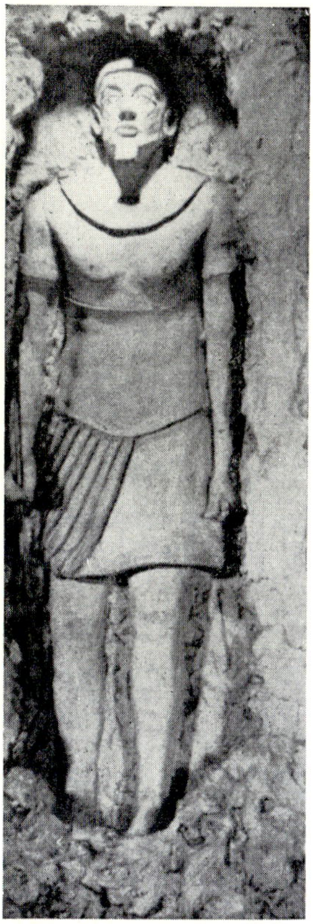

Fig. 21. Imhotep, circa 3000 B.C. (*MD Medical News* Magazine, June 1958. New York, MD Publications, Inc. [Photo Jas. Coyne, sculptor Doris Appel.])

upon their gods and goddesses who originated and also provided cures for diseases. Their outstanding divinity was Thoth, the reputed founder of medicine. (Thoth is confused with Hermes Trismegistos by some authors, but according to Findley they are one and the same.) Thoth presided at the Temple of Hermopolis, where he wrote the famous *Hermetic Books*, one of which is devoted to diseases of women. Egyptian mythology is replete with names of goddesses, whose chief concerns were with parturient women. There is 'Anuqet, goddess of fertility, Bes, protector of childbirth, Hat Hôr, patroness of pregnant women, Ubastet and her sister, Sekhmet, deities of warmth and germination, Heqet, goddess of the cradle, and Nekhbet, titulary goddess of parturition, puerperium and wet-nursing. Osiris (or Apis), the bull god and his wife, Isis (mother of Horus), were the patrons of therapy. Isis was also looked upon as the goddess of fertility and protectress of women in all the ailments peculiar to their sex. After Isis, they turned their attention to the demigod.[1] Imhotep (circa 2900 B.C.) was the true healing deity. Supposedly of divine origin, this legendary figure now appears to have been an actual historical personage who lived during the 3rd Dynasty.

These divinities may have been imitated by the Greeks subsequently, for we find parallel gods in the Grecian concept. The Greek Aesculapius, son of Apollo, the sun god, was the first great physician of the Hellenes; his Egyptian counterpart is Imhotep. We can identify the Egyptian 'Anuqet with the Grecian Hestia, the Egyptian Uzoit with the Greek Leto, and the Egyptian Nekhbet with the Greek Eileithyia.

The priest physicians did most of the practice of medicine. They began by treating the sick at the shrines of the various gods. The most famous shrine or temple was the temple of Isis at Philae. In a manner these temples were likened to present day hospitals; here they prayed, offered invectives against the demons of disease, made votive offerings and appeals to the divine patrons of restoration and health.

During the 1st Dynasty, which dated about 3400 B.C., it was customary to bury the dead by inhumation in the sands of the desert. They confided to nature not only the actual bodies of their dead, but all their equipment as well and the preservation of these has helped us to reconstruct their lives and culture. Because of the dry climate and the preservative effect of direct contact with the sand, it is possible to examine anatomically the soft and perishable parts of the body. These facts suggested to them the possibility of artificially preserving the body by making mummies. This evidence is found in the 1st Dynasty. The body was wrapped in many layers

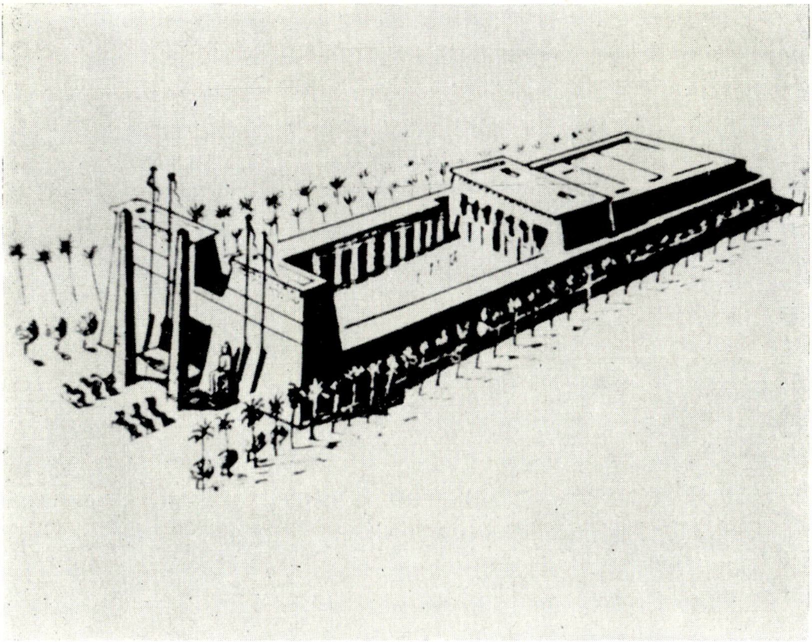

Fig. 22. Sketch of a Temple. (The Bettmann Archive.)

of fine linen bandages, the mummy was covered in resin which set to form a hard carapace. The details of the features were indicated by painting on the outermost wrappings, and the genital organs were modelled with linen and resin. This was done in order that the sex and personal likeness of the dead person might be perpetuated. This practice of mummification continued for 30 centuries. All the viscera were removed but the heart. The body was immersed in saline solution and then desiccated and anointed with a paste made of resin mixed with salt, soda and fat. The brain was removed through the nostrils, especially during the 18th Dynasty. The art of mummification familiarized its users with the internal structure of the body and with chemicals for preservation. More important, its long usage was important because it helped to overcome the prejudice against cutting the human body, and so made dissection possible. It was in Egypt that the Greek physicians first carried out systematic dissection and laid the foundation of the science of anatomy. Peculiarly, mummification, which played so important a part in the development of medical science, was in fact a religious

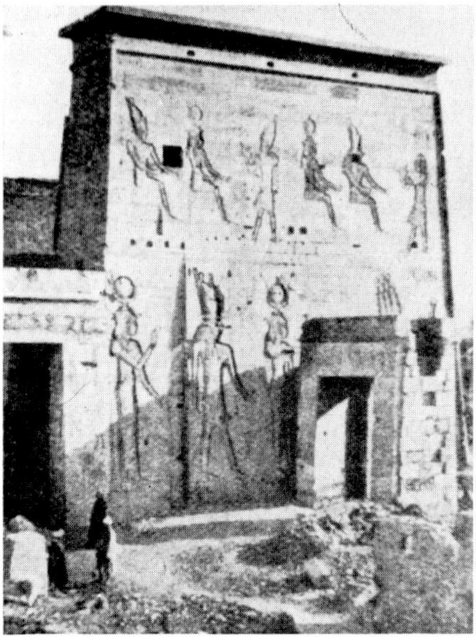

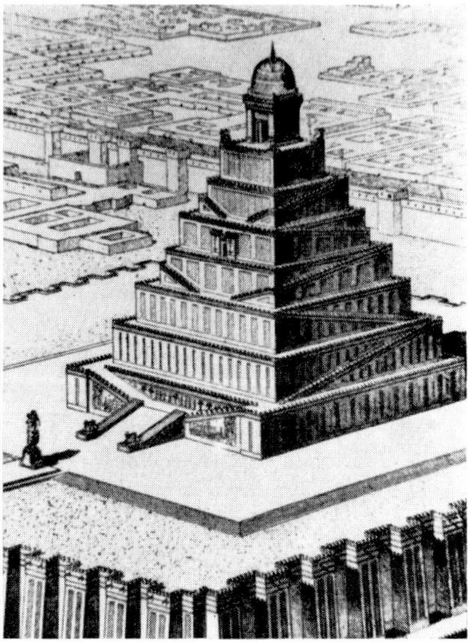

Fig. 23. Pilon of the Great Temple at Philae, Egypt. (Blum and Tatlock: *A Short History of Art.* London, Batsford, 1926.)

Fig. 24. Chaldean temple. (Blum and Tatlock: *A History of Art.* London. Batsford, 1926.)

observance, and its practice was not carried out by physicians.[2]

Because of the peculiar circumstances arising out of the Egyptian customs and beliefs, the Greek anatomists, in the 3rd Century B.C. were able to practice dissection of the human body in Egypt. The papyri show that the Egyptians themselves had some knowledge of the structure and functions of the body for many centuries. Though Egypt could not compete with Greece in scientific knowledge and thought, she at least inaugurated what others have developed; she offered the facilities for the advancement of knowledge and research. So we can well say that the debt of civilization to Egypt is incalculable.

Embalming and mummification provided opportunities to learn anatomy and some physiology, but most important, was the knowledge gained in comparative anatomy. The Egyptians became familiar with the appearance and mutual positions of the organs of the body. It afforded them the opportunity to compare human and animal organs. They evolved over 100 anatomical terms. The external genitalia, vagina, and cervix were named and differentiated

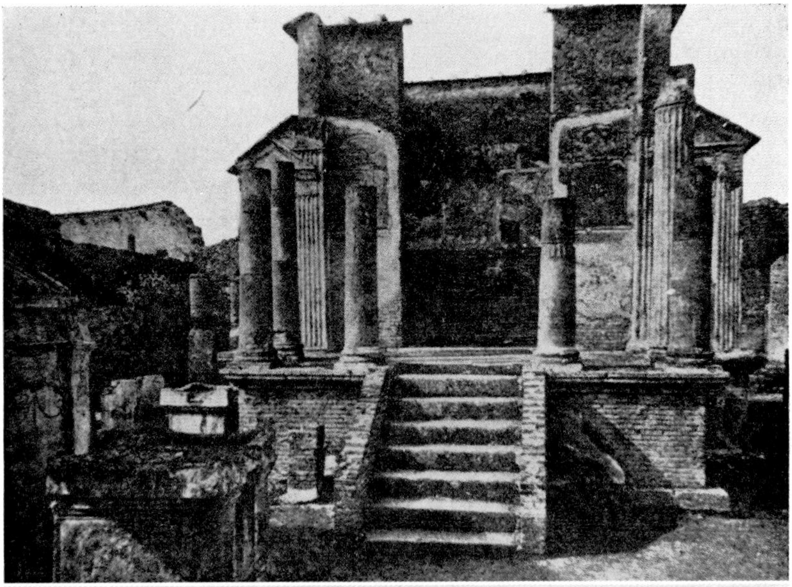

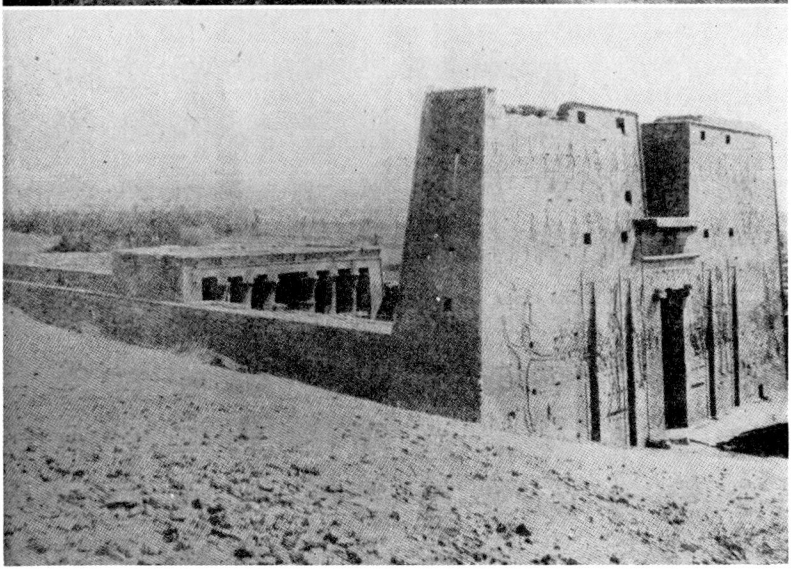

Fig. 25. Temple of Isis, in Pompeii. (Miller, Walter; ed.: *The Standard American Encyclopedia*, XV vols. Chicago, Standard American Corporation, 1916, vol. v.)

Fig. 26. The Temple of Horus at Edfu. (Miller, Walter; ed.: *The Standard American Encyclopedia*, XV vols. Chicago, Standard American Corporation, 1916. vol. v.)

in a discussion of prolapse, but the ovaries and tubes were never mentioned. Undoubtedly they possessed some knowledge of gynecology, but it was not at all clear or rational. Ulceration of the cervix, including neoplastic ulceration, is never mentioned, unless we consider as an instance of carcinoma uteri, cases with peculiarly disagreeable odor. Irregular menses and leukorrhea are mentioned without rationale. Prostitution existed and there is evidence that gonorrhea prevailed. But they did not recognize the complications that go with gonorrhea, such as bartholinitis, pyosalpinx, and the other complications. The Egyptians were the first to mention uterine prolapse in medical literature. Tampons and suppositories were introduced into the vagina, and enemata were known to be used. Gynecological surgery was unknown.

Physiology was confined to the heart as the center of a vascular system; they did not understand the circulation, but recognized the relation of the heart and pulse. As to the pathology contained in the papyri, they spoke of boils, carbuncles, suppuration and bilharzial infections.

Pharmacology of the Egyptians was crude and yet ingenius. They administered the excrements of animals, used the grease of eels, the wine of the he-goat, the intestines of the wolf, the dung of domesticated animals, the afterbirth of women, human blood and urine, the nails of fingers and toes, the wax from the ears; these and countless other remedies derived from human and lower animals were employed in the healing of the sick. But such substances differed only in their crudity from those employed as late as the 18th Century and foreshadowed the organotherapy of modern times.

The following prescriptions for female ailments are found in the *Ebers Papyrus*:[3]

1. To prevent leucorrhea in a virgin: Anoint the breast, body and limbs with a lotion prepared by crushing the dried liver of a swallow in sour milk.
2. To regulate the menses: Douche the patient with a mixture of garlic and wine. If this fails, douche with fennel, wonder-fruit, honey and sweet beer for 4 days.
3. To correct a displaced womb: Mould (film of dampness) from the wood of ships, rub in yeast of fermented beer and

let patient drink it. Or oil of earth (petroleum) with fedder (manure) and honey, rub the body of the patient. Or dried excreta and froth, use as a rubbing agent.

4. To induce labor: Fennel incense, garlic, sert-juice, fresh salt and wasp dung, make into a ball and place in vagina.
5. To increase the flow of milk: Bones of the swordfish warmed in oil. Rub the back bone of the patient.

Also in the *Ebers Papyrus*, there is evidence that the Egyptians were concerned with the diagnosis of pregnancy, with sterility, lactation and menstrual disorders. They were very desirous of having children and the same papyrus recounts methods to ascertain if a woman could give birth. To hasten delivery instructions were given to "burn turpentine resin close to the abdomen. If this means remains without effect, place a mixture of oil of saffron and sweet beer on the abdomen."

Specialization was very common, and yet there is very little in the history of Egyptian medicine that indicated specialization in gynecology and obstetrics. However, a college in the city of Sais was in existence, where women physicians taught the art of midwifery and gynecology. It was the first medical school.[4] However, the priest physicians considered it beneath their dignity to soil their hands with this "lowly art," and it seemed more fitting that women helpers should usher the babies into the world. The birth stool was in use and labor was attended by four midwives, and women died from inability to give birth, from infection and from hemorrhage; mummies 6000 years old bear mute witness to this.

In ancient Egypt, medicine was patronized by royalty. The Pharaohs surrounded themselves with staffs of physicians that their lives might be protected and prolonged. It was in this royal setting where specialization abounded, one served as the "keeper of the drugs," another as the "head of the fumigation department"; an ancestor of Tutankhamen, in his reliance on specialists, went so far as to appoint a medical guardian for his left eye and another for his right eye.

The Egyptians were excellent physicians and enjoyed an enviable reputation in foreign lands. But, in time, Egyptian medical tradition hardened into a series of rigid laws which the doctor was compelled to obey or suffer grave penalties, especially if a patient died.

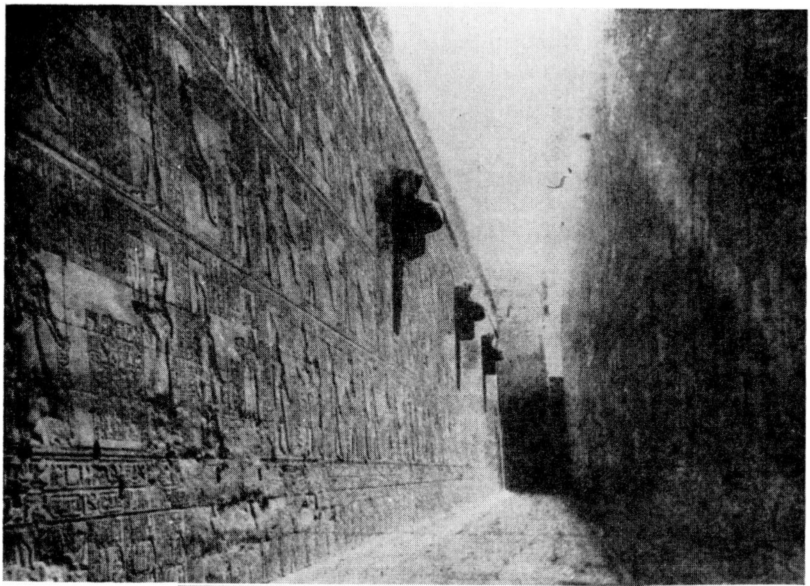

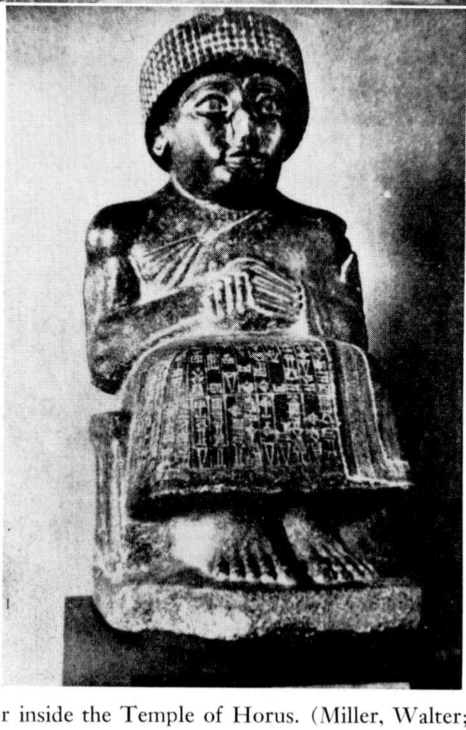

Fig. 27. A corridor inside the Temple of Horus. (Miller, Walter; ed.: *The Standard American Encyclopedia*, XV vols. Chicago, Standard American Corporation, 1916, vol. v.)

Fig. 28. Archaic votive statue. (Blum and Tatlock: *A Short History of Art.* London, Batsford, 1926.)

The result was that fallacious as well as factual medicines and therapy were passed along from generation to generation. Wisdom and stupidity piled up, with stupidity ultimately prevailing. Just as happened in all other fields of culture, medicine developed into formalism so that Egyptian civilization finally sank down and died of its own weight. But the Egyptian doctor, while he lasted, was "cock of the walk" in the ancient East. Later the Greeks were to draw heavily upon Egyptian findings to develop their own great medical system. In Roman times, Galen suggested that a sprinkling of Egyptian terms in a prescription would help to fortify the patient's belief in the remedy. And in the 18th Century, quacks in the streets of London could still lure crowds to their stumps by simply displaying "Doctor of Egypt" upon their shingles.[5]

Egypt, the birthplace of medicine, reigned supreme for 40 centuries, in the end to be usurped and replaced by Greek civilization.

Because the earliest sources of medical information came from the various Egyptian papyri, a cursory review of the writing of this period is presented in the following few paragraphs.[6] It was the Egyptians who discovered the papyrus and invented writing in the form of hieroglyphics, which have played such a great role in history.

The word itself means sacred writings. The Greeks' "hieros" means sacred, "glyphein," to carve. Earliest examples of Egyptian writing, memorial inscriptions from the 1st Dynasty, date from 3100 B.C. The last was set down in A.D. 394. It changed little in 2500 years in contrast to the huge mutations that have occurred in English in the 600 years between Chaucer and the present day. Hieroglyphics required such painstaking calligraphy that, in time, the scribes evolved a cursive, everyday handwriting called hieratic in which the elaborate hieroglyphics were reduced to wiggly lines representing only the barest suggestion of the originals. As the centuries passed, hieroglyphics was relegated entirely to sacred inscriptions on temples and funereal monuments, and hieratic became the dominant form. It was in hieratic that all correspondence, legal documents and business transactions were set down. It was in hieratic that the Egyptians left their legacy of medical science to the western world: the first medical books, the first anatomical and medical vocabulary, the first pharmacopeia (which included castor

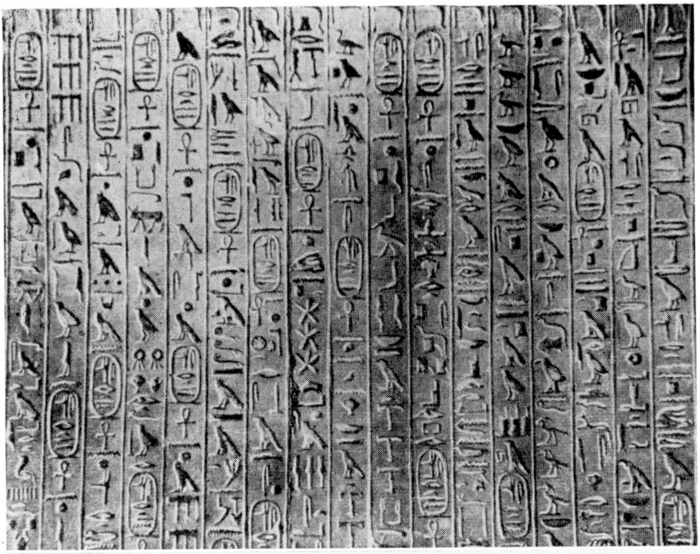

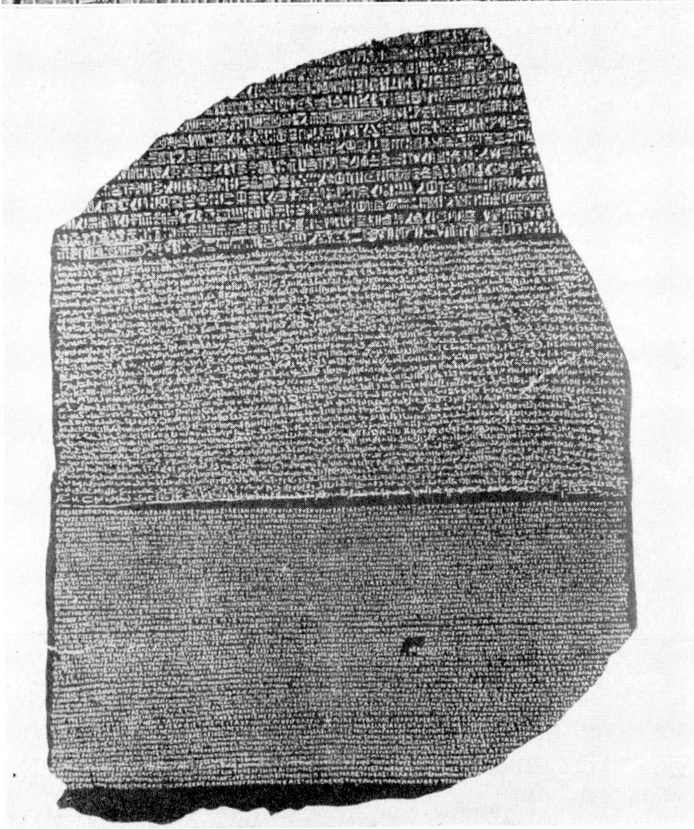

Fig. 29. Hieroglyphics. Inscriptions on the burial chamber of Sen-wosret-ankh. (Metropolitan Museum of Art, New York.)

Fig. 30. The Rosetta Stone. (Miller, Walter; ed.: *The Standard American Encyclopedia*, XV vols. Chicago, Standard American Corporation, 1916, vol. I.)

oil), the first instructions in surgery, in the diagnosis and treatment of disease and in the use of bandages, compresses, sutures and splints.

In time, however, hieratic gave way to a still more abbreviated script called "demotic." In the 2nd and 3rd Centuries A.D., demotic was swallowed up in turn by "Coptic," written in Greek letters with a few vestigial hieroglyphics interspersed. Although the Copts, who were early Egyptian converts to Christianity, ceased to write hieroglyphics, they continued to speak the language as late as the 16th Century A.D., and it is still read in Coptic church services in Egypt today.

Factual evidence of hieroglyphics, in the demotic and in Greek, is found in the *Rosetta Stone*, which was discovered in 1799 near the Rosetta mouth of the Nile in Egypt, by a Frenchman, M. Boussard. It is a tablet of black basalt 136 B.C. mentioning the reign of Ptolemy Epiphanes (circa B.C. 224-187). The inscription is in hieroglyphic, in demotic, and in Greek, and deals with the Egyptian priesthood gathered at Memphis in honor of Ptolemy Epiphanes. The stone was erected in 195 B.C. It was deciphered by Dr. Thomas Young and M. Champollion, and formed the key to the reading of the hieroglyphic characters. It was captured by the English on the defeat of the French forces in Egypt, and is now in the British Museum.[7]

While the Egyptians invented hieroglyphics which were, in a way, a sort of sign language and yet more complex, their pictures meant a great deal more than the objects they represented. It remained for Mesopotamia to improve hieroglyphics and give them more practicality, and the final evolution, that began as hieroglyphics, was the alphabet.[8]

The Egyptians used pictures, but the earliest inhabitants of Mesopotamia, the Sumerians, hit upon the idea of scratching their words in tablets of clay to evolve a system of V-shaped figures, which showed little connection with the pictures from which they had developed.

The Phoenicians, having become familiar with the art of writing invented by the Sumerians, regarded these pothooks as a clumsy waste of time. They were too practical as business men to spend hours engraving two or three letters. They set about and invented a new system of writing much superior to the old one. They borrowed a few pictures from the Egyptians and they simplified a number of the wedge-shaped figures of the Sumerians. They sacrificed the pretty appearance of the older system for the advantage of speed, and they reduced the thousands of different images to a short and handy alphabet of twenty-two letters.

In due course of time, the alphabet travelled across the Aegean Sea and entered Greece. The Greeks added a few letters of their own and carried the improved system to Italy. The Romans modified the figures somewhat and, in turn, taught them to the wild barbarians of Western Europe. These wild barbarians were our own ancestors, and that is the reason books are written in characters that are of Phoenician origin, and not in the hieroglyphics of the Egyptians or the nail script of the Sumerians.

First Occurrences and Outstanding Events

Principal and earliest actual records of our knowledge of medicine.
Thoth was the founder of medicine.
First systematic dissection by Greeks in Egypt.
First recorded anatomical terms of genitalia.
Egyptian pharmacology (in papyri) foreshadowed organotherapy.
Sais, the first medical school.
Egypt was the birthplace of medicine.
Other firsts by the Egyptians were medical books, anatomical and medical vocabulary, pharmacopoeia, instructions in surgery, diagnosis and treatment of disease, bandages, compresses, and sutures.
They invented hieroglyphics, our source of knowledge.
Phoenicians and not the Egyptians originated the alphabet.

References

1. Ricci, J. V.: *Genealogy of Gynecology*. Philadelphia and Toronto, Blakiston, 1950.
2. Dawson, W. R.: *Egypt and Assyria* (*Clio Medica*). New York, Hoeber, 1930, p. 73.
3. Ebers Papyrus: Quoted by Ricci, J. V.: *Genealogy of Gynecology*, Philadelphia and Toronto, Blakiston, 1950.
4. Gerike: *De Scolis et Institutis Medicis in Aegypto et Graecia*. Helmstadii, 1748.

5. Bettmann, O. L.: *Pictorial History of Medicine.* Springfield, Thomas, 1956.

6. *Life* Magazine: Chicago, Time, Inc., circa 1957.

7. *The Standard American Encyclopedia*, XV Vols., Walter Miller, ed. Chicago, Standard American Corp., 1916.

8. Van Loon, Hendrik: *The Story of Mankind.* New York, Garden City, Pub., 1938.

Chapter III

MESOPOTAMIAN (4000-331 B.C.)

WHEN Egypt was beginning to develop broad principles of medicine, the rest of the world, including tribes who were roaming the neighboring near eastern Orient, was practicing primitive medicine. However, evidence is available which shows that medicine in Mesopotamia began not too long after Egyptian medicine. In fact, some believe it started simultaneously in both lands, about 4000 B.C.

In Mesopotamia, unlike the rational medicine of Egypt, magic and religious practices held sway, and maintained their dominating influence to the very end. Mesopotamian medicine contained a volatile quality, probably due to a mixture of the races which inhabited its confines, and to the geographical disposition of these people which fostered continual warfare, resulting in an ever-changing supremacy among themselves. It was inevitable, therefore, that this influence eventually began to filter into the neighboring barbaric states. The history of Mesopotamia is much more complicated than that of Egypt because many people, tribes large and small, were involved.[1]

A. SUMERIAN (4000-2400 B.C.)

Toward the end of the 4th Millenium B.C., the country was populated by the Sumerians in the south and Semitic tribes in the north. The script they invented consisted first, like that of the Egyptians and Chinese, of ideograms of pictures. But it developed into a phonetic stage, with a sign for every syllable without, however, reaching the stage of the Egyptian or Hebrew scripts, which possessed signs for every consonant. Instead of papyrus and ink, the writing material was soft clay into which the cuneiform signs were drawn with a stylus made usually of a hard reed with a wedge-shaped end. This was later dried in the sun or baked in an oven; it became so hard that many thousands have survived to the present day. The Classical Sumerian Age from 3000 to 2400 B.C. made up the first period of Mesopotamian history.

B. SEMITIC (2400-1900 B.C.)

Eventually the Sumerian script was taken over by the Semites in the north and other peoples, and was used for the writing of a number of different languages. Around 2400 B.C. Sargon of Akkad (Semite) defeated the Sumerians and this became the first Semitic Empire.

C. BABYLONIAN (1900-1100 B.C.)

In 2000 B.C. Elam from the East and the Amorites from the west conquered Babylon (then Semitic), at that time a small and insignificant town. From here on, however, we have the beginning of a great kingdom, Babylonia. The greatest Amorite king, Hammurabi, ruled supreme in the very center of Mesopotamia. He was the greatest of all kings to reside in Babylon; he fought a thirty-years war in Elam. He built the great city of Babylonia. His greatest monument was his *Code of Laws.* The laws of the code state in plain words the rights and duties of the individual, regulate family and property relations and the entire social structure of the community. By the Code of Hammurabi (as well as the Mosaic Code) it was customary among social equals to retaliate for vengeance (*ius talionis*—"eye for an eye"). If, however, the victim was socially inferior, compensation in money took the place of vengeance. Thus the Code of Hammurabi prescribed:[2]

Art. 196. If a man has destroyed the eye of a patrician, his own eye shall be destroyed.

Art. 197. If he has broken the bone of a patrician, his bone shall be broken.

Art. 198. If he has destroyed the eye of a plebian, or broken a bone of a plebian, he shall pay one mina of silver.

Art. 199. If he has destroyed the eye of a man's slave, or broken a bone of a man's slave, he shall pay one-half the value. (In the Mosaic Code the man who injured his slave compensated by letting him free. *Exodus*, 21:26-7.)

Further, according to the Code of Hammurabi, adultery, if established beyond doubt, was punished by drowning. As almost everywhere in antiquity, there was no objection to the destruction of newborn children.

The golden age of Babylonia, like that of Egypt, did not last very long. The Hittites from the north and the Kassites overpowered it. This brought new blood, but no creative power, and so they were assimilated and civilization stagnated in Babylonia for a thousand years until the short flowering of the Chaldean Empire. It was before the establishment of the Chaldean Empire, that Babylonia was subjugated and conquered by Assyria.

D. ASSYRIAN (1100-606 B.C.)

Assyria was the northeastern bastion of Mesopotamia, a Semitic settlement in the upper valley of the Tigris. Assyrian influence began about 1900 B.C. These Semitic tribes were constantly at war with their neighbors, the Hittites in the north, Mittaini on the upper Euphrates, the Aramaeans in Syria, the Phoenicians on the coast, and the Babylonians on the south. From this hodgepodge of fighting, Syria came to the fore and reigned supreme from 750 B.C. until its total destruction in 606 B.C. Actually Assyria began to increase its momentum of power with the collapse of Egyptian influence in 1100 B.C. (Destruction of Syria is given as 612 B.C. by some authors.)

It was from Assyria that most of our knowledge of Mesopotamian medicine has been obtained from the thousands of clay tablets. The laws of the Assyrians were much stricter than those of the Babylonian Code. For instance, there are the stringent Assyrian regulations on injury to the genital organs and injury that caused miscarriage to a pregnant woman:[3]

> If a woman has crushed a man's testicle in an affray, one of her fingers shall be cut off; and if although a physician has bound it up, the second testicle is affected with it and becomes inflamed or if she has crushed the second testicle in the affray, both her nipples shall be torn off.

The most humane of the ancient Oriental codes was that of the Hittites, e.g.:

The penalty for causing miscarriage in a woman differed according to the age of the embryo. If it happened to a free woman in the tenth month the compensation was ten shekels of silver, but only five if in the sixth month, and it was five if the victim was a slave in the tenth month (moon months).

How Mesopotamia conceived disease to be, how it appeared to them, and what they did to ward it off and to restore health, is best exemplified in Babylonian and Assyrian medicine. Babylonian medicine was an integral part of religion. Whereas the Egyptians had papyri, the Mesopotamians used clay tablets. It is from these that we obtain much of the medical information. These tablets were medical books written by and for priest physicians, called "Ashipu." We learn that disease was caused primarily by demons, ghosts and evil spirits. Divination was the chief method of making diagnosis and prognosis. Prayers, incantations and other magic rites were the treatments most often employed. The literature of hepatoscopy was considerable and extremely interesting. Herodotus says that Babylonians had no physicians; more truthful would be the statement that they did not have the numerous physicians that Egypt had, but they did have some good ones. These physicians belonged to the most educated class of society, as priests; they specialized in the mysterious realm of inner medicine. The more obvious lesions were handled by the practical doctors called "Asu."

Actually any reference to gynecology is quite meager, and almost the same can be said for obstetrics. Women gave birth to their children as in Egypt, squatting on bricks or on a parturition chair, later lying on the bed. There would be several midwives and they were protected against evil spirits with amulets, prayers and magic rites.

E. CHALDEAN (circa 606-539 B.C.)

With the destruction of Syria in 606 B.C., a new Babylonian Empire, that of the Chaldeans, a Semitic state, took its place. This new empire continued for less than 100 years. About 588 B.C., Jerusalem was destroyed, and many Hebrews were taken as captives to Babylonia. An outstanding figure of this new empire was Nebuchadnezzar, who tried to recreate the golden age of Babylonia in the time of Hammurabi. When Nebuchadnezzar died in 561 B.C., the

Greeks had already colonized the coasts and islands of the Mediterranean and the Persians were coming to the fore.

F. PERSIAN (539-331 B.C.)

In the 6th Century B.C., the Persians conquered Babylonia (Chaldea) and Egypt. This marked the final eclipse of the Ancient Orient, and a decisive victory of the Indo-European peoples. They were to lead the destinies of the near East until the advent of Islam, and those of Europe and India to the present day. As long as Mesopotamian civilization was creative and strong, it assimilated foreign conquerors without difficulty; even in the 6th Century B.C. when it had long completed its course, it was strong enough to imprint its stamp upon the Persians, who wrote their triumphant inscriptions in cuneiform script and borrowed and adapted elements of Mesopotamian art. They used Aramaic alphabet, script and language; in fact Aramaic was becoming the international language of the Near East.[4]

When Persia came into the ascendancy about 539 B.C. and continued for 200 years, only few changes took place in customs and medicine. Medicine remained essentially demoniac. From such works as the *Zend-Avesta* and the portion of this called the Vendidad we learn that Thrita was the first man of the race to combat sickness and death. It was believed that disease was the result of evil spirits, which might, in the guise of flies, enter the body through its cavities, e.g., eyes, mouth, nose and genital openings. Corpses were shunned, and thus anatomical knowledge hindered. Menstruating and lying-in women were regarded as unclean and subject to isolation and purification. Djahi was the spirit of unchastity; it was she who first menstruated when kissed on the forehead by Angra Manjii (the evil one). Menstruating women were isolated for four days in a straw covered room with no fire and water (these were clean elements). The puerperal woman was isolated for forty days. Miscarriage was even more repugnant. There is practically no record of midwifery of the Persians of this period.[5]

First Occurrences and Outstanding Events

Sumerians invented a script similar to that of the Chinese and Egyptians.
Hammurabi, the greatest of Babylonian Kings, and his Code.

Most and first Mesopotamian knowledge of medicine came from clay tablets of the Babylonians and Assyrians.

When the Persians conquered Babylonia and Egypt, it marked the final eclipse of the ancient Orient.

References

1. Sigerist, Henry E.: *A History of Medicine, Primitive and Archaic Medicine.* Vol. I. London, Oxford, 1951.
2. Edwards, Chilperic: *The Hammurabi Code and the Sinaitic Legislation.* London, Truth Seeker, 1921, p. 38.
3. Driver, G. R., and Miles, John C.: *The Assyrian Laws* (Ancient codes and laws of the Near East, 2.) with translation and commentary. London, Oxford, 1935
4. Sigerist, Henry E.: *A History of Medicine, Primitive and Archaic Medicine*, Vol. I, Epilogue. London, Oxford, 1951, p. 492.
5. Findley, Palmer: *Priests of Lucina.* Boston, Little, 1939, p. 17.

Chapter IV

CHINESE, JAPANESE, HINDU AND HEBREW (3000 B.C.-A.D. 1765)

CONCURRENT with Mesopotamian medicine are the obstetrics and Gynecology of the Chinese, Japanese, Hindu and the Hebrews. Chinese medicine, influenced by India, had its many gods 3000 years B.C. Although it began much earlier than Japanese medicine it did not progress; its influence was transferred to the Japanese, who soon outstripped the Chinese, a status of medicine of the Far East that holds today. Indian medicine is definitely dated back to 1500 B.C. according to the *Veda;* some references are found of Indian medicine as far back as the 2nd Millenium B.C. and earlier. Hebrew medicine gives us clear-cut information in the Biblical Books, around 1300 B.C. The medicine of these empires, which began roughly about the same time as did Mesopotamian medicine, continued long after Mesopotamian medicine disappeared.

A. CHINESE (3000 B.C.-A.D. 1600)

Records of innumerable Chinese gods go as far back as 3000 B.C. They possessed healing power, and one of their first gods of healing was Shen Nung. Their medicine remained static for thousands of years, and had its origin in a demoniac conception. Retardation was due to religious dogma and the belief that the mutilated body of a Chinese may never meet its ancestors; and for the latter reason autopsies and, therefore, anatomy was a rarity. Autopsies were performed occasionally on executed criminals. Their medicine was based on a natural philosophy that the human body was itself a miniature universe, a microcosm whose every function had a larger counterpart in the external world. Since the universe was supposedly dominated by two cosmic principles called "Yang" (the celestial and beneficent spirit of life, heat and light) and "Yin" (the evil earthly goddess of death, cold and darkness), physiology became a simple matter of assigning body structure and function to either "Yang" or "Yin," and pathology contented itself with the theory that disease arose whenever the balance between these opposing forces was disturbed. Each of the primeval "Yang" and "Yin" worked ceaselessly for good or for evil. Everything originated from one or the other; there were "Yin" diseases and "Yang" diseases, "Yin" organs, "Yin" drugs and "Yang" drugs.

In the 6th Century B.C. a treatise on obstetrics and gynecology states that breech and transverse presentations were corrected by administering musk and heated powdered salt; that normally breech presented until the time of labor. If the hand presented, it was needled to make it withdraw, if the foot it was rubbed with salt. Chills meant the woman had too much "Yin," fever means too much "Yang." To hasten labor, boy's urine mixed with vinegar was sprinkled on hot bricks and inhaled. Sterility was abhorred; they loved children, especially the male child. A Moral Code forbade physicians to practice midwifery, so ignorant midwives were used. Maternal and fetal deaths were high. The squatting position was assumed in labor. A midwife undertook the most difficult manipulations in obstetric labor; she mutilated the baby, replaced prolapsed arm, and did extractions. Hemorrhage was controlled by irrigations with solutions of dried nettles. Retained placenta was not pulled away; a weight was attached to the cord in order to eventually deliver the placenta. Chinese medicine has remained primitive up to recent times.[1]

B. JAPANESE (0-A.D. 1765)

About the beginning of the Christian era, Chinese medicine began slowly to invade Japan by way of Korea and for nearly 1,000 years dominated the practice of medicine there. In the 16th Century, Japanese medicine acquired originality in the person of Nagata Tohuhan, the Japanese Hippocrates. The first scientific work on obstetrics was published by Kagawa Shigen in 1765. Under his leadership and stimulated by contact with the western world, Japan began her remarkable progress which soon outstripped China and all other Oriental nations.[1]

First Occurrences and Outstanding Events

A. Chinese

First Chinese God of Healing was Shen Nung.

First Chinese treatise on obstetrics and gynecology was in the 6th Century.

B. Japanese

First scientific work in Japanese was by Kagawa Shigen, in 1765.

References

A. Chinese

1. Findley, Palmer: *Priests of Lucina.* Boston, Little, 1939, p. 24.

B. Japanese

1. Findley, Palmer: *Priests of Lucina.* Boston, Little, 1939, p. 28.

C. HINDU (1500 B.C.-A.D. 500)

There is fragmentary evidence in the *Veda* or Holy Books that Indian medicine goes back to the 2nd Millennium B.C., and even earlier. Groups of Aryan tribes filtered into India conquering it (others laid the foundations of the Ancient Persian Empire and civilization), followed shortly by invading Greek and Nordic tribes, of ancient Europe, the Aryan immigrants of the 2nd and 1st Millennium B.C. In 1500 B.C., there is definite evidence of Indian medicine. The beginning of Indian medicine and civilization was called the Vedic period, so called because of the four Vedas or holy books dated between 1500 and 1000 B.C. The Rig-Veda and the Atharva-Veda contain most of the medical information. The other two are the Yajur-Veda and Sama-Veda. This period persisted until 800 or 500 B.C. During this, the Vedic period, medicine and particularly obstetrics and gynecology, was largely undeveloped, the importance of gods and the supernatural still prevailed. During this same period, medicine elsewhere, except in Egypt, was extremely primitive. Even in Rome, and perhaps to a less extent in

Greece, medicine was likewise undeveloped; certainly in Rome there were no known physicians.[1]

Toward the latter part of the Vedic period, 600 to 500 B.C., there must have been some influence bandied back and forth between India and Greece, for men like Pythagoras, Empedocles, and Plato influenced Indian thought; also Greek physicians in the 6th Century lived at the court of the Persian kings to whose empire India belonged. These facts imply that there must have been an interchange between the two civilizations.[2,3]

Then came the Brahmanistic era, which lasted to A.D. 1000, with the Arabian influence, dominance of the priestly cast and high scientific thought. Casaka, Susruta (Aesculapius of the Hindus) and Vagbhata were their great physicians. Anatomy did not exist because of religion. Their pathology and physiology were really primitive, their surgery fair, their obstetrics and gynecology meager and poor. The following information will give some idea of ancient Indian medicine: they believed the semen was derived from all parts of the body, as was menstrual blood, both originating in the "Chyle." The embryo was supposed to be the product of semen and menstrual blood. They also believed conception occurred anytime during the first twelve days after the period.[4] They believed, however, that conception occurred most readily during the menstrual epoch, for then the cervix was open "like the flower of the water-lily to the beams of the sun."[5] When the menses stopped in pregnancy it went to the breasts and produced milk. The sex of the child was dependent upon the preponderance of seminal or menstrual fluid and the latter increased in amount on odd days; the child was male if conception occurred on an odd day (after menstruation). Also if the right breast or right eye was larger, or if the mother desired food of a masculine type, the child would be a male.

They knew something of the uterus and tubes, and the formation of the embryo which was described in detail and various stages. The two dozens of diseases of women described, had to do with the menses, dysmenorrhea, pain in the genital organs, pathological conditions of the vagina, abortion, injuries to the vagina and perineum caused by coitus, and uterovaginal tumors. They used fumigations and irrigations of the rectum and vagina, and tapped ovarian cysts by trocar (there is some question about the truth of this latter statement).

In their deliveries, the following procedure took place: "In the ninth month of gestation, the woman was placed in a clean hut built for this purpose. Some gruel was given to hasten labor, fumigations were also used (smoke from the black skin of snakes). Neither cephalic nor podalic version was practiced; dismemberment of the dead fetus and cesarean after death were done. There was no such instrument as the forceps, as we know it." Kedarnath Das agrees with this.[6] The same author describes the use of a knife in such a way that he may not cut a living child with it, for if the child is injured he may destroy both mother and child together. In the same paragraph he says that he grasps in his hand a sickle-shaped knife and his description goes on to say how the child is dismembered, care being taken not to injure the mother. This entire paragraph is confusing because one does not know whether he is describing a forceps operation or an embryotomy.

Retained placenta was treated by pressure, shaking and emetics. Lying-in women got up in ten days, dieted rigidly for six weeks.

Indian practices were to impinge upon Western civilization many years later in the guise of Arabian medicine. They also extended themselves to the Far East, as the fringes of Chinese culture show. Of all the ancient systems except the Greek, that of India was the most influential.

First Occurrences and Outstanding Events

The beginning of Indian medicine and civilization was called the Vedic period.

Their gynecology and obstetrics was meagre and poor. They believed that conception was most apt to occur during the time of menstruation, and that when the menses stopped in pregnancy it went to the breasts and produced milk.

Of all Oriental influences in medicine, Indian was the greatest, except Greek.

References

1. Findley, Palmer: *Priests of Lucina.* Boston, Little, 1939, p. 19.
2. Sigerist, H. E.: *A History of Medicine, Primitive and Archaic Medicine*, Vol. 1. London, Oxford, 1951.

3. Zimmer, H. R.: *Hindu Medicine.* Baltimore, Johns Hopkins Press, Preface, pp. xlviii, 1 and 171.
4. Susruta: *Samhita.* English translation, edited by K. L. Bhishagratna, 3 vol. Calcutta, Bhishagratna, 1907-1916.
5. Wise, T. A.: *Commentary on the Hindu System of Medicine.* Calcutta, Thacker, 1845, p. 32.
6. Das, Kendarnath: *Obstetric Forceps; Its History and Evolution.* Calcutta, The Art Press, 1929.

D. HEBREW (1300 B.C.-A.D. 500)

Hebrew medicine can be traced back to the time of the Sumerians, two or three millenniums B.C., suffering all sorts of vicissitudes in their existence, but always surviving these ordeals of constant warfare of the Semitic races that made up a large part of Mesopotamia. If we examine their history from about 300 B.C. to the sixth Christian century, we can obtain as an excellent picture of the turbulent existence of the Hebrews.[1]

When Alexander the Great conquered Persia in 331 B.C. (Some authors give the date as 332 B.C. and even 336.) and established the city of Alexandria, Jerusalem opened her gates to him and he spared the city. But after a few years he died. It was not long before Ptolemy Soter, ruler of Egypt, captured Jerusalem and transported thousands of its people to Alexandria. Ptolemy was tolerant and the Jews enjoyed peace. In 170 B.C. Antiochus IV (Epiphanes) of the Seleucid Dynasty, King of Syria, the son of Antiochus the Great, who in his day had shelled Hannibal, wrested Jerusalem from Egyptian control. He tried to suppress all traces of Judaism. Oppression led to rebellion, and ultimately the Maccabean family efforts destroyed the Seleucid control, restoring them to the control of the Egyptians. The supremacy which Alexandria wrested from Greece lasted 400 years, and during all these years the Jews remained in close contact with Hellenistic influence, although dominated by Egypt, then Syria and then Egypt again. But in 63 B.C. Jerusalem succumbed to Pompey's (Roman) legions. With Roman aid Herod I of the Idumean Dynasty assumed control of Judea, however Jerusalem gradually rose to its former position of importance. Finally Titus, son of Vespasian, captured Jerusalem and subjugated it. For sixty years Jerusalem lived in comparative peace, when in the year A.D. 132 Hadrian wiped them out again; then, peace continued for Jerusalem until A.D. 306 when it became a Roman colony under Constantine the Great. Trouble began again in A.D. 326 when Macarius was ordered to recover the site of the crucifixion, and veneration for the relics associated with the life of Jesus began. In A.D. 460, by the efforts of Empress Eudocia Augusta, wife of Theodosius II, protection was afforded both Jew and pagan. Though paganism flickered out, Judaism kept glowing until the 6th Century A.D. when again the Persians and later the Mohammedans were preparing to attack Syria.[2]

Through centuries of persecution and during the numerous periods of subjugation to which they acceded tolerantly, they made many contributions. They seemed destined to play a particularly important part as transmitters of Oriental knowledge to the Christian West as well as to the Islamic East. In fact the medical views contained in the books of the Testament were passed on to the Medieval world in the West and in the East. It became a link between the Ancient Orient and the Middle Ages.

Their medical history began not too long after the origin of Hindu medicine, about 1300 B.C.; this is approximately 300 years after the *Kahun Papyrus*, and roughly 800 years before Hippocrates. By 900 B.C., David, author of the *Psalms*, and Solomon of the *Proverbs* appeared, and they had as a contemporary, the epic poet Homer. The Biblical Books, *Genesis*, *Exodus*, *Leviticus* and *Deuteronomy*, all of which contain traces of gynecological knowledge, were written about 1300 B.C. and were attributed to Moses. The great sacred books of the Hebrews called the *Pentateuch* and *Talmud* are further sources of their medicine.

The ancient Jewish conception of disease clung closely to that of the Babylonians, Assyrians and the Egyptians, but they remained aloof from the incantations, exorcism and astrology of these people. To the Hebrews, God was the only physician and at the same time the only source of disease. Therapeutics consisted largely of prayer and barbaric sacrifice. The efficacy of the faith and common sense methods employed by the prophets is exemplified by the prophet Elisha, who, when he was asked to restore to life the smothered boy of the Shunammite, took the child to the roof and revived him quickly with a form of artificial respiration. Bending over the child,

Elisha[3] blew air into his mouth and thereby set off seven sneezes. The sneezes removed an obstruction in the child's trachea, and recovery was almost instantaneous; a method used to this day to resuscitate newborns.

They made much of physical purity, the clean and the unclean. Their sex hygiene forbade them to have intercourse with a menstruating or parturient woman, and they were obliged to bathe after coitus. Sterility was looked upon by the ancient Hebrews as a shame. Abram's wife Sarah, after ten years of married life, was still without offspring. To determine which one was sterile she permitted Abram to cohabit with her young maid Hagar; Hagar was soon pregnant (*Gen.* 16:4) thus proving Sarah's sterility and as a result Hagar "lost her respect for her mistress" for according to Rashi (Rashi *Gen.* 16:2) such a woman is not properly built but is rather thrown together in a haphazard manner.[4]

A knowledge of the anatomy of female genitalia was limited for the most part to the visible parts, though the uterus, cervix and bladder were mentioned. The *Talmud* mentions the mons veneris, the vulva, vestibulum vaginae, orificum urethrae, hymen, vagina, septum vesico-vaginalis, septum vagino-rectalis, uterus, canalis cervicalis, cavum uteri. In the *Gemara*, the following treatment (pure superstition) for menstrual disturbances appears:

> Take of Persian onions thrice three measures, and boil them in wine and give it to her to drink, saying "arise from thy flux." But if it does not prevail, set her in a place where two ways meet, and let her hold a cup of wine in her hand, and let somebody come behind her and affright her, and say "arise from thy flux." But if it does not benefit, let her dig seven ditches, in which let them burn such wines as are not yet four years old, and let her take in her hand a cup of wine, and make her sit down over that, and make her sit down over another. And in every removal, you must say to her "arise from thy flux."

In the *Nidda*, a section devoted to menstruation states that vaginal bleeding is unclean and therefore a ritual bath was used at the cessation of the bleeding, except when due to defloration, when it was not considered "impure" and therefore did not necessitate bathing. They used many queer methods of differentiating flows that were due to defloration or otherwise, e.g., sitting on wine barrels, to see if the breath showed the odor of the wine. It was customary to have two witnesses examine bed sheets after marriage for evidence of ruptured hymen; medico-legal entanglements often resulted. One Samuel, rabbi and physician, was of the opinion that defloration could occur without the loss of blood. They believed the hymen could regrow if injured before the age of three. In light of modern evidence this is not so.[5]

A woman remained unclean for one week after the birth of a male child, two weeks if female. There followed a period of purification, thirty days after birth for a male child and sixty days for a female. In the *Mishna,* a section devoted to miscarriage, the same purification ritual held. As noted by the Egyptians and Greeks, the uterus was supposed to be very sensitive to odors, and the Hebrews also believed this. They said that miscarriages were due to the smell of flesh, but also added trauma, sudden fright and psychic influences, which could all be controlled by charms. The proper preventive (Sabath "66") was an amulet known as the "upright stone" ("ewen thekuma").

They recognized the signs of puberty and the symptoms of menstruation. Of great interest is their recognition of extramenstrual bleeding as being of serious pathological consequence. There is some reference to the occasional practice of cesarean section. Hebrew women understood the use of the vaginal speculum, a crude instrument that was inserted by the patient herself or midwife. Male physicians were not permitted to openly examine a female patient.

Though they relied on God to heal the obscure diseases, the lay physician treated the self-evident cases. In *Ecclesiastes*, 38, written about 200 B.C., the patient is advised to "pray unto the Lord . . . then give place to the physician, for the Lord hath created him and thou hast need of him." Before he could practice, the Jewish doctor had to obtain his permit from the law courts. Fortunately he was spared from the cruel Babylonian practice of retribution for failure to cure. He even was urged to charge a proper fee, since as the *Talmud* puts it "free cures seldom work," and "a physician who charges nothing is worth nothing."

Mosaic Law contained both the essence of the Jewish religion and at the same time an impressive system of pre-Hippocratic medical thought. Though Moses did not originate this code all by himself, he remains to this day one of the most farsighted proponents of preventive medicine. Besides preventive medicine, forensic medicine has developed from the Hebrews. The concept of the purification of the body in the sight of God and "a day of rest" are the greatest contributions of the Ancient Hebrews to medicine.[6]

First Occurrences and Outstanding Events

First to recognize extramenstrual bleeding by the use of a tubular speculum

First to use the speculum (as above).

First record of cesarean operation.

Originated preventive medicine, forensic medicine and the day of rest.

References

1. Sigerist, H. E.: *A History of Medicine, Primitive and Archaic Medicine*, Vol. 1. London, Oxford, 1951.
2. Ricci, J. V.: *Genealogy of Gynecology*. Philadelphia and Toronto, Blakiston, 1950.
3. Bettmann, O. L.: *A Pictorial History of Medicine*. Springfield, Thomas, 1956.
4. Raschi or Rabbi Schlomo Izchake (A.D. 1040-1105) wrote about this, probably from Rashi *Gen.* 16:2.
5. Sachs, Aron: *Die Gynakologie im der Bibel und im Talmud*. Leipzig, E. Lehmann, 1909.
6. Bettmann, O. L.: *A Pictorial History of Medicine*. Springfield, Thomas, 1956.

Chapter V

GRECO-ROMAN ERA (500 B.C.-A.D. 500)

A. GREEK (500 B.C.-0)

THE STORY of Greek medicine usually begins with the pre-Hippocratic years. Actually, however, Greece must have felt the influence of Egyptian and Mesopotamian cultures much earlier. We have only meager references to this very early period because of the lack of historical information available. But we do know that an Oriental influence was at work, and became more noticeable when the Mesopotamian civilizations began to make actual contact with its neighbors overseas, the first of these was by the Phoenicians during the time of Homer (circa 800 B.C.). Eventually the Greeks began to travel to these western Oriental outposts, in order to satisfy their thirst for more knowledge, and by the 6th Century B.C. Egypt was officially opened to foreigners. Philosophers and learned physicians travelled extensively; Hippocrates, Galen, Aretaeus and Dioscorides, Plato and Eudoxus can be numbered among them if we are to believe their writings which contain a fair amount of papyral medical lore. The awareness of this new culture, Grecian culture, really began when Alexander the Great defeated the Persians and Assyrians in 331 B.C., although it had existed for hundreds of years before by slow infiltration. Of all the Oriental influences on Greece, the most effective source was Egypt, Babylonia, and from the Minoans and possibly from the Hindus.

The Greeks, like the Egyptians (possibly copied from them) had their gods of healing, e.g., the Greek Apollo and the Egyptian

Thoth, Aesculapius and Imhotep and countless other similar representations of parallel gods. The mythical and spiritual aspects of this early Greek culture in medicine which was derived mainly from the Babylonians began to lessen as early as 1250 B.C. Machaon, one of the sons of Aesculapius, and physician-in-chief of the Grecian forces at the battle of Troy, removed arrow heads, stopped the bleeding, medicated wounds and cared for the sick in a business-like fashion without the slightest use of magic. Though this was true in the treatment of wounds resulting from obvious physical causes, the unexplainable diseases were still subjects of theurgy.[1]

From the Minoans, besides sanitation and hygiene, they learned of the Serpent Symbol which the Minoans originated.[2] The Aesculapian staff has often been confused with the Caduceus otherwise known as the "Herald's Wand" used by Hermes (Mercury) to open

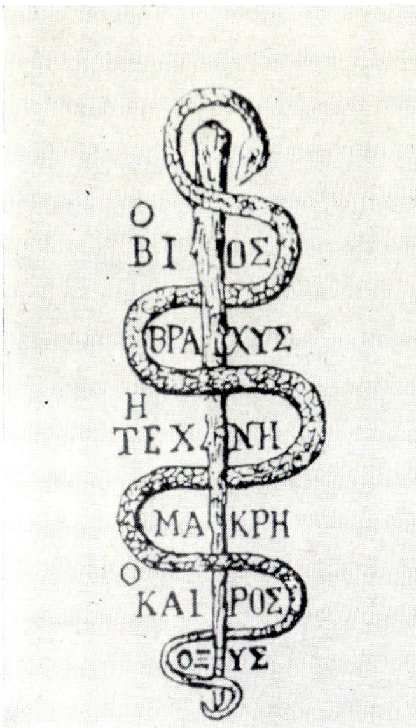
Ο
ΒΙ ΟΣ
ΒΡΑ ΧΥΣ
Η
ΤΕΧ ΝΗ
ΜΑ ΚΡΗ
Ο
ΚΑΙ ΡΟΣ
ΟΞ ΥΣ

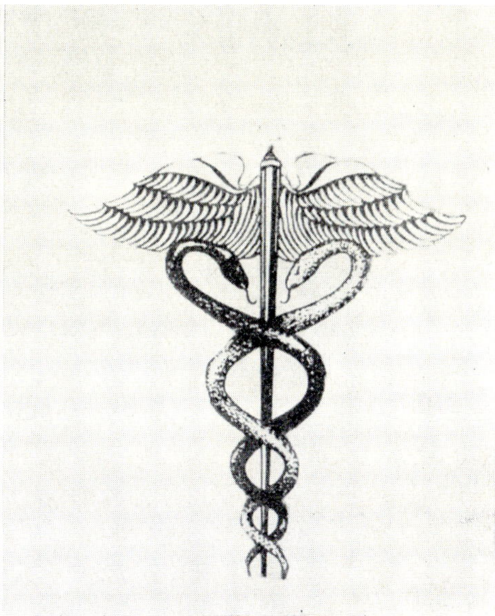

Fig. 31. Aesculapian wand. (The Bettmann Archive.)
Fig. 32. Caduceus.

doors between gods and men (a sort of business calling card). The Aesculapian staff entwined by one snake, instead of two as in the Caduceus, is regarded by classists as the true symbol of the profession.

The interesting question of who came first, Aesculapius or the serpent, has been settled in favor of the serpent. Reptiles have been considered synonymous with wisdom since time immemorial. The snake, in particular, coming out of the ground, which holds many curative substances, was believed to possess secret healing powers. Consequently, the ancient Greeks ate snake meat to acquire proficiency in the healing arts and even immortality.

From the Egyptians the Greeks obtained the wholesome and sound practices of their medicine. A few authors claim that Aesculapius carried Egyptian medicine to Greece, that he was Egyptian, that he wrote the papyri and that he was one and the same person as Imhotep, who also was supposed to have written the papyri, however most writers agree that the authors of the papyri are anonymous.

This period in the history of medicine could be called the Aesculapian era. It was the sacerdotal order in primitive Greece that practiced medicine as an art, and it is quite possible that the practice of medicine had its beginning in this manner and at this time, and Aesculapius was the patron god of the science of medicine.

The birth of Aesculapius might be the first cesarean section because, according to legend, Coronis, his mother, had betrayed Apollo, his father, who destroyed her by fire on the funeral pyre after taking the premature infant from her uterus. The child was then left to Chiron to be raised and educated. Chiron the Centaur, of Thessaly, is credited with teaching Aesculapius the art of healing. The idea of a cesarean birth of Aesculapius comes from the Greek poet Homer in the 13th Century B.C. Other authorities think Aesculapius was born before his mother died of puerperal sepsis. According to them the "burning" Homer speaks of probably refers to fever.[3, 4]

When we read that Aesculapius was the son of Apollo and Coronis we should keep in mind that mythology played so great a part in the lives of the Greeks of this period that they often named great people as gods or sons of gods. By now our ideas may be somewhat confused as to the reality of such persons. Aesculapius, however, was real, and except that he was a great healer and had temples built for him and had at least two sons, we really know very little.[5]

The first Greek temple erected to his worship was a temple at

Titane, dedicated about 50 years after the fall of Troy, 1250 B.C. It was not long before celebrated temples spread world wide, we find them at Cnidus, Pergamus, Cos, Epidaurus and elsewhere. They served as health resorts and schools of medicine. One of the oldest such temples was named after Amynos, an Athenian god of healing. It was founded at Athens as early as 1000 B.C. Another named after Amphiaraos, a prehistoric warrior, was founded near Oropus in Attica at the end of the fifth century B.C.[6]

The famous temple at Epidaurus erected to the memory of Aesculapius was equipped with a hospital ward and with a lair for sacred serpents who played an important part in therapy. These patients underwent the process of temple sleep or incubation to await assistance from a god or from the sacred serpents in the form of an illuminating dream or vision which the priest would later interpret for them. With the aid of heat and soft flute music, tame reptiles were coaxed to lick the patient's wounds. A snake biscuit was on sale in the temple; patients bought it and fed the serpents with the hope of improving relations between patients and the reptiles.[7]

Neither birth nor death was allowable in a temple. If a pregnant woman were in the temple for a reason other than her pregnancy and suddenly developed labor pains, she would be expelled forthwith. A patient obviously dying would be mercilessly expelled so that many died on the hillside, probably alone and unattended. Besides the practice of incubation, patients were bathed, massaged and given applications of soothing ointments in these temples. Sometimes surgery was attempted. Above all, fresh air and recreational activities (the theater at Epidaurus seated 12,000) helped to insure some kind of relief. Thus the patient left the establishment refreshed and strengthened in his faith. In the light of modern psychotherapy, the Aesculapian temple compares favorably with the sanitarium or rest home. In the beginning the temples were sustained by gifts, later fees became necessary.

The priests, who were called Aesclepiads, were individuals of average mental faculties; they were solely concerned with cures; in a sense they were the clinicians. Medicine as a higher branch of thought and as a science occupied the minds of great intellects of Ionian Greece, namely the philosophers, and, in a way, they were the basic science group of today. They aimed at an explanation of

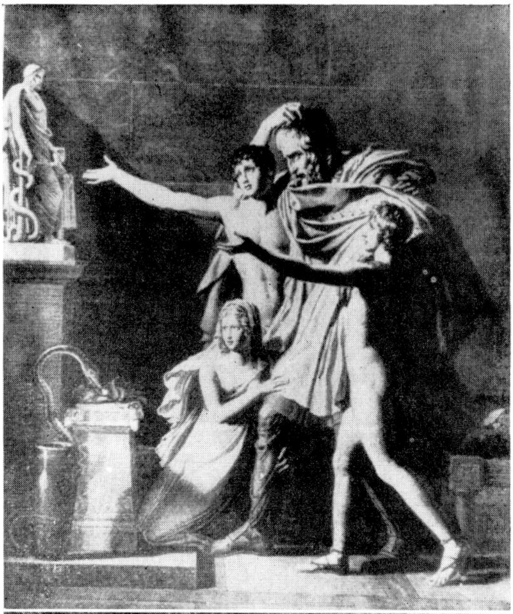

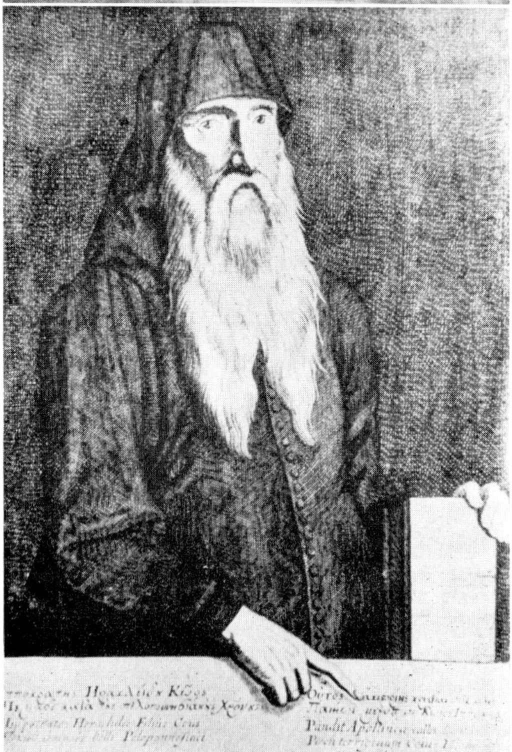

Fig. 33. Imploring Aesculapius for a cure. (The Bettmann Archive.)
Fig. 34. Hippocrates. (LaWall, C. H.: *Four Thousand Years of Pharmacy*. Philadelphia. Lippincott, 1927.)

physiological and pathological phenomena. These subjects together with anatomy were neglected by the physicians. This separation continued as late as the 2nd Century A.D., e.g., Soranus, the greatest gynecologist of the ancients did not think it necessary to consider the anatomy of the female genitalia. On the other hand Galen (circa A.D. 130-200) insisted on physiology and anatomy as indispensable. Likewise Pythagoras of Samos (circa 580-496 B.C.), Diogenes of Apollonia (circa 430 B.C.), Democritus of Abdera (b. circa 460 B.C.), Parmenides of Elea (circa 450 B.C.) and Empedocles of Agrigentum, considered by Galen as the founder of the Italian School of ancient medicine, were definite and specific in their physiology, particularly in their calculations of generation. Much animal experimentation was done to obtain physiological data. Alcmaeon of Crotona (500 B.C.) the most famous physician just before Hippocrates said that the fetus nourished itself through its body, like a sponge. Anaxagoras of Clazomenae (b. circa 500 B.C.) teacher of Pericles, maintained that the fetus was nourished through the umbilical veins.

If any progress were to be made in medicine this separation of practitioner and thinker would need to be repaired; the basic scientist and the clinician would have to work in unison. This transition began with Euripides (circa 480-406 B.C.), Anaxagoras (b. circa 500 B.C.), Pericles (490-429 B.C.), pupil of Anaxagoras, Socrates (469-399 B.C.), pupil of Plato (circa 427-347 B.C.), Sophocles (494-406 B.C.), Aristophanes (448-385 B.C.), Herodotus (484-425 B.C.), the historian, and his equal Thucydides (circa 460–400-395 B.C.), and Phidias (500-434 B.C.), the sculptor. Then came:

HIPPOCRATES (circa 460-377 B.C.) and with him came the turning point of medicine. It was he who put medicine upon the foundations of rigid scientific observations and high morality. He not only brought the scientist and the clinician together, but by so doing he wrested medicine from the temple physicians of the cult of Aesculapius and effected a separation so complete that the fundamentals of Hippocratic medicine continued for over 2,400 years. Hippocrates was born on the island of Cos, according to Soranus. Legend has it that he was a direct descendant of Aesculapius, but we must remember that the old Greeks had a way of deifying their heroes. He studied medicine in Athens, practiced and taught for many years in various cities of Thrace, Macedonia and Thessaly. He was interested in general medicine mainly, his interest in gynecology as such was minor. He was the first to record his views on disease and treatment, and so has the distinction of being "the father of medical literature" as well as "the father of medicine."

The important medical centers or schools of this period were developments of the temples of health, the outstanding ones were those of Epidaurus in Argolis, Greece; Cos, off the coast of Asia Minor, where Hippocrates learned some of his medicine; his father being one of his instructors, and Cnidus on the coast of Caria. In the Cnidian school, Euryphon, an older contemporary of Hippocrates but not as great, was the leader and particularly interested in gynecology and obstetrics. He treated prolapse by suspending the woman tied to a ladder by her feet. It was at about this period of history that male physicians began to partake of the practice of gynecology and obstetrics, often assisting the women who still did most of it.

Hippocrates' knowledge of anatomy and also physiology was really not so profound. Displacements of the uterus as high up as the liver or the heart is mentioned; this was probably the result of the failure to do bimanual examinations, although they did vaginal and abdominal examinations. The vaginal examinations were usually done by midwives.[8] They noted menstruation and conception quite accurately but did not understand its physiology. The Greeks coined the word menstruation, meaning catharsis, the name being indicative of the prevailing sentiment that the blood of the menstrual flux is impure. Pliny called the menstrual blood a "fatal poison, corrupting and decomposing urine,[9] depriving seeds of their fecundity, destroying insects, blasting garden flowers and grasses, causing fruit to fall from branches, dulling razors, etc." He found it to cause a dog to go mad, though later it was employed as a cure for the bite of a mad dog. The menstrual blood has been used as a therapeutic agent for a variety of diseases, such as puerperal fever, gout, erysipelas, goiter, hemorrhages, headaches, worms, and epilepsy. For this purpose the dried blood on the menstrual pad was mixed with wine or vinegar. The first napkin worn by healthy virgins was highly prized for its curative virtues and was believed to be particularly effective in the treatment of gout. Again, Pliny writes:

> If a woman strips herself while she is menstruating and walks around a field of wheat, the caterpillars, worms, and beetles and other vermin will fall off from the ears of corn. . . . a mare, big with foal, if touched by a woman in this state, will be sure to miscarry; nay, even at the very sight of a woman, though even at a distance. So pernicious are the properties of the menstrual discharge that woman, themselves the source from which it is derived, are far from being safe from its effects. A pregnant woman, for instance, if touched with it, or if, indeed, she so much as steps over it, will be liable to miscarry.

Because of the blighting effects of a menstruous woman, punishment was meted out to a woman who failed to make known her condition. This prohibition led to the custom of wearing a bandage about the head. Others had customs of fasting. For the menstrual period to be unduly prolonged was regarded a crime and was punishable with a hundred lashes of a whip.

The study of menstruation by the Grecian school concludes that the menses lasted at least three days, and in most women even longer. In healthy women the blood was like that of "a sacrificial animal" and flowed quickly. At the beginning and end of menstruation the blood was thinner and in less quantity. They even measured the amount of menstrual blood and the quantity from a healthy woman was given as "two Attic cotylae."

As to the duration of pregnancy, the Hippocratic school offered opinions that were not consistent, and showed the importance of numerology. There are figures of 182 days from one author while another goes up to 300 days as the length of pregnancy. This last is admitted, however, to be the longest possible pregnancy because by this time the child cannot get enough food from the uterus, so it becomes hungry and starts a series of violent movements which ruptures the membranes and start the process of delivery. Most authors of this school held to the more conventional 280 days but disagreed about whether this should be regarded as four groups of 70 days or seven groups of 40 days. The former grouping was more popular because it checked with the belief that a seven months child (three groups of seventy) would live, whereas an eight month child would not. This sort of thinking can be traced back to the Babylonian Assyrian numerologists with emphasis on the number seven.

There is an interesting passage in *The Nature of the Infant*, reputedly by Hippocrates, which reads: "they suffer in the whole body, but especially in the lumbar region and ischia; for their ischia separate." For hundreds of years this was read literally and taken to imply that in labor the bones of the pelvis underwent a physical separation, particularly at the pubic symphysis. The result was that for centuries the importance of disproportion between the mother's pelvis and baby's skull went unrecognized. Obstructed labor with the death of the fetus and possibly also of the mother was never due to a contracted pelvis. It was merely that the child was too weak to separate the pelvic bones of the mother.

About 400 B.C. there was a law in Athens that stated "midwives (Greek) had to be past the age of childbearing themselves but it was essential that they should have borne children." There were two classes of midwives and it was quite usual for them to call in a male doctor to assist at the birth. One group were the ordinary workaday midwives. If the case was normal they could conduct the delivery. Then there was the senior group of midwives who in reality were doctor midwives. They were permitted to prescribe drugs, induce abortion or bring on a birth prematurely. These senior midwives were also responsible for intoning the hymns which invoked help of birth goddesses, Artemis and Hera and Eileithyia. A goddess called upon not nearly so often was Actemia. She was terrified by her mother's suffering at her own birth and so she besought from Zeus the favor of eternal virginity. But she changed her mind completely for she gave birth to fifty daughters. These goddesses and particularly Eileithyia were believed to assist at childbirth and bring children into the world, and at the same time they could increase the pains of labor as a punishment for want of chastity.

One of the duties of midwives was to advise eligible men which young girls would be likely to produce the best offspring for them. Midwives received no special instruction; they depended on experience almost entirely. One of the commonest maneuvers they practiced was to bind a cloth around the swollen abdomen of the woman in childbirth and with each pain they would tighten the binder.

They used an obstetric chair later in this period; earlier they used the husband's shield for the place upon which the confinement took place (Lacedaemonian women).[10]

Superfetation was considered a common manifestation. Malpositions of the uterus were noted, especially prolapse. Malpositions in young women were considered more serious, and immediate marriage was suggested, for in general, women who cohabited enjoyed better health. Whether or not speculae were used is not certain. Some allusion to its use is found occasionally. In such instances the patient herself, or another woman, inserted the speculum. Puerperal fever, septic abortion, ulcerations of the womb were recognized. Stenosis of the cervix and lacerations were noted. Cancer as such was not recognized.

Therapeutically, fumigation was the commonest mode of therapy. It soothed, softened and opened the genital parts.[11] The uterus was considered a "wandering organ" and fumigation by fragrant odors was supposed also to attract the aberrant uterus to its normal site; offensive odors repelled it. Tamponades of astringent drugs were used. Sounds and dilators were used to stretch the cervix and correct displacements.

Much of the information we have of this time and particularly about Hippocrates is obtained from the famous *Hippocratic Collection*. These writings were by different men at different historical periods. The treatises containing gynecological references were edited at the beginning of the 3rd Century B.C. by scholars of the Alexandrian school at the express request of Ptolemy Soter. There still remains some confusion and doubt as to the authenticity of some of these writings, but it will be of interest to quote from some of these references in order that we might get a better appreciation of gynecology as it was understood and practiced in the 4th and 5th Centuries B.C. Of the writings that contain gynecology there are The *Prognostics*, the *Epidemics*, the *Aphorisms*, *Airs*, *Waters*, *Places* and *The Oath*. We shall quote only briefly from some of these. These collections contain both generalizations and case histories. For more completeness we suggest reference to Adams, The Genuine Works of Hippocrates.[12]

THE OATH, quote from:

In the "Oath" is stated "I will not give to a woman an abortive

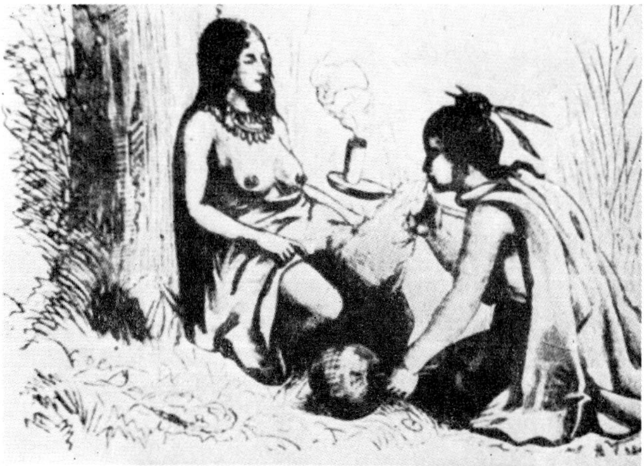

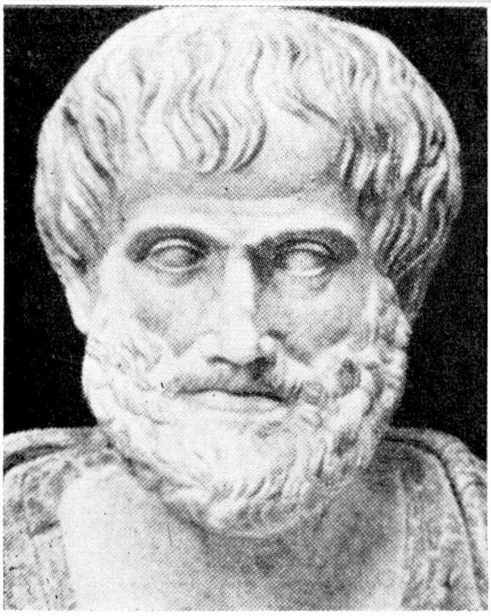

Fig. 35. Fumigation in delivery. ([Witkowski] G. Steinheil, Paris.)
Fig. 36. Aristotle. (Culver Service.)

remedy." As a matter of fact during this era there was little moral feeling about abortion, nor was it an offense against the state. This feeling of unscrupulousness about abortions continued for about two centuries.[13]

The Oath, as we know it, is the Christianized version and it forbids abortion by any process. In the original pagan reading of the oath it was specifically the use of the pessary to induce abortion that was forbidden, a free rendering being: "I will not give to any woman a pessary to produce abortion." Plato and Aristotle stated that abortion was permitted for the purpose of limiting the population. Permitted or not, it seems that it was extensively practiced and the disastrous after effects in some cases were described by one writer of the Hippocratic School:

> If the womb becomes ulcerated, both blood and pus are discharged; there is a strong odour, acute pains in the loins, groins, and lower part of the abdomen. The pains gradually ascend from the flanks to the sides and the shoulder blades, and sometimes they reach to the collar bones, and there is intense headache and delirium. After a time the woman swells and grows weak, faints and is feverish and chilly. Her legs especially become swollen. The disease occurs after a woman aborts; the fetus is found to be putrid, and the lochia do not appear and the womb is very hot to the touch.
>
> If called upon to treat such a case while the pains are present, bathe the patient with much hot water and apply hot fomentations to the painful parts. If the woman is strong, make a uterine injection. The ulceration is to be treated with oxide of lead, gall nuts, myrhh, and calcined Egyptian alum.

THE PROGNOSTICS, quotes from:

> Women may be judged of whether they are in a fit state for conception or not by attending to the following circumstances: In the first place to their shapes. Women of smaller stature more readily conceive than taller persons; the thin than the fat; the white than the ruddy; the dark than the pale; those who have prominent veins than the contrary. In oldish women it is bad to have much flesh, but a good thing to have swelled and large breasts. In addition, inquiry should be made whether or not the menstruation be regular as to time and quantity. And it should be ascertained whether the uterus be healthy, of a dry temperament, and soft; neither in a state of retraction nor prolapsus; and its mouth neither turned aside, nor too close, nor too open. When any of these obstructions come in the way, it is impossible that conception can take place.
>
> In such cases as cannot conceive, but appear green, without fever, and the viscera are not in fault; these will say that the head is pained, and that the menstrual discharge is vitiated and irregular. But such of these as have the proper color, are of a fat habit

of body, the veins are inconspicuous, they have not pains, and the menses either never appear at all, or are scanty and intense, and this is one of the most difficult states of sterility to remove. In other cases the health is not to blame, but the fault lies in the position of the womb. The other contingencies in this place are attended with pains, discoloration, and wasting.

In cases of false conception, in which women are deceived by the nonappearance of the menses, and by the increase of the belly and movement in it, they will be found to have headache and pains about the neck and hypochondria, and there is no milk in the breasts except a little of a watery character. But when the swelling of the womb passes away they will conceive, unless there be any other impediment. For this affection is beneficial in so far as it produces a change in the uterus, so that afterwards the woman may prove with child. Women with child have not these pains unless the headache be habitual to them, and in addition they have milk in the breasts. Women affected with chronic discharges are to be asked whether they have pains in the head and loins, and in the lower part of the belly, and whether their teeth be set on edge, and if they have dimness of sight, and noises in their ears. Such women as vomit bile for several days while in a fasting state, though they are not with child nor have fever, are to be asked whether they have vomited up round lumbrici, and if they say not, they should be warned that this will happen to them. This affection happens principally to married women, then to virgins, and less seldom to other people.[14]

THE APHORISMS, section 5, quote from:

28. Fumigation with aromatics promotes menstruation, and would be useful in many other cases, if it did not occasion heaviness of the head.
33. In a woman when there is a stoppage of the menses, a discharge of blood from the nose is good.
34. When a pregnant woman has a violent diarrhoea, there is danger of miscarrying.
37. In a pregnant woman, if the breasts suddenly lose their fullness, she has a miscarriage.
41. If you wish to ascertain if a woman be with child, give her hydromel to drink when she is going to sleep, and has not taken supper, and if she be seized with tormina in the belly, she is with child, but otherwise she is not pregnant.

42. A woman with child, if it be a male, has a good color, but if a female, she has a bad color.
44. Women who are very lean, have miscarriage when they prove with child, until they get into better condition.
46. Such women as are immoderately fat, and do not prove with child in them, it is because the epiploon (fat) blocks up the mouth of the womb, and until it be reduced, they do not conceive.
47. If the portion of the uterus seated near the hip-joint suppurate, it gets into a state requiring to be treated with tents.
48. The male foetus is usually seated in the right, and the female in the left side.
50. If you wish to stop the menses in a woman, apply as large a cupping instrument as possible to the breasts.
59. If a woman does not conceive, and wishes to ascertain whether she can conceive, having wrapped her up in blankets, fumigate below, and if it appear that the scent passes through the body to the nostrils and mouth, know that of herself she is not unfruitful.
60. If woman with a child have her courses, it is impossible that the child can be healthy.
61. If a woman's courses be suppressed, and neither rigor nor fever has followed, but she has been affected with nausea, you may reckon her to be with child.
62. Women who have the uterus cold and dense, do not conceive, and those also who have the uterus humid, do not conceive, for the semen is extinguished, and in women whose uterus is very dry, and very hot, the semen is lost from the want of food; but women whose uterus is in an intermediate state between these temperaments prove fertile.[15]

When Hippocrates died in 377 B.C. the famous medical schools at Cos and Cnidia were still flourishing.

Polybos (circa 360 B.C.), son-in-law of Hippocrates, had assumed leadership on the basis of his treatises *On Diseases of Women* and *On Sterility*. This may be considered one of the earliest texts on gynecology. At Cnidia,

Diocles of Carystos (circa 350 B.C.), the last of the Hippocrateans was one of the few Greek anatomists and embryologists. Among the many organs of the body that he discovered were the oviducts, of the sheep.[16] (Rufus also was credited as the first to recognize the Fallopian tubes in animals, Fallopius in man.)

In 331 B.C., after defeating the Persians, Alexander the Great, pupil of Aristotle, founded the city of Alexandria. In 307 B.C., approximately seventy years after the death of Hippocrates, the Alexandrian School in Egypt was established.[17] With the aid of Ptolemy Soter, a library and museum was founded that became world famous; as long as eight hundred years later Aetius used this library to compile important sections of his famous work, *Diseases of Women*. The school became the seat of one of the celebrated medical schools of antiquity.

ARISTOTLE (384-322 B.C.). Through the efforts of Aristotle and his pupil Theophrastos, at this institution, clinical medicine was superseded in importance by zoology, botany and comparative anatomy. What Aristotle really did was to forge a bridge between biology and medicine, comparable to the philosophers and practitioners of an earlier period.

Aristotle was not a physician, he was a great naturalist and zoologist and gave to medicine many fundamentals relative to menstruation, conception, sterility, and the gravid state of humans. He said that women menstruated more than all female animals; animals that lay eggs do not menstruate, the menstrual blood is converted into scales, feathers, and hair. He noticed that incompatability between ovum and sperm is an important part of sterility. He was the one who described superfetation.

In Alexandria dissection of dead bodies was freely allowed, hence an increase in the knowledge of anatomy. Two celebrated anatomists and founders of systematic human dissection were Herophilus (4th Century B.C.) and Erasistratus (300-250 B.C.) They are considered, by some, as the founders of the medical school at Alexandria. They demonstrated that all peripheral nerves are linked to the spinal cord. Herophilos described the ovaries in detail. Erasistratos was the first to maintain that women had diseases peculiar to their sex. He came close to discovering the circulation of the blood.[18, 19]

The death of Hippocrates in 377 B.C., the founding of the city of Alexandria in 331 B.C., and the beginning of the Alexandrian School in 307 B.C. was a time which coincided with the decline of

Greek culture; this culture was directed to Egypt, where it lasted for more than 400 years. Toward the end of this period, this Grecian culture in Egypt outdid itself by contributing to medicine two of the greatest gynecologists and obstetricians of antiquity, Soranus and Rufus, who studied in Alexandria and practiced in Rome. When Greek culture ran its long course in Alexandria, it changed its direction toward the rising Roman Empire, so that by 47 B.C., through the efforts of Caesar, medicine passed from the Nile to the banks of the Tiber.

First Occurrences and Outstanding Events

Beginnings of medicine came from the sacerdotal order in Greece.

Aesculapius was the patron God of the science of medicine.

First temple of worship of Aesculapius was "Titane" in 1300 B.C.

The greatest gynecologist of ancient times was Soranus.

Hippocrates put medicine on rigid scientific foundations and high morality.

Hippocrates was the first to record his medical views, therefore he was called the father of medical literature and father of medicine.

This was a period of history when male physicians began to partake of the practice of obstetrics and gynecology.

The word menstruation was coined.

One of the earliest texts on gynecology by Polybos circa 360 "on diseases of women and on sterility."

Herophilus and Erasistratus, 4th century, were the founders of the medical school at Alexandria and of systematic human dissection.

Erasistratos was the first to maintain that women had diseases peculiar to their sex.

References

1. Bettmann, O. L.: *A Pictorial History of Medicine*. Springfield, Thomas, 1956.
2. Bethel, J. P., ed.: *Webster's New Collegiate Dictionary*. Springfield, Mass., Merriam Co., 1949.
3. Haggard, H. W.: *Devils, Drugs, and Doctors*. New York, Harper, 1929.
4. Frazier, J. G.: (edit. and trans.) Apollodorus: *The Library*, 2 vols. London, Loeb Library, 1921.
5. Da Costa, J. C.: *Trials and Triumphs of the Surgeon*. Philadelphia, Dorrance, 1944.

6. Lamb: (edit. and trans.) Plato: *Symposium.* London, Loeb Library, 1932.
7. Bettmann, O. L.: *A Pictorial History of Medicine.* Springfield, Thomas, 1956.
8. Littré Émile: (edit. and trans.) *Oeuvres complétes d'Hippocrate,* 10 vols. Paris, Baillière, 1839-1861.
Nature of Women, 40, vii, p. 385.
9. Bostock, and Riley, H. T.: (edit. and trans.) Pliny: *Naturalis Historia,* 6 vols. London, Bohn's Classical Library, 1855-7.
10. Graham, Harvey: *Eternal Eve.* London, Heineman, 1950, p. 40.
11. Littré, Émile: (edit. and trans.) *Oeuvres complètes d'Hippocrate,* 10 vols. Paris, Baillière, 1839-1861.
Diseases of Women, II, 133, viii, p. 285-287.
12. Adams, F.: *The Genuine Works of Hippocrates,* 2 vols. London, Sydenham Society, 1849.
13. Edelstein, L.: *The Hippocratic Oath: Text, Translation and Interpretation.* Baltimore, Johns Hopkins Press, 1943.
14. Adams, F.: *The Genuine Works of Hippocrates,* Vol. 1. London, Sydenham Society, 1849, p. 220.
15. Adams, F.: *The Works of Hippocrates,* Vol. 2. London, Sydenham Society, 1849, pp. 240-246.
16. Bostock, and Riley, H. T.: (edit. and trans.) Pliny: *Naturalis Historia,* 6 vols. London, Bohn's Classical Library, 1855-7.
17. Leonardo, R. A.: *History of Gynecology.* New York, Froben, 1944.
18. Ricci, J. V.: *Genealogy of Gynecology.* Philadelphia and Toronto, Blakiston, 1950.
19. Leonardo, R. A.: *History of Gynecology.* New York, Froben, 1944.

B. ROMAN (0-A.D.500)

While Greece slipped into obscurity and the Alexandrian school continued to develop the arts and sciences, Rome was forging ahead and had practically arrived at its imperialistic zenith. It began back in 63 B.C., when Pompey's legions, with Roman aid, Herod I, assumed control of Judea; the Jews remaining under Roman "supervision" until A.D. 600. With this beginning in 63 B.C. Imperial Rome commenced its march forward, and by 146 B.C. Sicily, Jugurtha and Numidia, Carthage and Corinth were destroyed. Greece thus became a Roman byway to the Orient. The threshhold of Egypt was thrown open to Latin plunderers, Caesar decimated the German tribes and subjugated Gaul. Finally Augustus conquered the land of the Nile. By the last pre-Christian century all roads led to Rome.[1]

In the early period of Roman history, immorality and sexual excesses (and much gynecology of an infectious nature) abounded because of the poor leadership of the rulers, some of whom were either old and feeble or mad, coarse, beastly, profligate, mean, dissolute, vicious and inhuman. These depraved leaders were Tiberius, Caligula, Claudius, Nero, Galba, Vitellius and Vespasian. A century later the rulers were able leaders, and good rulers, and Rome realized its maximum expansion and prosperity. These capable men were Nerva, Trajan, Hadrian, Antoninus Pius and Marcus Aurelius. It was at this time in its history that Rome produced the greatest gynecology and obstetrics of antiquity. In medicine the great names of Soranus, Rufus, and Galen were the gifts to the world by these Romans.

Rome, like the Greeks, had its goddesses; in fact it got them from Greece. The most powerful divinity protecting the Roman woman in labor was Lucina who was comparable to the Greek Eileithyia. Then, of course, there were the lesser goddesses such as Juno who was responsible for menstruation; pregnant women brought her flowers to guard against abortion. Midwifery came to Rome from the Grecian and from the Alexandrian schools. It was Herophilus who wrote a book on midwifery in 300 B.C. He and Erasistratus were the greatest teachers, among other subjects, of midwifery in Alexandria. They were therefore the most important source of midwifery of the Romans.

Pliny says that the Romans had no physicians for 600 years, the heads of the household had their own treatments. Cato, like Pliny, had little time for the Greeks; Cato became known as "the Carthage must be destroyed Cato." But in 219 B.C., despite the terrible popular disapproval of Greek Physicians, there came to Rome a Greek named Archagathus, who was trained in Alexandria. In Rome the reliance on household gods soon began to give way to Greek physicians so that it was not long before other Greek medical men followed Archagathus. Pliny wrote ruefully: "it is a well known fact that those physicians, who, without being able to speak Greek, attempted to build up a practice in Rome, failed to gain the confi-

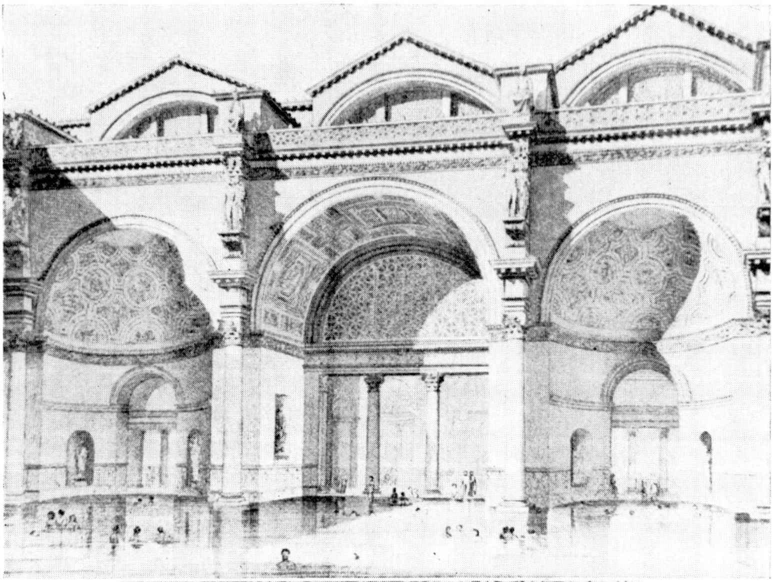

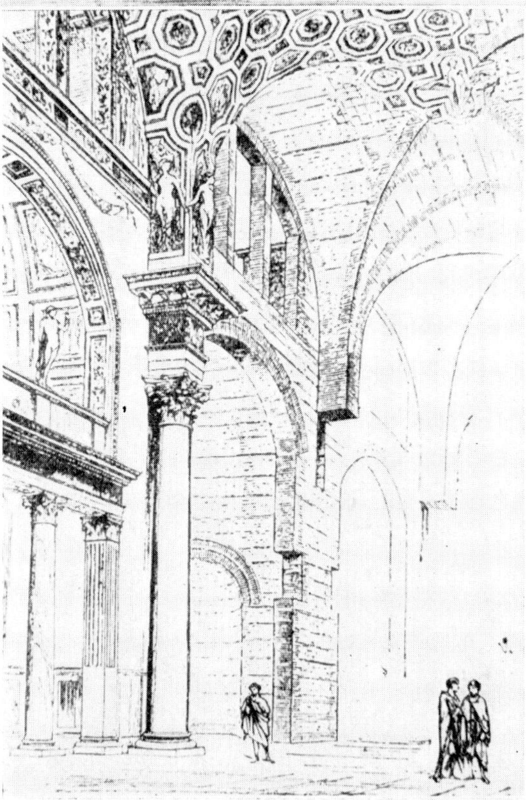

Fig. 37. The Frigidarium, Baths of Caracalla. (Blum and Tatlock: *A Short History of Art*. London, Batsford, 1926.)

Fig. 38. The Tepidarium, Thermae of Caracalla. (Blum and Tatlock: *A Short History of Art*. London, Batsford, 1926.)

dence of their patients, even those who were not at all familiar with that language."

Because of the successes of Archagathus, Asclepiades (128-56 B.C.), born at Prusa in Bithynia, came to Rome in 90 B.C. He treated many distinguished Romans, among them Cicero and Caesar. He was the first to found a medical school in Rome. He was immensely successful even though he was disliked intensely by the majority of Romans, as were all things Greek, and in spite of the fact that he considered Hippocratic doctrines as a "meditation upon death." His chief therapeutic weapons were a careful diet adjusted to every ill, a liberal prescription of wine, together with massage, bathing and bleeding.

The power of Rome was increasing steadily along with its victories in the field of battle. A degree of luxury and vice never before known prevailed among the four million Romans, and eventually the sober republican rule gave way to an imperial immorality. If the "ruling class" and particularly the Emperors were lustful, their wives were no better. Faustina, Agrippina, and Messalina preferred the stews to the palace and Agrippina used to spend many nights in the Roman brothels accepting as many men as came her way. Promiscuity was the order of the Roman day and reached its peak in the famous baths where both sexes shed their garments along with any lingering inhibitions.

Venereal infections must have been rampant, although no literature of this period remains that comes even close to a description that might be gonorrhea. However, orchitis and phimosis are accurately described.[2]

In Rome the practice of medicine was open to all, there were no restrictions and no laws to stop them; if anyone felt he possessed the necessary knowledge to practice medicine he was at liberty to carry on. In pagan Rome there were schools but no hospitals. According to St. Jerome, the first hospital in Rome opened its doors about A.D. 380. A Christian matron, Fabiola by name, donated her home for this purpose. All the clinical bedside teaching was given at the homes of the patients.[3]

At the time of the last pagan century, which is the first part of the history of Roman medicine (the 1st Century B.C. and shortly thereafter) three names are prominent in medicine. They are Aurelius Cornelius Celsus, Gaius Plinius Secundus and Pedacius Dioscorides.

AURELIUS CORNELIUS CELSUS (27 B.C.-A.D. 50). Celsus was not a practicing physician. He wrote in Latin rather than the customary Greek used in medicine. His gynecology adhered closely to the Hippocratic viewpoint. He wrote a treatise called *De Medicina.*

He was the first to show any glimmerings of the procedure of podalic version.[4] By the 3rd Century A.D. he was completely forgotten. He used over ninety authors to compile his book. His gynecology is indeed very sketchy. He described the womb as very small, not much larger than a body that may be embraced by one's hands. He used pessaries and gave medication for menstrual disturbances such as wild cucumber pulp in breast milk to promote the menses. One chapter is devoted to the uses of massage and friction generally as applied to the diseases of women. It is recommended particularly for diseases of the womb, which, according to Celsus, is, after the stomach, the organ most frequently attacked by disease (the incidence of occurrence of disease of the stomach and the uterus is the same today). He states that women with diseases of the womb may lose their reason and, to prevent this, cold compresses should be applied just above the pubes. Prolapse of the womb calls first for a careful inspection to see whether it is healthy or diseased. According to its appearance it is to be treated with astringent washes and the like before being placed in its normal position. To retain it there, a medicated pessary is pressed firmly into the vagina and the thighs are then bound together. He advised that a vagina constricted by inflammation should be incised, and suggested a crucial incision for imperforate hymen.

GAIUS PLINIUS SECUNDUS (Pliny the Elder) (A.D. 23-79). Pliny the Elder, who was born in northern Italy and educated in Rome, was not a physician. He consulted more than 2000 books in compiling his *Historia Naturalis* and many of these books used were written by physicians. The material was interesting, but of little value in gynecology. It was the one book of classical antiquity read steadily throughout the Dark Ages.

There are still more than a hundred manuscript copies of it, and after the invention of printing it passed through more than eighty editions. He gives us one of the earliest accounts of hermaphrodites.

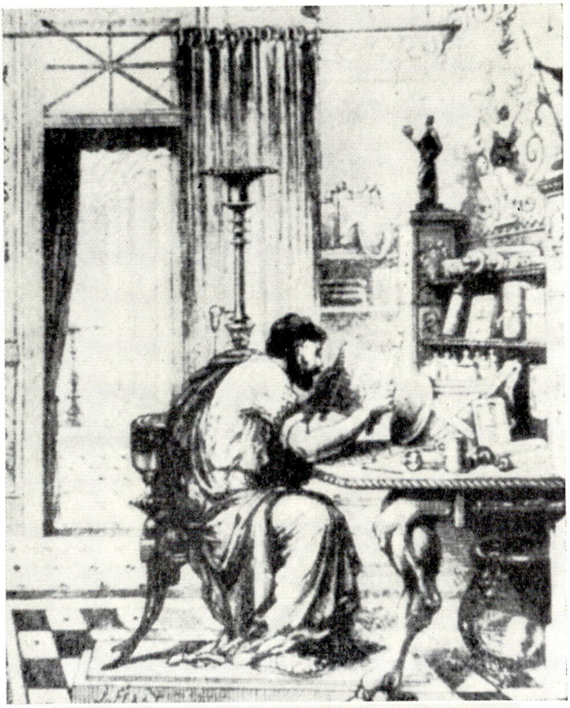

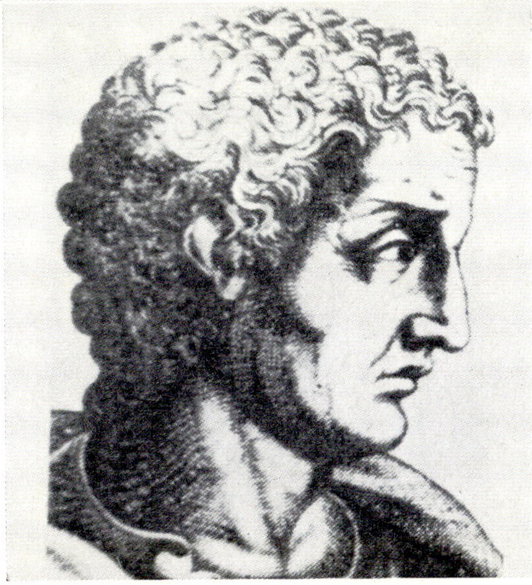

Fig. 39. A. Cornelius Celsus. (The Bettmann Archive.)
Fig. 40. Gaius Plinius Secundus (Pliny). (The Bettmann Archive.)

The Greek custom of depilation was taken up by the Romans. Domitian used fine tweezers to pluck out the genital hairs of his many mistresses. Martial described pubic epilation as a facet of male homosexuality. Pliny accepted the custom as a vagary of taste and protested against it. Pliny prescribed certain drugs to be applied for "keeping a woman's breasts firm and desirable," and to allay offensive odors from the armpits "apply blood from a lamb's amputated testicles." He is one of the earliest authors to refer to cesarean section.

Historia Naturalis:[5] In book VII, Chap. VI, on evidence of early pregnancy, we read:

> If ten days after a woman hath had the company of a man she feel an extraordinary ache in the head, and perceive giddiness in the brains as if all things went round; find a dazzling and mistiness in the eyes, abhorring and lothing meat, and withall a turning and wambling in the stomach, it is a sign that she is conceived, and beginneth to breed; if she go with a boy better colored will she be all the time, and delivered with more ease, and by the fortieth day, she shall feel a kind of motion and stirring in her womb. But contrary it falleth out in the breeding of a girl, she goeth more heavily with it, and findeth the burden heavier, her legs and thighs about the shape will swell a little. And ninety days it will be before she absolutely perceiveth any moving of the infant.

In Book VII, Chap. XIII, an interesting opinion on infertility is given:

> Some bodies there be by a secret of nature so disagreeing that they are unfit for generation one with another. And yet as barren as they be so coupled together, fruitful they are enough being joined with others. . . . Some women are barren all their youth; and others again bear but once in their whole life. Some never go their full time with their children; and such women, if peradventure by help of physick or other good means, and choice keeping, they overcome this infirmity, bring daughters ordinarily and no other.

The most brilliant period of Ancient Medicine began with the latter part of the first century following the age of Celsus, and extending to the end of the second century.

Rufus of Ephesus[6] (b. A.D. 99) was born twenty years after the death of Pliny. He wrote a book called *On the Names of the Parts of the Body* in which he describes the female viscera, internal and external. Because he knew about the vas deferens in the male, he dissected the sheep and found what he described as varicose vessels on either side of the uterus going to the ovaries and into the uterus and not to the bladder as was believed at that time; these, of course, were the oviducts. Galen, Aetius, and others mentioned them but he was the first to describe them in detail (in animals). He differentiated clearly the uterus from the vagina, and vaguely, the cervix from the fundus. He named the clitoris, the labia (nympha) and the myrton (myrtiformis).

He wrote on the bony pelvis, but did not differentiate between the male and female. He also wrote a treatise on *Diseases of the Kidneys and Bladder*, particularly about calculi.

Really, there is very little known about Rufus other than that he was trained in Alexandria and practiced in Rome during the reign of Trajan. Soranus, a fellow townsman of Rufus, has left us much greater volumes of information in medicine, especially in gynecology and obstetrics.

SORANUS OF EPHESUS[7] (A.D. 98-177), studied in Alexandria and practiced in Rome. His medicine lived on for many centuries; the Byzantine compilers wrote of him repeatedly. His works were often pillaged; he was the most plagiarized author of antiquity.

Soranus was opposed to the all too prevalent practice of abortions in Rome. He fought against mysticism and superstition. He wrote on dystocia and podalic version. Gynecology and obstetrics reached its highest stage of development with Soranus, and yet some of his inaccuracies are hard to conceive. For instance he did not believe there was a hymen and that during intercourse the cervix elongated like the male organ. His description of the vagina is quite accurate except for the hymen:

> The length of the vagina is in most adults four inches. It is certainly closed and narrower in virgins, being furnished with folds held together by vessels taking origin from the uterus; these cause pain in the first sexual intercourse, when the folds are opened out, for they are broken and discharge the blood usually seen. For the view is false that a thin partition membrane has grown up, barricading the vagina, and that this is broken, and causes pain at a first coitus.[8]

His examination of cases was thorough and detailed; his failure to note the hymen is probably due to the lack of acquaintance with young virgins who were rarely examined. He declared that an enlarged clitoris was a "shameful thing" which could be "erected like a penis and used for Lesbian coitus." The cure was simple, cut away the excess; his illustration of "children in a womb" is another example of his erroneous conceptions.

Soranus used a speculum to examine the cervix. He recognized infections of the uterus such as puerperal infections which were treated by hot baths, hot drinks, counter-irritation, cupping, leeches, sitz-baths, fomentations, and injections of hot oil into the uterus. He also describes under the heading "The Debilitated or Atonic Uterus" what today we call subinvolution, and for this he recommended exercises, general tonics and uterine injections. His treatment for prolapse was very definitive and apparently much more logical and scientific than some of the prevalent methods such as inserting half a pomegranate into the vagina, which served as a plug besides its astringent action. His treatment was as follows:

> Catheterization to be followed by an enema, the patient was then placed on her back with the buttocks raised and thighs flexed and separated. The prolapsed parts were to be well smeared with hot oil, while a plug of wool the size of the vagina and tied round with thread was being soaked in a warm decoction of myrtle. The prolapse was then to be borne upwards by gentle pressure until the uterus had reverted to its normal position. The plug was then introduced to maintain the correct position. A pad of wool soaked in astringent wine was applied to the vulva, and sponges soaked in vinegar to the abdomen. Finally, with both thighs crossed firmly, bandages were to be applied encircling the loins, the pubes, and both thighs. On the third day the patient was to be carried to a sitz-bath of warm dark astringent wine. After this the vaginal plug was removed and replaced by a new plug. This treatment was to continue every third day until the condition was cured.[9]

In deliveries Soranus advocated the use of the birth stool. He maintained that the pelvic bones separated. One of the finest works of ancient medicine that has been handed down to us, is his chapter on menstrual disorders. He distinguished between primary and secondary amenorrhea, said the treatment could be either local or

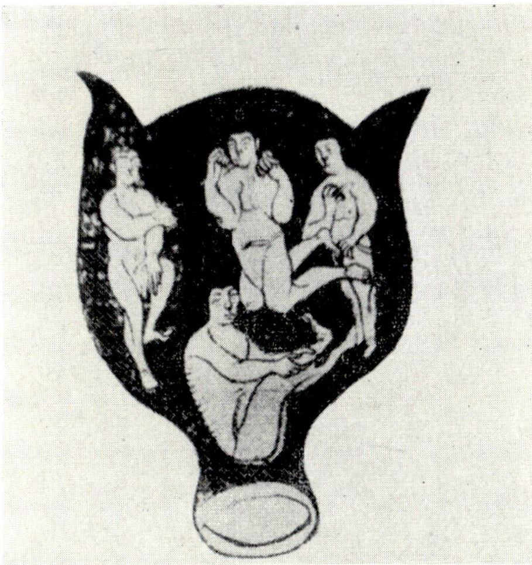

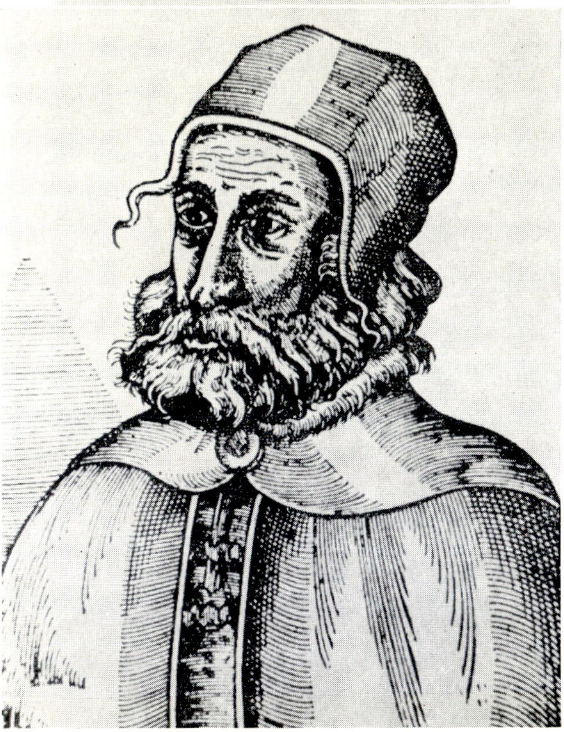

Fig. 41. Soranus' idea of children in womb.

Fig. 42. Galen. (Woodcut in Les Oeuvres de Ambroise Paré, 1575.)

systemic (for which one must search in attempting to treat these cases). He did go wrong on the most favorable time for conception which he said was just after menstruation.

The etiology of prolapse was discussed by Aretaeus the Cappadocian, a Greek physician who did not practice in Rome, but in the Roman province of Cappadocia in Asia Minor. He believed procendentia to be the result of the relaxation of the ligaments of the uterus. He was the first to mention ligaments, and compared them (the broad ligaments) to the sails of a boat.

Soranus' text on *Diseases of Women* has been summarized into sixty-six chapters by the Frenchman Francois Herrgott. The names, which I will only enumerate, will give us some idea of the subjects of this period when gynecology was at its height. They are "Anatomy of the Vagina and External Genitalia," "Signs of Impending Menstruation," "Is Menstruation Advantageous?" "Is Sexual Abstinence in the Female Conducive to Good Health?" "Until What Age Must a Woman Remain a Virgin," "Signs by Which We Can Tell Whether a Woman Is Fertile or Not," "What Is the Most Favorite Time for Conception?" "Signs of Pregnancy," "Signs of Impending Miscarriage," "Are There Diseases Peculiar to Women?" "Suppressed Scanty Menstruation and Dysmenorrhea," "Inflammation of the Uterus," "Anatomy of the Uterus," "Hard Tumors of the Uterus," "Prolapse," "Hemorrhage," and "Leucorrhea."[10]

Not too many years before the death of Soranus, there came into prominence in the medical world of Rome, a man whose accomplishments remained alive many years longer than any of his Roman predecessors. His name was Galen.

GALEN (b. A.D. 130; d. circa A.D. 200). The city of his birth was Pergamus in Asia Minor. He studied medicine at Pergamus and subsequently at Alexandria. The medical school at Alexandria was still in the ascendancy. Galen remained there for most of the nine years since his departure from Pergamus, after which he returned to his birthplace. He was there only four years going to Rome where he ultimately achieved immense success.

In the history of gynecology and obstetrics Galen never attained the greatness of Soranus; his greatest interests were toward experimentation, anatomy and writing. He derived much of his knowledge in anatomy and physiology from domestic animals. So far as gynecology is concerned, Galen left nothing that was original and little that was of interest even from the works of others. He was dogmatic, infallible, pious and very often merely theoretical. The omniscience that he assumed suited perfectly the mental indolence of those who preferred the dictates of authority to the difficulties of reason. They continued to believe such doctrines of Galen's as "the moon controls the monthly period in women" to those of Soranus whom they eventually forgot. He wrote more than 200 separate articles, only a few containing gynecology. Besides some contributions in sterility, he wrote rather interestingly in his *De Locis Affectis* that displacements (of the womb) were due to the retention of the menses which causes a congestion of the ligaments. More accurately he states, in his book, that "if menstruation stops and, among other symptoms, the patient complains of nausea and a deranged appetite, then the midwife must examine the neck of the womb with her finger. If the cervix is closed but feels soft then the woman is pregnant. If it is closed but hard to the touch, then the uterus is diseased and will probably be found to be displaced."[11]

Up until Galen's time there had never been any definitive description of cancer. He was very interested in tumors and discussed malignancy for the first time with any clarity. The following paragraph is a good example of Galen's style and gives us probably the first description of an operation for cancer of the breast:

> If you attempt to cure cancer by surgery, begin by cleaning out the melancholic tumor by cathartics. Make accurate incisions surrounding the whole tumor so as not to leave a single root. Let the blood flow and do not check it once, but make pressure on the surrounding veins, so as to squeeze out the thick blood. Then treat it as any other wound.
>
> We have cured cancer in the early stages, but after it has reached a large size no one has cured it without operation.
>
> We have often seen in the breast a tumor exactly resembling the animal called the crab. Just as the crab has legs on both sides of his body, so in this disease the veins extending out from the unnatural growth take the shape of a crab's legs. We have often cured this disease in its early stages, but after it is grown to a noticeable size no one has cured it without surgery. In surgery we attempt to excise the tumor in a circle in the region where

> it borders on the healthy tissue. On account of the size of the vessels, especially when they happen to be arteries, there is immediate danger of hemorrhage, but if you use ligatures, extension of the disease to the surrounding parts takes place. If we elect to cauterize the roots of the tumor, there is also no small danger connected with this when the cauterization takes place close to important organs. But in its beginning, as I have said, we have often cured this disease, especially when the melanicholic tumor is not excessively thick.[12]

Galen was not particularly interested in practical gynecology and obstetrics, his importance to our specialty comes indirectly. His influence in medicine, which continued for fourteen centuries, is so great, that he cannot be ignored in our history and in the proper era—Roman medicine. However, it is not necessary to go into this part of our presentation in too much detail, since it is a "short history of gynecology and obstetrics."

At this point we come to the end of the Classical Period of Ancient Medicine, the Greco-Roman era of obstetrics and gynecology. A culture in medicine that had its origin in Egypt and Mesopotamia.

Medicine shuttled back and forth in its long history, as we have noted. It started in Egypt and Mesopotamia, continued on to Greece, then back again to Egypt (Alexandria), and a little later it (Greek medicine) proceeded to Rome. We shall see how Roman medicine, basically Greek, eventually directed itself back to the Orient again: Byzantine.

First Occurrences and Outstanding Events

Lucina was the goddess of women in labor.

Herophilus and Erasistratus were the most important source of midwifery in Rome.

Asclepiades was the first to found a medical school in Rome.

The first hospital in Rome, A.D. 380, was donated by Fabiola.

Celsus was the first to show any knowledge of Podalic Version.

Pliny gave the earliest account of hermaphrodites.

Most brilliant period of ancient medicine, from the latter part of the first century to end of second century.

Rufus of Ephesus (b. A.D. 99) and Soranus (A.D. 98-177) were the greatest obstetricians and gynecologists of antiquity. They learned in Greece and practiced in Rome.

Galen (A.D. 130-circa 200) whose accomplishments remained alive longer than any of his Roman predecessors.

Galen discussed malignancy for the first time with any clarity.

References

1. Ricci, J. V.: *Genealogy of Gynecology*. Philadelphia and Toronto, Blakiston, 1950, p. 102.
2. Graham, Harvey: *Eternal Eve*. London, W. Heinemann, 1950, p. 58.
3. Ricci, J. V.: *Genealogy of Gynecology*. Philadelphia and Toronto, Blakiston, 1950, p. 99.
4. Fairbairn, J. S.: *Gynecology with Obstetrics*, London, Milford, 1928.
5. Bostock, and Riley, H. T.: (edit. and transl.) Pliny: *Naturalis Historia*, 6 vols. London, Bohn's Classical Library, 1855-7.
6. Daremberg, C. V., and Ruelle, C. E.: *Rufus Ephesius*. Oeuvres; text collationné sur les manuscrits, traduit pour la première fois en francais, avec une introduction. Publication commencée par Ch. Daremberg, continuée et terminée par C. E. Ruelle. Paris, Baillière, 1879.
7. Temkin, Owsei: *Soranus' Gynecology*, transl. with an introduction by. Baltimore, Johns Hopkins Press, 1956.
8. Dietz, F. R., ed.: *Soranus of Ephesis, Concerning Diseases of Women, etc.* Königsberg, 1838. Regiomontii Pr., Graefium, 1838 (Greek text).
9. Ermerins, F. Z.: *Soranus of Ephesis, Concerning Diseases of Women.* Utrecht, Traiecti ad Rhenum, 1869.
10. Herrgott, F. J.: *Soranus d'Éphèse, accoucher.* Contribution à l'étude de la version podalique. Paris, H. Lauwereyns, 1882.
11. Kuhn, C. G.: Galen: *medicorum graecorum opera quae exstant*, 28 vols. Lipsiae, Cnoblochii, 1821.
12. Graham, Harvey: *Eternal Eve*. London, Heinemann, 1950.

Chapter VI

BYZANTIUM (A.D. 400-700)

As a result of its many conquests the Roman Empire became so widely spread out that control became difficult from its capital in Rome; it was necessary to divide it into an eastern and western section in order to maintain proper surveillance. Thus was laid down the foundation of her imperial rival, Byzantium. So, after more than three hundred years, Roman medicine moved to the shores of the Bosphorus. There were other reasons for this shift in supremacy; most important were the Goths from the north persistently sweeping southward and Asia pressing westward. These barbarian tribes from the north, the Huns, Goths and Norsemen, according to Van Loon, maintained a steady and destructive attack upon civilization for twelve generations, committing murder, war, arson and plunder that laid waste to everything in its path. Through the intervention of the Church, Europe was eventually saved; this began when Emperor Constantine became converted to Christianity and selected Byzantium for his capital in the 4th Century A.D. Because the east was primarily under Grecian influence, we find medicine back in its place of origin, Greece, devoid of all Roman influence. Established at Ravenna in the 5th Century A.D. was Theodoric, King of the Visigoths, the second barbarian ruler of Italy.

For over 200 years Byzantium remained triumphant while Rome deteriorated. In the 6th Century A.D., the east (Byzantium) under Emperor Justinian closed the medical schools at Athens and Alexandria. The west became Christianized, so that Rome was again rising by virtue of its Church instead of the military. In A.D. 579, St. Augustine landed at Thanet, thus bringing England under Roman rule. By the 7th Century A.D., Christianizing influence spread in every direction; this Christian influence enveloped the Goths, Vandal, German, Frank and the Anglo Saxon.

In A.D. 630, the Mohammedans began their merciless campaign of aggression, beginning with Byzantium. This new "culture" (Moslem) was sweeping westward, destroying and acquiring everything in its path. Byzantium and the west were united by the common bond of Christianity, so that the Mohammedans were temporarily checked when they reached the center of France, from whence they were pushed back into Spain. Byzantium continued on for seven centuries more, all the while suffering innumerable assaults, and in the end ceased to exist as the dominant eastern influence.

According to Neuburger[1] it was the Church that prevented the complete wreck of ancient culture. As paradoxical as it sounds, while the Church saved the ancient civilization, including medicine, it also struck a virtual death blow to scientific medicine. This was the indirect result of the Church's attitude. While it should not be said that the early Christians were antagonistic to science, they did manifest a blighting indifference that stifled scientific research and subordinated medicine to religion. They replaced the rational therapeutics of Galen and Hippocrates by charms and amulets, faith healing, miracles and prayers. A bond between the early Christian martyrs and the people at large lay in the suffering which they shared. During their holy ordeals, martyrs had been subjected to torture of the most infernal kind. As saints they later assumed patronage over those parts of the body that had been molested, e.g. St. Agatha, deprived of her breasts in anti-Christian outbreaks helped nursing mothers and cured pectoral pain.[2]

The greatest blow to scientific medicine was received when the Christians forbade human dissection. But a redeeming feature of this Christian influence, according to Gibbon, was the establishment of the first hospitals for the care of the sick and the aged.

The first Christian infirmary was founded by Fabiola in Rome, soon to be followed by charities by St. Basil in Caesarea, and hospitals for the exclusive care of women and foundlings were established in Treves, Odessa, Angers and Milan. The care of the sick became the sacred duty of the early Christians.

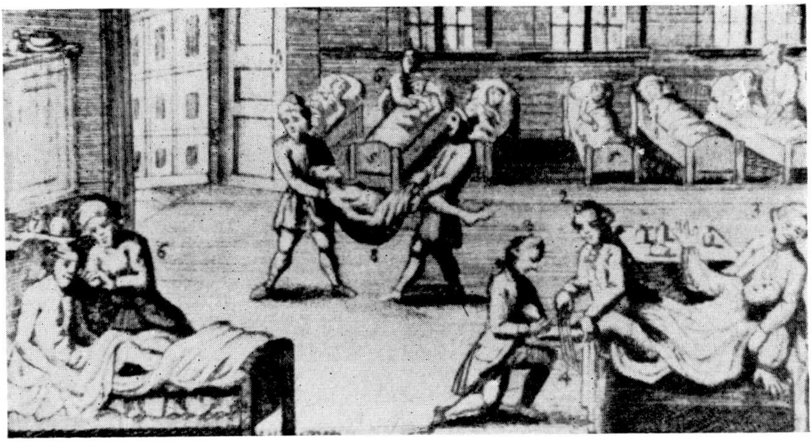

Fig. 43. Physician-staffed hospital. They started as monastic infirmaries for the poor and the sick. (The Bettmann Archive.)

When the supremacy of medicine shifted to Byzantium and even up to the time it reached Arabia, the rest of Asia and Europe and the Anglo Saxons were still woefully ignorant in medicine. They had no schools or educational centers of their own, so that a few of their more ambitious emissaries came to Rome, Greece and particularly Byzantium. It is in this period then, that the rest of the world and Europe especially, began to partake of medicine.

The Byzantine period produced three outstanding compilers of medical literature; they were Oribasius, Aetius of Amida and Paulus of Aegina. They reflected the teachings of the classical period of Hippocrates to Galen. They added nothing new, they simply rewrote the medicine of the Graeco-Romans. The enormous task involved in their compilations is not only interesting, but will show what difficulties they countenanced in order to produce these compilations; a crude art of the period in question which they no doubt improved immensely. For clinical purposes they used tablets of wax, made from the leaves of trees, and later made copies on more convenient materials for preservation, and in special cases the priest, the physician, or the patient had the history carved on stones and placed in the temple. Papyrus reed was the chief article on which to write, but frequently there was interleaved with each four sheets of the papyrus, a sheet of costly parchment, to give stability to the whole. A roll or volume usually consisted of skins of the goat or calf joined one to another until often they reached 100 feet in length.

The instruments used in writing varied with the material chosen for the manuscript. For waxen or leaden tablets, a needle, or stylus, was employed, often made of iron. For writing with ink, a calamus, formed from the reed of the Nile, was much in use; the calamus sometimes, however, was made of silver. Quills also were used in very ancient times. The ink was made either from a dark fluid from the cuttle fish, from the finest soots, or the coal of ivory or wood, mixed with gum and diluted with acids, ink that kept its pristine blackness for centuries. Titles of the chapters were sometimes written in colored inks. Writers folded three or four sheets together, had them stitched separately and then connected with similar sheets already stitched, and the whole covered by linen, silk or leather. Such was the formidable task in writing a book in ancient times.

ORIBASIUS (circa A.D. 325-403) was born in Pergamum, the birthplace of Galen, studied at Alexandria and settled in Byzantium. He so epitomized Galen, who thus continued as a dominant medical figure until the advent of Vesalius, that his encyclopedia of medicine consisted of seventy books. His books contain descriptions of quite a varied therapy. Baths, sweating, purging, blood-letting, enemas and fumigations. Among many other purposes, fumigation was used for prolapse of the uterus. The technique as described by McKay:

> A cover of wood, pierced in the center, was placed on the vessel where it is fixed by means of potter's clay, or by a paste of flour. Into the opening in the lid a pipe is fixed, very exactly, so that no air can enter the vessel. To the extremity of the pipe (that is projecting from the vessel) a small tube of lead is fixed. The woman is placed on an accouchement chair which has an opening in the center. Under the chair a small flame is placed, and over this flame the fumigating vessel is adjusted, and the pipe is intro-

> duced into the hole in the chair, after which the leaden pipe, which reaches beyond the opening in the chair, is passed by the patient into her vaginal orifice. The vessel being heated, the fumes pass up the pipes and fumigate the vagina.[3]

Also used for prolapse, were a number of disagreeable drugs; included was castor oil mixed with vinegar.

Fourteen drugs were enumerated that were used to increase the menstrual flow or the flow of milk, both of these conditions were supposed to have a common source, the blood stream.

Oribasius had an enviable reputation as an obstetrician. He described what he termed a "mole" which enlarged the womb and resembled pregnancy, but did not end in labor when the time for delivery came. So far this sounds like the mole we know. But as he goes on with his description "the belly remains distended for three or four years, then diarrhea sets in and delivers a fleshy mass. In some cases the mole becomes so hard that it cannot be cut with an ax." This sounds like a fibroid, perhaps calcified and a submucous one. We believe enough quotes have been given to permit us an inkling at least of his medicine. After all much of it is simply a reiteration of that of Galen. He was born three centuries after the death of Galen, and was the last and greatest of the pagan compilers.[4]

Aetius of Amida (A.D. 502-575), as his title implies was born in Amida, a town in Mesopotamia in the beginning of the 6th Century. He studied medicine in Alexandria and practiced in Byzantium. He wrote sixteen books, mostly on general medicine and surgery, the latter based on Rufus, while his obstetrics and gynecology is after Soranus. His books have served as an epitome of gynecological knowledge of the ancient Graeco-Romans. He abstracted his work from the Alexandrian library. Even though gynecology remained unchanged for a thousand years, until the brilliant contributions of Vesalius, Aranzio, Fallopius and Eustachius in the 16th Century, the summary of gynecology by Aetius was abstracted by Paulus of Aegina in the following century, the seventh; in the eighth it was translated into Arabic and accepted unchanged by the celebrated Arabian physicians of the 9th to the 12th Centuries. Further it was from this summary that the Salernitan masters lectured on gynecology. In the 14th Century, Joannes Actuarius, the last of the Byzantine physician authors (A.D. 1350) abstracted it for his treatise *Methodus Medendi.* In the 16th Century it was the basis of Caspar Wolff's *Harmonia Gynaeciorum.*

He discusses complete cervical stenosis, as a result of a congenital malformation. Also stenosis as a result of inflammation and ulceration, lacerated and eroded cervix, and cancer of the uterus (as Galen). Prolapse and malpositions are also discussed. In order to get a clearer idea of his presentations, we shall present one paragraph from his Chapter LXXXVI devoted entirely to vaginal examinations with the patient in various positions and the uses of the speculum. He goes on to say:

> Place the woman in a supine position (posture), let her flex her thighs on the abdomen and separate the knees, placing her hands in the popliteal space, and support the thigh by the use of a suitable band tied around the neck. Do this in bright light. Let the surgeon sit at the right of the patient, and by means of a speculum, of a size suitable to the age of the patient, let the surgeon observe. By the use of a probe, let him measure the depth of the vagina so that he may not compress the uterus with the blades of the speculum. If the blades of the instrument are longer than the vaginal canal, balls of wool may be placed at the vaginal orifice so that the instrument may not enter beyond the given point. It is advantageous to introduce the blades with the screw turned to the uppermost part; it is best for the surgeon to hold the instrument while an assistant turns the screw so that the vagina may distend and the vaginal folds separate.[5]

For palpations one finger examinations were done, e. g., Chapter LXXXIII: "If a finger be placed in the os, the condition of the cervix may be noted." Bimanual examination was not used except when a bladder stone was to be expressed.

Byzantine obstetrics and gynecology which extended from the 4th to the 7th Centuries were actually very unproductive. This era can be closed with a short résumé of Paulus.

PAULUS AEGINA (A.D. 625-690). The text of Paul which was a repetition of the best work of the *Graeco-Roman Period*, served as a link between Soranus and the Arabian authors. Rhazes, Haly Abbas, Avicenna, Albucasis and Averroes quoted him, in fact their works are tinged throughout with his concepts. He is credited with seven books. Though he was regarded as the "first man-midwife," we find nothing original in his works. He was especially interested in pessaries, these however bear no relationship to pessaries as we know them today, instead pessary meant simply a tampon. They were made of licorice, rue, scammony and the juice of cabbage and were employed to stimulate the menstrual flow and to overcome obstruction to the womb. Then, too, there were pessaries of an astringent nature made of wool dipped in the medicine and applied to the mouth of the womb, to "restrain the female discharge, contract the womb when it is open and impel it upward when it is prolapsed." He prescribed pessaries to open the mouths of blood vessels (womb), pessaries made of tuscan wax, the oil of lilies, the fat of geese, unsalted butter, burnt resin and stag's marrow, devised for relief from "inflammation of the womb, ulceration and coldness of it, in ascension upwards, eversion and inflation thereof." He gave injections of aromatics and fomentations to open the mouth of the womb in sterility. He removed the clitoris in nymphomania. He employed the speculum, which became virtually forgotten until discovered by Recamier in 1801 who was then regarded as its originator.[6]

First Occurrences and Outstanding Events

First to found hospitals, in Rome by Fabiola.

Period when Europe and rest of world began to partake of medicine.

Paulus of Aegina, of the 7th century, was regarded as first man-midwife.

References

1. Neuburger, Max: *History of Medicine, Vol.* 1, Engl. transl., London, Oxford, 1910.
2. Bettmann, O. L.: *A Pictorial History of Medicine*. Springfield, Thomas, 1956.
3. McKay, W. J. S.: *History of Ancient Gynecology*. London, Baillière, Tindall and Cox, 1901.
4. Bussemaker and Daremberg, C. V.: *Oeuvres d'Oribase*, texte Grec., traduit en Francais, Paris, Imprimerie Nationale, 1851-76.
5. Ricci, J. V.: *Genealogy of Gynecology*. Philadelphia and Toronto, Blakiston, 1950, p. 160.
6. Adams, F., transl.: *Paulus Aegineta, The Seven Books of*. London, Sydenham Soc., 1844.

Chapter VII

SALERNITAN (A.D. 700-1200)

THE DETERIORATION of Byzantium marked the true beginning of the Dark Ages, a state of utter negligible progress, particularly in obstetrics and gynecology, lasting until the Renaissance which began in the 15th Century. During this period dominion of the Mohammedan world prevailed; Christian influence began to dwindle. What little remained was monastic and came mainly from Byzantium and a very small amount from Rome.

Concurrently with Arabic medicine, there developed in Salerno, in southern Italy, a medical school. Salerno is near Monte Cassino, an old monastery; monastic medicine was still influential and there is no doubt that in some way the close association of this monastery had something to do with the beginning of the medical college at Salerno. The actual date that this school began is not known, but it must have been around A.D. 650, because it was known even at that time as a health center throughout Europe. One version states that its inception was about A.D. 900, founded by four doctors, a Greek, a Jew, an Arab and a Christian. It wrested leadership from the Arabs. The Crusades, the Saracens and the Normans had much to do with the establishment of Salerno, for when the Normans took over Sicily and southern Italy through infiltration and open conquest, they merely catalyzed the latent cultural fusion between Arabic, Jewish, Greek and Latin elements. At the medical college in Salerno both teaching staff and student body were coeducational. Greek concepts of medicine were adhered to; in the middle of the 11th Century, Constantine attempted to alter the concepts of the

Graeco-Romans by introducing Arabic subtleties. After Constantine died, the teachers at Salerno who followed showed their dislike for Arabic influences, for there were religious differences, stories of the Crusaders and forays of the Saracens on Italian shores, all of which made Mohammedan medicine very unpopular. By the middle of the 11th Century, Salerno became well established, and the most productive epoch in medieval medicine began. So during the 12th Century we have medicine of the Greek and Byzantine influence again; toward the end of the 12th Century, when the fame of Salerno began to wane, schools based on Salerno as their model began to emerge at Naples, Bologna and Montpellier.

Some of the outstanding scholars of Salerno besides Constantine, are Bartholomaeus, Archimatheus, Platearius, the Younger Cophon and Praepositus. Cophon is supposed to have written the first book in anatomy *Anatomia Porci* (Pig Anatomy) in Christian Europe.

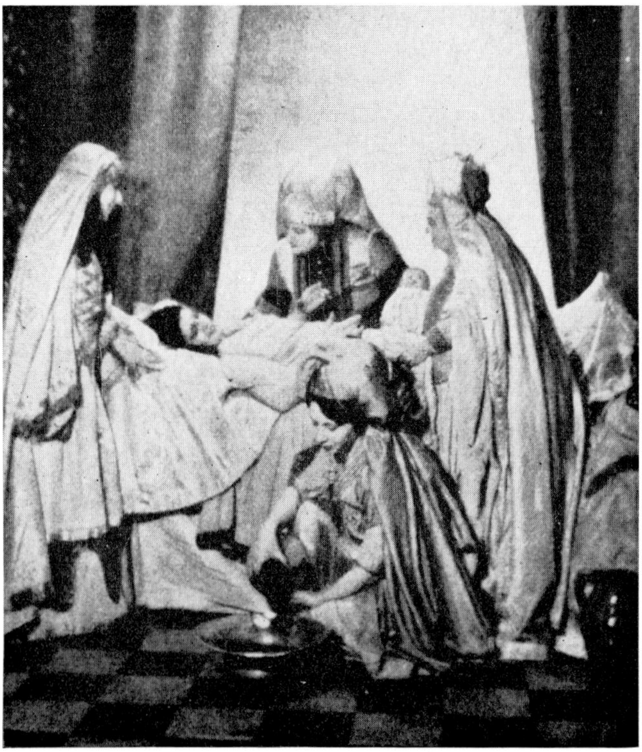

Fig. 44. Trotula. (Davis and Geck, Inc.)

Of greater interest is the long list of women physicians of that school, such as Rebecca Guarna, and Louise Trencapilli, Abella and Mercuriade and lastly and most remembered Trotula.

During this period of few books and almost universal illiteracy, it was most natural to make medical precepts easy to remember by turning them into verse. The famous poem *Flos Medicinae*, or *Regimen Sanitatis Salernitaum*, translated into many languages and used for hundreds of years, constitutes the backbone of all practical medical literature up to the time of the Renaissance. This poem, which includes within itself all the essential didactic characteristics of the Salerno school, was committed to memory by thousands of physicians for whom each of these verses had the quality of Holy Writ.[1]

The best known English text of this poem is that of Sir John Harington, a godson of Queen Elizabeth. The three most quoted couplets are:

Use three physicians still: first Doctor Quiet,
Next Doctor Merry-man, and Doctor Diet.

Joy, Temperance, and Repose
Slam the door on the doctor's nose.

Wine, Women, Baths, by Arte or Nature warme
Us'd or Abus'd do men much good or harme.

These verses are full of Elizabethan ribaldry, but the advice to use such simple remedies as garlic, pepper, sage, rue and others makes these verses laden with sound common sense. A few such examples are:

If in your drink you mingle REW with SAGE,
All poyson is expeld by power of those,
And if you would withal Lusts heat asswage,
Adde to them two the gentle flowre of Rose.

Rew is a noble hearbe to giue it right,
To chew it fasting, it will purge the sight,
One quality thereof yet blame I must,
It makes men chaste, and women fills with lust.

Faire Ladies, if these Physicke rules be true,
That Rew hath such strange qualities as these,
Eate little Rew, lest your good husbands (REW).

There was rarely any reference to obstetrics in this poem, one of the very few references:

> The worms that gnaw the wombe and neuer stint,
> Are kil'd, and purg'd, and driuen away with MINT.

The literature on Trotula is extremely confusing. It is not even certain that such a person existed, and if she did her real name was not Trotula. Some authors believe that Trotula was the title of a book written by a Roman freedman of the Empress Julia. A certain Baccio thinks that her name was Ruggieri. K. Campbell Hurd-Mead,[2] states that Trotula was a physician, authoress and wife of Platearius. Elizabeth Mason-Hohl says that Trotula died, according to church record, in 1097. According to Singer, the compilations credited to Trotula are really those of one Trottus, a male.

Dame Trot, of nursery-rhyme fame, was traditionally believed to be Trotula, a woman of noble family who was a teacher at Salerno in the middle of the 11th Century, and who wrote a series of works known as The Trotula. The Trotula were not very good books; for example the procedure recommended for the treatment of difficult labor:

> When there is difficult labor with a dead child, place the patient in a sheet held at the corners by four strong men, with her head somewhat elevated. Have them shake the sheet vigorously by pulling on the opposite corners, and with God's aid she will give birth.

Madame Trotte de Salerno, in her *De Passionbus Mulierum, Ante. in, et Post Partum*,[3] gave much advice on normal pregnancy and the puerperium. There was nothing new in these instructions that was not known by the Greeks and the Romans, in fact whatever was good in obstetric teaching at Salerno had a familiar ring about it (from the Graeco-Romans).

In this same volume is the instruction, taken from Soranus, to support the perineum with a linen pad while the head is advancing, and a very full description of the disastrous effects of neglecting this precaution. But what is original, and credited to Trotula, is the repair of the resulting complete perineal tear by primary suture. Here it is:

> The uterus, if prolapsed, must be softened by hot wine compresses and replaced, and the tear itself sutured. A tampon soaked in hot wine and butter should be placed in the vagina to retain the uterus, while deep stitches with silk thread were to be taken at the anus, and in three or four other places, and the whole dusted with powder. Then a linen cloth soaked in tar water was to be tightly bandaged against the wound, and the patient's feet held "higher than her head." She was kept in this position for eight or nine days, without bathing. She was not allowed to cough or vomit, and her diet was very simple. Pads were placed against the anus or in the rectum, to prevent any contact with feces. The perineum will be stronger than before it was torn, but it would have been better to avoid such injury by greater care at the birth of the baby.[4]

In Chapter XXV there is an interesting paragraph under the heading of "On the Manner of Tightening the Vulva so that a Woman who has been seduced may appear as a Virgin." It reads thusly:

> Unless it were permissible to deal with the tightening of the vulva for an honorable reason we should make no mention of it. But since sometimes conception is hindered by this, it is necessary to aid this impediment thus: "Take snake's blood, Armenian clod, pomegranate bark, egg white, mastic, and oak galls, an ounce or two of each or as much as you like. Reduce to a powder and let them all be cooked together in heated water. Put some of this combination into the vagina. Or take oak galls, sumac, plantain, larger black briony, alum, and dwarf olives. Let them be cooked in rain water and let the private parts be fomented with this decoction."[5]

One of the theories that the Salernitan doctors used as a basis for their medical practice, was that of "humoral balance." This was simply an alteration and addition to a very old concept whose foundation was laid down by Empedocles (600 B.C.) which stated that the world, the macrocosm, consisted of four elements: fire, water, earth and air. Hippocrates and Galen applied this theory to man saying that man was a microcosm composed of four "humors," which resembled the elements: blood (fire), phlegm (earth), black bile (water), and yellow bile (air). If these humors were properly mingled, health prevailed; if the balance was upset, sickness followed, and it was the physician's problem to restore the equilibrium. The Salernitan theory was almost the same except that they said that in every person one humor dominated the others to form a new balance, and further this dominant humor determined a person's physical and emotional characteristics, his temperament. Thus, the sanguine fellow "fat, and prone to laughter" was surcharged with hot, moist blood; the phlegmatic person, given to "rest and sloth," was dulled by cold phlegm; a choleric chap, "easily angered," had hot yellow bile for his dominant humor, and lastly, cold, dry black bile depressed the melancholy man ever "pensive, peevish and solitary." This theory of fluids persisted until 1858, when Virchow published his *Cellular Pathology*, replacing fluidism by solidism, regarding the cell as the body's main entity. From this theory of humors evolved two of the commonest practices in medicine, the observation of urine and bloodletting. The urine became, in a way, a convenient window for observing the humors at work. Uroscopy became the very keystone of medical diagnosis. Bloodletting or phlebotomy was hit upon as the most expedient method for ridding the body of the excess and therefore injurious humors. Doctor and layman alike rejoiced at bleeding the body at every opportunity, for even the most trivial reasons. Doctors were responsible for developing bloodletting, but barbers performed the actual task, a performance which was considered too menial for the doctor. It became, however, the first wedge advancing the barbers to barber-surgeons, and finally to full-fledged surgeons.[6]

First Occurrences and Outstanding Events

Salerno was the first European medical school.

First book on anatomy (*Pig Anatomy*) in Christian Europe, by Cophon.

Trotula was the first to repair a complete perineal tear by primary suture.

Barbers did the bloodletting; too menial for the doctors, therefore the first wedge to barber-surgeons and eventually to full fledged surgeons.

References

1. Gurlt, E.: *Geschichte der Chirurgie*, Vol. 1. Berlin, Hirschwald, 1898, p. 695.
2. Mead, Kate Campbell (Hurd): *A History of Women in Medicine*. Middletown, Conn., Haddam Press, 1938.

3. Mason-Hohl, Elizabeth: *The Diseases of Women*, by Trotula of Salerno, a tr. of Passionibus Mulierum Curandorum, Los Angeles, Ward Ritchie Press, 1940.
4. Mason-Hohl, Elizabeth: *Ibid.*, Chapter XX, p. 167.
5. Mason-Hohl, Elizabeth: *Ibid.*, Chapter XXV.
6. Bettmann, O. L.: *A Pictorial History of Medicine.* Springfield, Thomas, 1956.

Chapter VIII

ARABIAN (A.D. 700-1200)

In the 7th Century A.D., when Byzantine influence practically disappeared, the Mohammedans began a relentless attack on their neighboring countries extending all over Europe as far as Spain. They captured Damascus, Persia, Jerusalem, Mesopotamia, Egypt with its Alexandria, and the land far beyond Carthage. They even threatened Byzantium. They also captured Toledo, Cordova and Granada, all Christian cities of Spain. In the 8th Century they invaded Gaul, but were soon routed by the Franks there, after which they retreated keeping only their Spanish conquests. At this time Franks, Byzantines and Moslems were vieing for European control. Bagdad began to lose control of a Mohammedan empire that had spread itself too thin and too far. Spain was the first to revolt, Egypt followed suit. In the 10th Century unity collapsed, and Spain became the center of influence.

In the 7th Century A.D., when Mohammedan (Arabian) influence first began, a number of significant historical changes in medicine (and civilization) took place. Besides the establishment of the first European medical school, at Salerno, there were the decline of monastic medicine and the beginning of European medicine. Universities began to rise all over Europe. Philosophy, theology and canon law were the main courses studied in the intellectual centers of Paris, Oxford, Cologne and Bologna during the middle ages. Presumably the Church, which was dominant in the early part of this period, would not tolerate investigation and experimentation; but, it seems that any group that would promote theology, and the other subjects taught from the very inception of the universities, would hardly omit medicine. However, the Mohammedans, through the court of the Norman rulers of Palermo invited Arab, Jew and Gentile to proceed with intellectual development unhampered. They did this by calling attention to the European translations of the massive Arabic medical manuals, which were in reality tomes of second-hand Greek medicine. Eventually medicine, as stressed at Salerno, was brushed aside, while Arabic texts became standard and incontrovertible. The European physician became scholastic in his outlook. He made no sharp clinical observations; he simply translated Arabian medicine. It was the Arabian medicine of Rhazes, Serapion, Albucasis, Avicenna and Isaac Judaeus.[1]

A medical school which played an important role in the transmission of Greek medicine to the Mohammedans was a school at Jundi-Shapur, founded in the latter 5th Century. It had been previously established three centuries earlier by Greek physicians. The real birth of Arabian medicine began between A.D. 750 and 850 in Bagdad. Since there was no Mohammedan medical tradition, they began with imitation of the Greeks, who were admittedly the greatest physicians of the time. What the Mohammedans accomplished in the way of medical schools and hospitals in Bagdad, their rivals, the Fatimites in Egypt and the Ommiades in Spain, soon imitated. The same applied to the establishment of libraries, for the Mohammedans were unsurpassed as collectors of manuscripts and texts, mostly Greek. By the time they assumed leadership in medicine, Greek science was in a decrepit state. But the medicine of the Arabs was never really a science, and yet it was not all plagiarism for they exceeded their predecessors in clinical medicine as a result of their keen powers of observation. They did not leave a single treatise on gynecology; whatever gynecology and obstetrics they bequeathed was found scattered and mixed with other phases of medicine.

Rhazes (A.D. 850-923), a master clinician of this era, was born in Rei, Persia. He studied in Bagdad, and later became a director of a Bagdad hospital. He wrote more than 200 books. He wrote a ponderous work on medicine generally called *Continens*. In this book his gynecological references are the Greek and Byzantine authorities. He discussed all the diseases they wrote about, and as an example of his therapy in gynecology he states in his *Continens*:

> For retention of the menses he advised bleeding at the ankle, purgation, hot baths, massage, suppositories of savin, black hellebore and hiera. For prolapse you replace the organ, and pack the vagina with tampons soaked in astringent solutions. For sterility in fat women, prescribe exercise, regulation of diet, tampons of honey, oil of myrrh, clysters and venesection. For an imperforate hymen you perform incision and follow by daily coitus to keep the orifice open, in place of the use of leaden tubes. If the uterus is displaced you grasp the cervix and pull it in the opposite direction.

In his *Liber Helchavy*, a book devoted mostly to midwifery, he says:

> Head presentations require no manual interference, but all other presentations the midwife should insert the hand in the womb and turn the baby. If this fails, the child should be dismembered and delivered piecemeal. If an arm or a leg presents, and delivery cannot be effected, cut them off. In severe postpartum hemorrhage, use cold astringents and bandage the extremities. In all complicated deliveries a physician should be called.

Rhazes predicted the number of babies yet to be born by counting the knots in the "navel string," also that labor is initiated when the blood vessels in the wall of the womb begin to loosen, that at maturity the child cannot obtain sufficient nourishment and air in the womb. To stimulate labor pains he massaged the abdomen and dilated the cervix.

While Rhazes was known as "the Father of Arabian Medicine," another rather dominating figure in Arabian medicine known as the "Prince of Physicians" was Avicenna.[2]

AVICENNA (980-1037) was born in Afshena. He led a roving life in the courts of the Persians, was suspected of treason and imprisoned, but soon escaped. He spent fourteen years in research and writing. He trod the primrose path and died in the prime of life at 58. He wrote on law, astronomy, mathematics and medicine, prose and verse, in Arabic and Persian. He wrote at least twenty major treatises on medicine; his *Canon* dominated European medi-

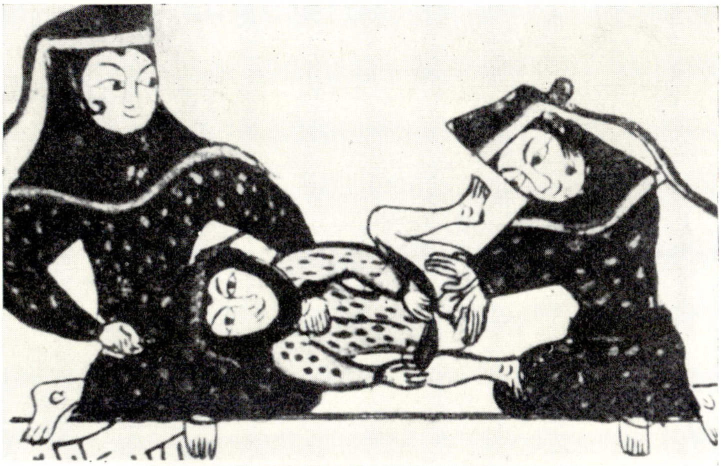

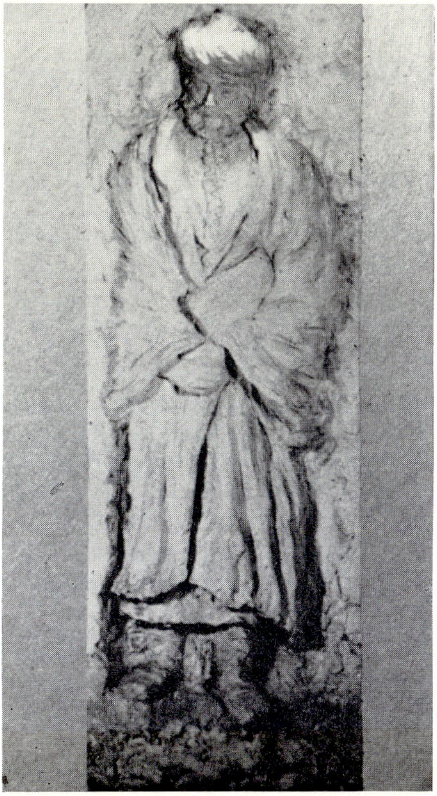

Fig. 45. Reducing a prolapse. (The Bettmann Archive.)

Fig. 46. Maimonides. (*MD Medical News* Magazine, June 1958. New York, MD Publications, Inc. [Photo Jas. Coyne, sculptor Doris Appel.])

cine for six centuries; however, most of it was Galenish. A few quotes from it shall not be amiss:

> Sterility is due to causes involving both the male and female, diseases of their respective sperms, maladies of their genital organs, psychic disturbances, such as melancholia, fear and apprehension. Sterility may be detected in several ways: one is if the sperm floats in water, it is defective. Another, the urine of a sterile woman when poured at the roots of lettuce will dry up the plant. Still another, some say that if a sterile woman voids on grains of wheat, barley and on beans placed in an earthen pot, no sprouting will occur by the end of seven days.
>
> But the older method of fumigating the vagina with aromatics and directing the fumes into the matrix by means of a funnel is preferable; if the aromatic odor does not exhale from the mouth or nose, there is sufficient indication that the woman is sterile. Abortions may be due to a blow, to excessive exercise, a severe fall, violent temper, fear and melancholia. Abortion may be produced, by those who abhor pregnancy, by prolonged baths and increased respiratory effort. The fetus is deprived of fresh air and consequently dies. Abortion may also be induced by drugs, fasting, purgation, excessive coitus and massaging of the cervical os.

Avicenna applied hooks to the dead baby and was fearful of leaving it long in the uterus, and yet nowhere does he mention septic infection by any term. Smellie calls him a copyist, having borrowed from Paulus the embryotomy operation, from Philumenos the technic of extracting the secundines and from Rhazes the use of the fillet. And although he contributed nothing original, Sir William Osler called him the greatest in the history of medicine.

Some of the other outstanding Arabians of this period are Serapion the Elder, Haly Abbas, Albucasis, Avenzoar, Averroes.

The Arab doctors were incompetent in gynecology (and surgery), because modesty kept them away from female patients, and because the proscriptions of Allah against cutting human flesh, dead or alive, made dissection or surgery virtually impossible.[3] At the same time a similar attitude existed in Western Europe; the cleric physician refused to shed blood, and by 1163 the Council of Tours had resolved that surgery should be abandoned by schools and by all decent physicians.[4] The rescue and revival of medicine (surgical) occurred when

ALBUCASIS (936-1013) taught his students to treat diseases by fire and as a result the cautery became a national instrument in Arabia. He aided obstetrics by advising what is known now as the Walcher position (a position in which a woman lies at the edge of a table with her legs dangling). In one of his books he illustrated obstetrical instruments, forceps with crossed blades and dilators.

AVENZOAR (1092-1162) of Seville and AVERROES (1126-1198) of Cordova were good friends; they dismissed the *Canon* of Avicenna as "mere waste of paper." Instead they turned to Galen, Paulus and Aristotle.

Another famous name of this period was MOSES MAIMONIDES (1135-1204), also born in Cordova. He was a Jewish scholar and physician. He was repeatedly persecuted and kept moving–to Morocco, Jerusalem and then to Cairo. He was court physician to Saladin, a Moslem sultan. Maimonides was highly esteemed by the Arabs as well as his own people. The Jews led a peaceful life among the Arabs, much more so than among the Christians. The Caliphs used them to translate medical classics into Hebrew and Latin. Jewish physicians even brought these translations to Central Europe exercising an accelerating influence on medicine.[5]

First Occurrences and Outstanding Events

Mohammedans were unsurpassed as collectors of manuscripts and texts; no origination of their own.

Rhazes was the father of Arabian medicine.

Avicenna was the Prince of Physicians.

They were the first to use the position now known as the Walcher position.

References

1. Ricci, J. V.: *Genealogy of Gynecology*. Philadelphia and Toronto, Blakiston, 1950.
2. Browne, E. W.: *Arabian Medicine*. Cambridge Univ. Press, 1921.
3. Browne, E. W.: *Arabian Medicine and Surgery*. London, Oxford, 1922.
4. Campbell, D.: *Arabian Medicine and Its Influence on the Middle Ages*. London, K. Paul, Trench, Trubner, 1926.
5. Bettmann, O. L.: *A Pictorial History of Medicine*. Springfield, Thomas, 1956.

Chapter IX

EUROPEAN (A.D. 1200-1450)

The medieval period contained a number of extremely interesting facts that had to do with the progress of medicine. It was in this period of history, when the Crusaders protected Europe from Moslem invasion and carried war into the enemy's camp that they learned of the existence of hospitals much more advanced than the Roman military hospitals, or the hospitals founded in India centuries before. The crusading Franks were comparatively barbarous, and were amazed at the medicine they were able to witness and "pick up" from the Saracens.

Hippocrates said, "Surgery (which included gynecology and obstetrics) was the very right arm of internal medicine," and Galen said, "Surgery is only a mode of treatment." From Avicenna onwards, the Arabs distorted this dictum, perhaps because it fitted perfectly their religious obsession that it was unclean or unholy to touch the human body. Arabians pushed this doctrine so far that the Christian Church swallowed it whole. The result was that the Council of Tours in A.D. 1163 forbade surgery, so the barbers, bathkeepers, and sow gelders were the sole practitioners of surgery. Toward the end of this period, through the grace of a few men of unusual stature such as Magnus, and Mondinus and Richard of Salerno, the light of day began to show through; gynecology and obstetrics and medicine generally began to take on at least a resemblance to a scientific approach to problems medical.[1]

Albertus Magnus (A.D. 1193-1280) was born in Laubingen in Swabia, educated at Padua where he absorbed Aristotle. He lec-

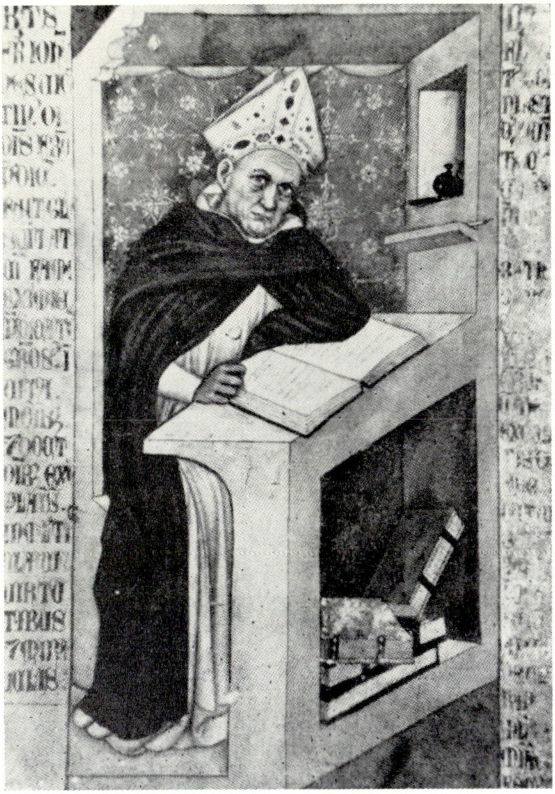

Fig. 47. Albertus Magnus. (The Bettmann Archive.)

tured throughout Germany and in Paris; he represented the best in this classical era of Medieval culture. His achievements in theology, scholastic philosophy and the natural sciences won for him the title of magician and because his writings were so all encompassing he was known as "Doctor Universalis," and like most of the learned men of his time he was an astrologist. He believed and taught that the planets presided over the development of the unborn fetus. He said:

> The fetus became very active in the seventh month of gestation, that it rested from its exertions in the eighth month and at the end of the ninth month it comes into the world healthy and strong. If, perchance, it was born in the eighth month having been exhausted from its strong movements in the previous month, it would surely die because of fatigue.

The Dominican monk Magnus further adds:

> It is a grave mistake of nature to hinder a woman from coition and to forbid her from cohabiting with one she loves though it be a sin in morals. Women possess a great quantity of corrupt and venomous menstrual blood, whether young or old should have copulation with men often to chase away that corrupt substance.

He wrote the *De Secretis Mulierum* and in Chapter III he deals with the influence of the planets on the formation of the fetus.

A remarkable bit of information when we remember that he was not permitted to actually practice, is the following:

> It sometimes happens that during delivery the perineum may tear through the rectum making one opening out of two. This occurs because the perineum is rigid, and the fetus is large.

Actually, Magnus contributed little that was original to medical science. He was ignorant of obstetrics. To him the stars and planets were very real factors in obstetrics. His greatest contribution to the natural sciences was his interpretation of the teachings of Aristotle, and in this role he has proven himself an indispensable link between ancient and modern learning.[2]

Among the surgeons who flourished in this period, the thirteenth century, were Rolando Capezzuti,[3] Teodorico Borgognoni who disbelieved the dogma of laudable pus, Bruno da Longoburgo, Guglielmo da Saliceto and his follower Lanfranchi of Milan. Finally there was Richard of Salerno, who wrote *Anatomia Vivorum*, the only volume with a smattering of gynecological anatomy.

A few short quotes are given in order to acquaint us with the state of their gynecology and obstetrics, specialties which neither of the men, who are quoted, practiced as entities. In fact their obstetrics and gynecology was only a small segment of their general surgical practice.

Guglielmo da Saliceto says in his *Summa Conservationis et Curationis*:

> Cancer of the matrix is difficult to cure but the symptoms, always distressing, may be mitigated by the use of decoctions of opium, camphor and rose water. Moles (fibroids evidently) produce abdominal enlargement simulating pregnancy, but there is

an absence of fetal movements. For women who have difficult labors he advocates contraceptions. One of the methods is "when the female completes the coitional act, she separates her thighs, rises and takes several steps backward hopping on one foot; in this manner she descends a flight of stairs so that all the spermatic fluid leaks out." Another method is to "tie a twig of Scolopendrian around the thighs, and keep there during coitus."[4]

RICHARD OF SALERNO: His *Anatomia Vivorum* shows a rising consciousness of female anatomy, and can be construed as a forerunner of anatomy as an important step in the field of gynecology; this was really more seriously begun by Mondinus of Bologna shortly afterwards. We quote from Chapter XL just sufficiently to give us the picture:

> God created the uterus to be the instrument and the place of generation in women. Its neck is to be compared with the penis, and its internal cavity to the "oschium" or scrotal pouch; and it bears the same relation to the male generative organ as a seal bears to its impression in wax. The female organ is inverted or turned inward; the male is everted or turned outward. The neck of the uterus has pouch-like membranes and folds, resembling the neck of the bladder, so that it may be dilated and constricted according to necessity. . . . Inside, at the middle of the uterus, there are two horns or nipples, to which two fetuses adhere, a male on the right side, a female on the left. Just as nature has prepared two breasts as external organs of nutrition, so are there two internal organs of attachment. Some mistakenly say that there are five cells in the uterus and others say seven, because a corresponding number of fetuses can be carried in the uterus at once; but it must be said that even as many pears may be seen hanging from one tree, by which they are nourished, so may several fetuses adhere at once to one process in the uterus. On account of the fact that one of these two processes is connected with the right nipple, the other with the left, Hippocrates says that if the right breast shrinks a male fetus will be aborted. . . . . the passage of the female sperm from the "testicles" to the uterus is short; and the sperm enters the uterus at once at the lower part of the uterus on each side and not through the os itself. For this reason it does not unite with the male sperm until both reach the uterus. Below the internal os there is another opening, that of the bladder, which enters the neck of the uterus, and thus the

urine is discharged by the same channel through which the sperm enters.[5, 6]

Mondinus of Bologna (1275-1326) was born in Bologna where he studied and later occupied the chair of medicine. His first dissection took place in Bologna in 1315, and this event was a tremendous step in the development of medicine. His fame rests upon the fact that he started dissection of the human body again, after a lapse of 1500 years and not from any clarity in his descriptions in anatomy. As a matter of fact his descriptions are less clear than those of da Saliceto and therefore less clear than those of Galen since the latter was copied almost verbatim by da Saliceto. It might be well to compare a part of the quotations of Mondinus in his *Anathomia* with those of Richard of Salerno quoted above in order to emphasize Mondinus' lack of descriptive ability.

> You must know that the organs of generation in man and woman are similar in certain respects and differ in others. The origin of the spermatic vessels is the same in both sexes. The difference lies in their terminations and distribution. In woman these vessels end at the matrix, close to the testicles (ovaries); and to be exact, they arborize outside the matrix. From these veins two branches are given off which penetrate the abdomen, lie under the dermis and, traversing upward, reach the breast. This long vessel is absent in animals which have the mammae in the abdominal area. The matrix is situated in the pelvic cavity; it is surrounded by ligaments . . . it is joined to the sides by means of two large ligaments which hold the matrix in place. The matrix is quadrangular and somewhat round in contour with a long neck. It consists of seven cells. In volume it varies, depending on the age of the individual, the number of gravidities, coitus and virginity. . . . The matrix of a sow which I dissected in 1316 was larger than any I have seen in women; but to be sure it contained thirteen little pigs.

From the above quote one gets the idea that the amount of human dissection was very much less than animal dissection, and this latter fact may account for the "seven cells of the uterus." Glaring errors that go way back to Hippocrates that the uterus normally extended to the umbilicus (non-pregnant), and that it wandered to the region of the diaphragm in cases of "uterine suffocation" were corrected by Mondinus. His quotation to this effect, also from his *Anathomia* follows:

> The matrix is subject to a variety of diseases; but one thing is certain from an anatomical point of view—the matrix does not wander upward in the region of the heart, liver and throat as some believe, in cases of uterine suffocation. This is impossible. Suffocation is due to a condition whereby the matrix does not expel the superfluities; and consequently they are carried to the upper organs. If these vapors reach the stomach by arterial communication, the patient sobs and is subject to gastric upset, and it is said that she has a uterus in her stomach; if the vapors reach the lungs and diaphragm, panting developes, and it is said the woman has a uterus in her throat; but if the vapors reach the heart, suffocation and syncope occur.[7,8]

Papers which contained gynecology and obstetrics by some of the other and less famous physicians of this period such as Henri de Mondeville (1260-1320 A.D.) point very definitely to animal dissection mainly and human dissection occasionally; he, too, states that the uterus has two compartments. He goes on to say that the uteri of animals have as many compartments as they have breasts in order to be able to feed the entire litter, assuming that the average litter is the same as the number of breasts. Since the female of the human species has two breasts, it is deduced that the uterus has two compartments; a highly theoretical deduction of course, which apparently is based on animal dissection. Or they may simply have propagated the information obtained from the Classicists, for it was Galen who taught that the uterus had two horns, and this bit of information, like the rest of the teachings of that period, was never questioned.[9,10]

The Medieval Period began with Byzantine supremacy in medicine and ended with the period that may be considered a beginning renaissance due mainly to the new approach to anatomy. The entire Medieval Epoch was comparatively sterile and non-productive, particularly in its middle portion. It is often designated the Dark Ages. Their medicine was aptly phrased when they proclaimed that "to know the texts of Galen, Avicenna and Hippocrates was to be a physician."

The early history of this period can be credited with being the source of stimulation of European medicine, mainly through the efforts from Byzantium. Later, during the Moslem supremacy, we note that the Arabians also engaged in the spread of medicine through Europe. They fostered medicine that was not original, actually it was Greco-Roman, and mostly Greek medicine that the Arabians conveyed to the new European medical institutions.

At the end of the Medieval Period one may discern the increased interest in medicine, the beginning or revival of a semi-scientific approach, through the subject of anatomy. This effort at medical reform or revival reached its zenith in the next period of history—the Renaissance.

First Occurrences and Outstanding Events

Albertus Magnus was known as Doctor Universalis.
Started human dissection again after a lapse of 1500 years—by Mondinus.

References

1. Crump, C. G. and Jacob, E. F.: *The Legacy of the Middle Ages*, London, Oxford, 1927.
2. Ferguson, J.: *On a copy of Albertus Magnus' De Secretis Mulierum* . . . , Westminster, Nichols and Sons, 1886.
3. Carbonelli, G., ed.: *La Chirurgia di Rolando da Parma detto dei Capezzutti,* Reproduzione del Codice Latino n. 1382 della R. Biblioteca Casanatense Roma, Roma, 1927.
4. Scharschmidt, F. O.: *Die Anatomie des Wilhelm von Saliceto. Diss.*, Leipzig, 1914.
5. von Toeply, R.: *Studien zur Geschichte der Anatomie im Mittelalter.* Leipsig u. Wien, F. Deuticke, 1898.
6. Corner, G. W.: *Anatomical Texts of the Earlier Middle Ages.* Washington, Carnegie Institution of Washington, 1927.
7. Fischer, G. J.: Mondino de Luzzi, in *Ann. Anatomy and Surg.* Brooklyn, 1882.
8. Pilcher, J. E.: Mundinus and the Anatomy of the Middle Ages, in *Columbus M. J., 17*: 1896.
9. Bos, A.: *La Chirurgie de Maitre Henri de Mondeville.* Paris, Fermin Didot, 1897-98.
10. Nicaise, E.: *Chirurgie de Maitre Henri de Mondeville,* French transl. Paris, F. Alcan, 1893.

Chapter X

RENAISSANCE (A.D. 1450-1600)

ACCORDING TO Riesman it is difficult to accurately delineate the Renaissance period, that is, its beginning and its termination. "For all we know," he says, "the centuries following the specified dates of the Renaissance may be changed in years to come to include the centuries up to the present time."[1] Because of this lack of sharp division, some events are credited to the middle period, while others are placed in the Renaissance era by some authors. For example, acknowledgment of the venereal disease that we know as syphilis (1495) is ascribed to either the close of the medieval period or the beginning of the Renaissance; in fact as early as the 12th Century in France, mercurial inunctions were used, even though it was near the end of the 15th Century before anyone had a clear idea of syphilis. Also, there were the anatomy of Mondinus in 1315, more than a hundred years before the usually accepted date (1450) of the start of the Renaissance, and the amphitheatres of anatomy at Padua and Bologna a few years later, all of which were supposed to give the impetus to medicine that up to this time was totally lacking, since Galen in fact. These events have been considered transitional elements which eventually led to a full awakening of medicine when such masters of anatomy as Vesalius came into full bloom at the end of the 16th Century.

The wane of Church power, the freedom of the intellect in all matters, the rearrangement of government and geography and the discovery of printing were the underlying reasons for the progress of medicine that took place during the "Renaissance," a period

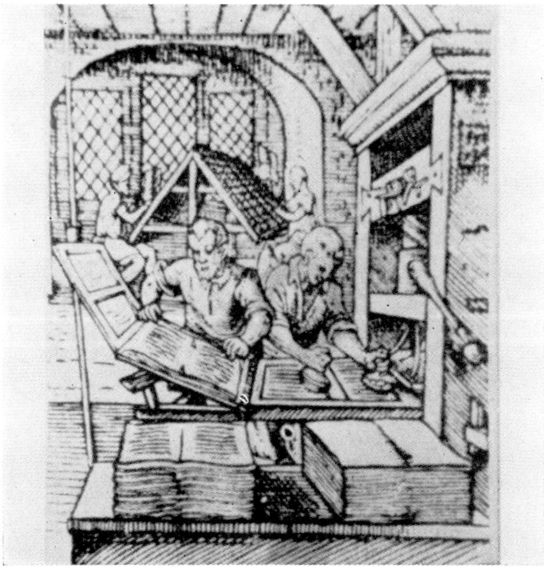

Fig. 48. Printing, newly invented. (The Bettmann Archive.)

usually given at 1450-1600. I am inclined to concur with Dr. David Riesman in his views that it is difficult to assign the Renaissance to such a limited period. We must admit that great changes were occurring at this time in the nature of a preparation for the tremendous advances in medicine to come, and would it be entirely wrong to say that a renaissance continued until 1800, the date when medical advance became appreciably evident as shown by the sudden jump upwards of the line in our graph which shows the progress of medicine at a glance? Actually the Renaissance may be considered a formative era, a time when scientific approaches were established which led to medical practices along entirely different, new and more scholarly methods, continuing until 1800 at least, at which time the efforts of the previous few centuries came to fruition.

In the previous pages we have discussed the history of gynecology and obstetrics up to A.D. 1400, the end of the period we designated as the Middle Ages, an era when stagnation prevailed. Regardless of what we call the subsequent eras, whether we say late Medieval, Renaissance, Transition or Formative, we shall continue our story by examining events that followed the Middle Ages, in other words let us go on to the 15th Century, and as a start it might be well to appraise the status of the "world" at this time and thereby see how it relates to the progress of medicine which began to take on a new look.

In 1453, Byzantium fell to Mohammed II, the Crusades were ending and Church influence had waned. All of Europe became politically and nationally minded except Italy which was only interested in her artists and scientists. England lost her French provinces, France became a kingdom under Louis XI and his son Charles VIII. Portugal became sovereign as did Spain under Ferdinand and Isabella, and at the same time Spain acquired new lands in America. In the East the Turks came alive. In central Europe, Germany was dominated by the remains of the Roman empire, and all Italy was bickering among its numerous states.

The Medieval tradition of Pope and Emperor ruling as a unit was replaced, with the result of continual conflict among the newly formed countries. England, France and the Netherlands fought against Spain. The continental countries fought themselves to exhaustion, and England rose to dominance, and then attacked Spain which began to deteriorate by the end of the century, as did the Papal power by the rise of Luther in the Protestant Reformation. Such was the state of affairs when the intellectual movement, the "Renaissance" began and the old culture and religion were slipping. Added to the forces involved in this change was the invention of printing and new world discoveries. During the 16th Century, Protestant Reformation and Catholicism continued to collide head on, and all over Europe there were persecution, murders, exiles and burnings. This conflict existed everywhere, but had less effect in Italy, where the Renaissance movement started, and as a result Italy excelled in the Arts and in medicine, this tremendous lift in medicine having been started by the teachings of Mondinus, in 1315, of anatomy by the dissection of human bodies.[2]

One of the scourges that became better understood during this period was syphilis. Toward the end of the 15th Century or the beginning of the 16th Century, a new plague or epidemic broke out in the form of widespread skin eruptions and ulcerations, with great destruction of all the tissues, causing many deaths, or persisted for years in those who were able to survive the initial illness. This new disease was said to have been brought to the Spaniards in Naples by the sailors of Columbus, who had acquired it in the West Indies. The Spaniards passed it on to the French invaders. The French called it the Neopolitan disease, the Spaniards named it the French disease, and Fracastoro was the first to coin the name "syphilis," which it retains to this day. Before this time syphilis was quite unknown as such, and it probably existed in a mild form. At any rate it was reactivated in the siege of Naples, where it at once assumed epidemic proportions and a severity which has never since been equalled. Such is one of the many stories handed down to us about syphilis. However, it seems more likely that this story (in Naples) is that of a typhoid epidemic.

Recognizable syphilis was first mentioned in an *Edict Against Blasphemers* issued by Emperor Maximilian I. Among other references to this condition that followed soon afterwards, was a book printed in Nuremberg called the *Vaticinium* of a Frisian poet-physician, Theodoricus Ulsenius. This contained a colored print of a syphilitic by the young and comparatively unknown Albrecht Dürer. Whatever country the disease attacked, the symptoms and spread was the same, although different names were appended. The first suggestion that syphilis had originated in the West Indies and had been carried from the New to the Old World by the sailors who accompanied Columbus, was in the *Tractado Cotra El Mal Serpentino*, which was written by Diaz de Isla about 1510 and published in 1539. He said that in Barcelona it was a new and unheard of affliction which Columbus' sailors had contracted in Haiti and brought to Spain in April 1493. The disease also became prevalent at Seville where a special hospital had to be built for syphilitics. Every country suffered and every country blamed it on some other country. Thus the first three names were "mal franzoso," "morbus gallicus," and "mala napoletana." Later it became in Polish, or German, or any other country, "Pock." Whether or not syphilis was brought by Columbus by contact between civilized and primitive races is not known definitely. Astrologers tried to explain it by the conjunction of planets. Paracelsus said, "The French disease derives its origin from the Coition of a leprous Frenchman with an impudent whore, who had venereal Bubos and after that infected everyone that lay with her; and thus from the Leprosy and Venereal Bubos the French Disease infected the whole world with its contagion." Another theory was that the disease could float from one person to the next without any physical contact. Thus Cardinal Wolsey was accused of giving syphilis to Henry VIII by whispering in his ear.

Also, the suggestion that Henry VIII suffered from syphilis is based largely on the obstetric histories of his first two wives. There were nine pregnancies with only two children surviving; this could be strong presumptive evidence of syphilis in the husband. His ulcerated "sore legge" which Thomas Vicary treated was probably gummatous; therefore, it is not surprising that the unfortunate Mary had a large projecting forehead, thin patchy hair, short sight, poorly developed breasts, and a grating voice.

One of the best descriptions of syphilis was that by Girolamo Fracastoro who was born in Verona (1484-1553). He graduated from Padua; Copernicus was one of his fellow students. He wrote a poem *Syphilis sive de Morbo Gallico*, published in Venice in 1530. Syphilis was the hero of a legend that Fracastoro invented. He was a Greek shepherd or swineherd who, when his pleas to the gods for a rain went unanswered, set up altars to King Alcithous. The gods dealt swiftly with this impiety.

> Forthwith a pestilence unknown before sprang up on the unhallowed earth. And first among them all, Syphilis, who had established the worship of the King with blood sacrifices, and raised altars to him among the mountains, manifested the foul sores in his own body; he first knew sleepless nights whilst his limbs were racked with pain. And from him, first to suffer it, the disease took its name and was called Syphilis by the native race. Before long the deadly infection spread itself among the folk in all the cities, nor in its virulence did it spare the King's person.

Giving the disease the name of a fictitious hero of a manufactured legend satisfied every nation's aspirations. Syphilis it was and syphilis it has been ever since. Fracastoro's description points out that symptoms did not arise immediately after infection and often did not appear till the moon had "four times circled the earth," during which time the disease lies dormant and gains strength.

Treatment, according to legend, resulted in time because a benign goddess cured a young man by bathing him in an underground lake of silver (quicksilver). They used bear grease, horse fat or pig fat with certain resins and gums mixed with quicksilver. Regardless of the vehicle used, they knew that mercury was the essential ingredient, applied by inunction.[3]

The upsurge of anatomy, which began in the early 14th Century with Mondinus, brought into prominence, in the 15th Century, men like Bartolomeo da Montagnana, who, in 1460 gave the clearest ideas of female anatomy by dissections, to date. There was Gabriele Zerbi da Verona, 1468-1505, Professor at Padua who divided the uterus into an upper and a lower part. His successor Alessandro Benedetti da Legnano (1460-1525) was the first to use the word perineum, cervix and procedentia. Also, he is supposed to have written on abdominal pregnancy.

At Bologna, Alessandro Achillini (1463-1512) not only kept anatomy to the fore, but he is credited with fresh notations on the hymen.[4] At the University of Ferrara, Luigi Bonacciuoli redescribed in detail the "mons veneris," the "clitoris" and the "hymen." The gynecology of this period was still very crude in spite of the advances especially in anatomy, e.g. in the *Fasciculus Medicinae* (1491) by Ketham we find the following description to cure sterility:

> Have both the husband and the wife drink the saliva of a rabbit, secreted while chewing greens." Also efficacious is the use "of a tampon soaked in a solution of oil with the powdered right testicle of a weasel." Or "drink mares milk immediately before coitus."[5]

In this book the writer quotes as his authorities Hippocrates, Aristotle, Pliny, Serapion, Avicenna, Galen and Albertus Magnus.

Immediately prior to Vesalius, there were two famous anatomist surgeons who should be considered; Da Carpi and Massa.

Jacopo Berengario Da Carpi (1460-1530), Professor at Bologna and Pavia, physician to Cellini among other greats. He was the first physician to state clearly that the fundus consisted of one cavity (this was long after Da Vinci's discovery). He is supposed to be among the first to do a vaginal hysterectomy. His father and nephew also performed this operation. The operation consisted of a technique in which a piece of stout twine was placed around the

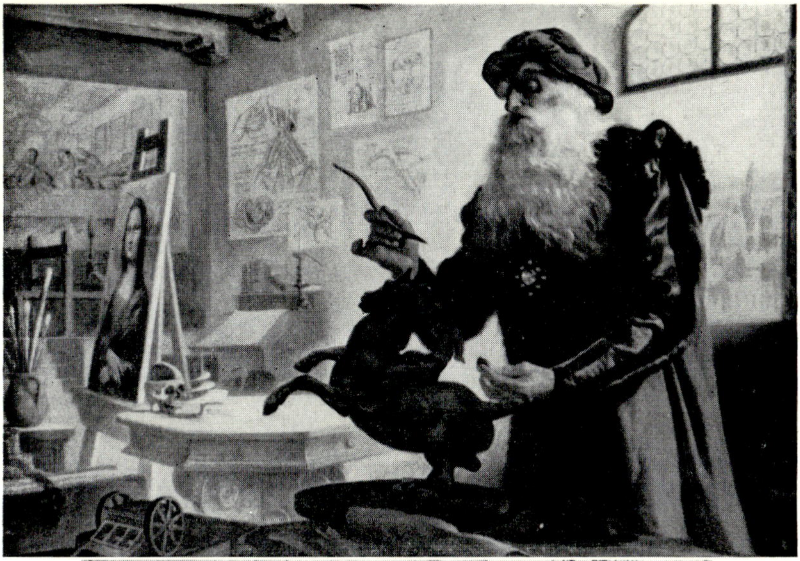

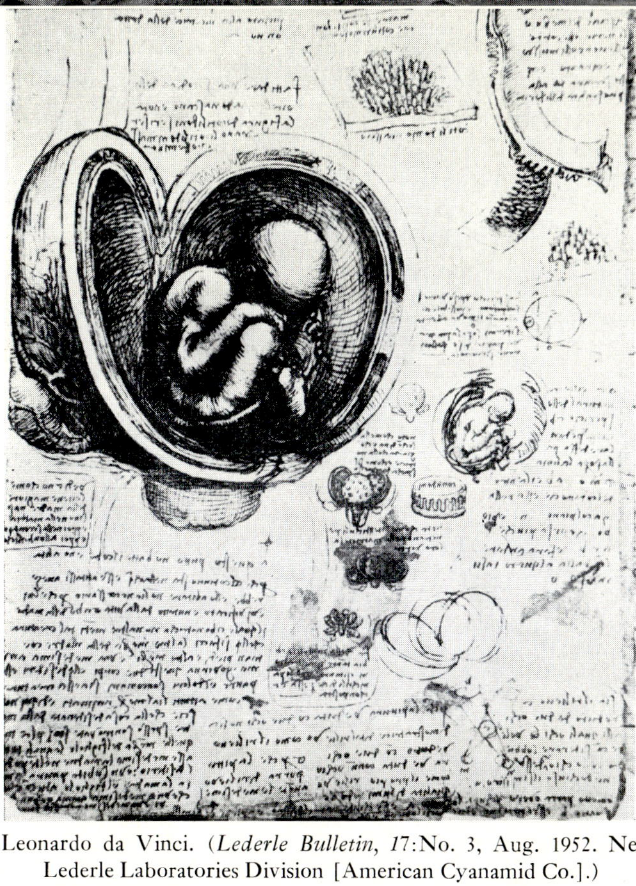

Fig. 49. Leonardo da Vinci. (*Lederle Bulletin*, *17*:No. 3, Aug. 1952. New York, Lederle Laboratories Division [American Cyanamid Co.].)

Fig. 50. Fetus in utero. (Drawing by da Vinci.)

prolapsed organ, gradually made tighter until the organ was severed; applications were then made to the area, of wine previously boiled with honey and aloes. This procedure was followed by fever that disappeared after two days.

Berengario was skeptical about the anatomy of his predecessors; he made numerous dissections and corrections in the work of the older anatomists, among them Galen and Mondinus. He was the first after Leonardo to make anatomical drawings entirely from nature. He was the first to describe the appendix, and he reported a case of ruptured uterus noted at a postmortem cesarean.[6]

NICOLAUS MASSA (1499-1569) was Professor of Anatomy and Surgery at Padua. For the most part he imitated Berengario, his anatomical drawings were much clearer though similar. An interesting contribution is his description of the uterus in which he states that there are three layers, which, of course, is the same as our present day findings, e.g., the peritoneal covering, muscular layer, and an inner lining.[7]

It was not to the physicians, as so often has been the case, that we are indebted for the revival of anatomy. It was to the Florentine artist and to Leonardo da Vinci in particular that we owe our gratitude. Michelangelo and Benevenuto Cellini were among many artists who contributed numerous drawings from anatomical dissections.

LEONARDO (1452-1519) was educated by Verrochio, the leader of the Florentine artists. His mother was a peasant but his father was a notary to great Florentine families. Leonardo was accomplished in scores of fields, such as painting, sculptoring, physics, anatomy, engineering and what not. He dissected about thirty bodies, and filled more than a hundred note books with sketches of anatomical notations. These books were not studied until 200 years later, at which time it was noted how far ahead of his contemporaries he had been. Among his many sketches is one of a fetus in the womb, uncanny in its utter accuracy of delineation. He represented the uterus as unilocular, instead of identifying it with the two-horned uteri of other mammals, as was customary. He also described accurately the fetal membranes.

Anatomy reached its fullness with the advent of an anatomist whom Garrison believed to be "the most commanding figure in

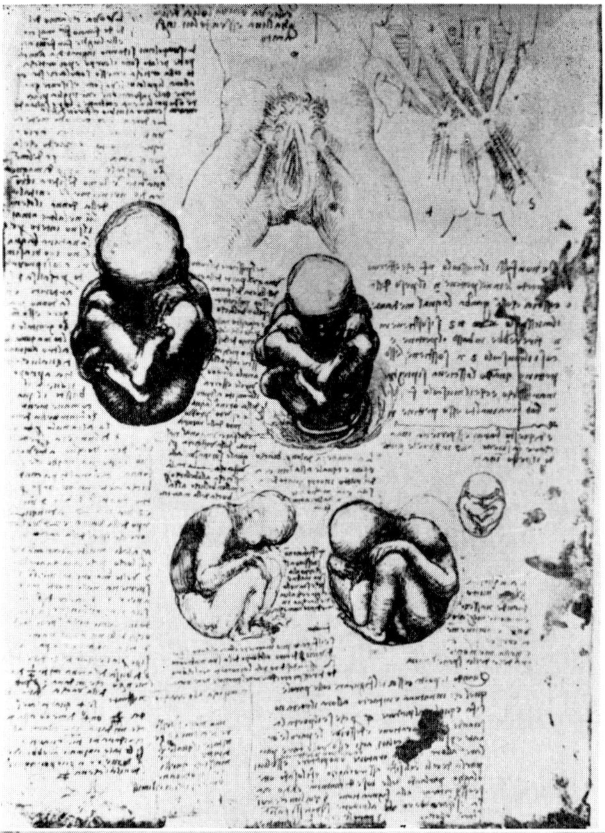

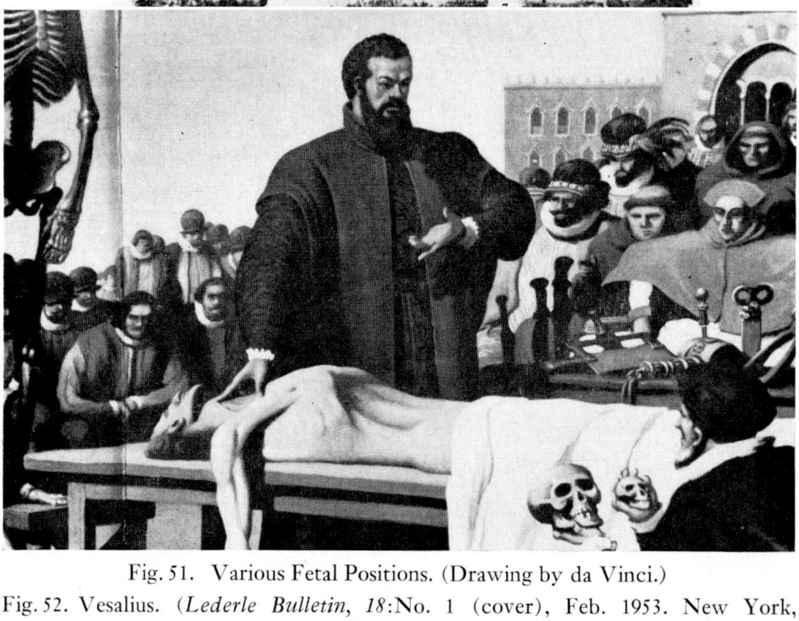

Fig. 51. Various Fetal Positions. (Drawing by da Vinci.)

Fig. 52. Vesalius. (*Lederle Bulletin, 18*:No. 1 (cover), Feb. 1953. New York, Lederle Laboratories Division [American Cyanamid Co.].)

European medicine after Galen and before Harvey," a man who completed the atlas of human anatomy that Leonardo planned but never finished.

ANDREAS VESALIUS (1514-1564) was this man. In Venice, he met Jan Kalkar, a pupil of Titan's. With Kalkar's drawings from dissections and Johann Gunther's translation of Galen's *Anatomical Institutes*, they produced the *Tabulae Anatomicae*. He was born in Brussels, of German parents. He studied in Louvain. He taught in France and ultimately became Professor at Padua. He spent five years dissecting bodies which he "snatched," if otherwise unable to procure, and went so far as to bribe judges in criminal cases to prevent undue injury to the bodies of convicts to be hanged. In 1543, at twenty-nine, he published the work with which he and Kalkar founded modern anatomy, the *De Humani Corporis Fabrica*. This work criticized much of Galen's work as being confused by conjectures based on the dissection of animals. In the *Fabrica* he gives a very accurate description of all the pelvic organs separately, the veins and the ligaments. He is the first to state the uterine cavity was not round, and although he agreed with Berengario that the fundus contained only one cavity, his drawing of the uterus shows an indication of a septum. It surpassed the works of Berengario because he (Vesalius) was a greater anatomist, and Kalkar a greater artist. His book is the first to show the left ovarian vein entering the renal vein.

Fame came to Vesalius early in life, so he spent the remainder of his existence as court physician to Charles V and Philip II, where, of course, his research anatomy ended. He died in 1564 of an unknown malady. Among other things he settled unequivocally the argument about the separation of the pubic bones in labor and the point of differences between men and women. He showed that the pubic bones, both in men and women, are joined by cartilage, and in the parturient women these bones do not become separated, nor do they in the lower animals. Realdo Colombo, one of his pupils who confirmed this, claimed that these bones were joined together so strongly that it was almost impossible to separate them with a knife. Vesalius made anatomy an exact science again rather than a ritual.[8, 9]

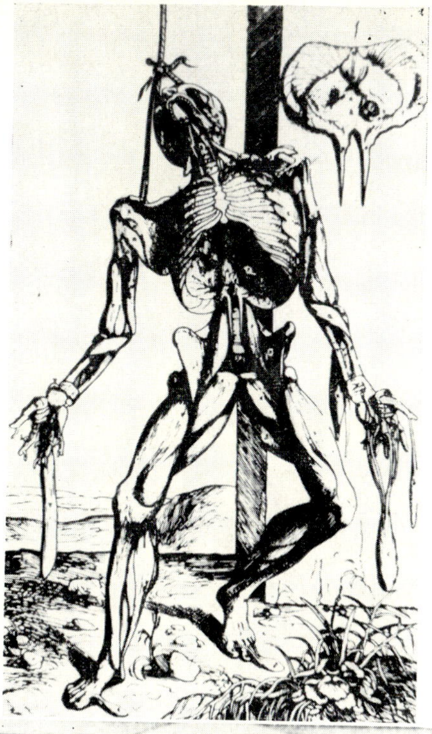

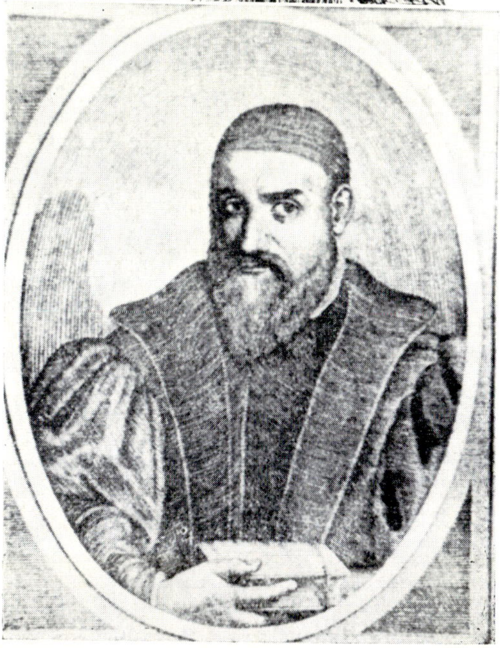

Fig. 53. Muscle dissection. (From Vesalius' *Fabrica.*)

Fig. 54. Gabriel Fallopius. (*Obstetrics and Gynecology*, *6*:No. 4, p. 467, Oct. 1955. New York, Hoeber.)

FALLOPIUS (1523-1562) The most brilliant and the most faithful of Vesalius' pupils, was Fallopius, who also held the chair at Padua. He died at the early age of forty, in 1562, at which time his teacher was recalled from Jerusalem to retake the chair, but never did for he died on his way to Padua. A year before his death he wrote *Observationes Anatomicae*, published in Venice in 1561. It contained the first really precise description of the clitoris. He gave the first accurate description of the tubes and ovaries. He called the tubes "uteri tubae," but they have since been called the Fallopian tubes. Rufus, Soranus and Vesalius had previously described the tubes, but none of them as accurately and thoroughly. In fact they used the tubes of animals (sheep), while he describes the human tubes. (Vesalius probably dissected and described the human tubes.) His description of the tubes and ovaries is interesting enough to repeat:

> All the anatomists assert with one voice that semen is made in the female testes, and that they are found full of semen, which I could never see although I gave no small labor that I might learn this. I have seen in them indeed some vesicles as it were turgid sometimes with water or a watery fluid, sometimes yellowish, sometimes limpid; but I have never seen semen except in the spermatic vessels themselves or those called "excretory." They affirm also that those spermatic vessels spring from the ovaries and are united completely to them, and end in the so called horns of the uterus, which is not at all the case, since I could never see those seminal tubes united to the ovaries unless the uterus was diseased.
>
> That slender and narrow seminal duct rises, fibrous and pale, from the horn of the uterus itself; becomes, when it has gone a little bit away, appreciably broader, and curls like a branch until it comes near the end, then losing the horn like curl, and becoming very broad, has a distinct extremity which appears fibrous and fleshy through its red color, and its end is torn and ragged like the fringe of well worn garments, and it has a wide orifice which lies always closed through the ends of the fringe falling together; and if these be carefully separated and opened out, they resemble the orifice of a brass trumpt. Wherefore since the seminal duct from its beginning to its end has a likeness to the bent parts of this classic instrument, separate or attached therefore it has been called by me the "Uteri Tuba."

> These are present not only in the human bodies, but also in the sheep, cows, and all other animals which I have dissected.

Fallopius named the vagina and also the placenta. Fallopius was known for his lack of ill feeling toward anyone, and often went out of his way in order not to hurt anyone. In describing the placenta he mentions Hippocrates who called the placenta "cotyledons," and used only the most graceful corrections in this instance, thus:

> Therefore the cups (or cotyledons) are those things of which Aristotle spoke, and truly are not found in the human or canine uterus, but only in that of horned animals and only in pregnancy.
>
> This being settled, what shall we say if Hippocrates mentions "cups"? May the Manes of so great a man, a man who was the presiding deity of the medical art, spare me when I say that he spoke the truth in words that deceiveth.

The same attitude recurs throughout the works of Fallopius. He always gave credit of an honest error to earlier authorities whose mistakes he corrected, such as cases where animals were used when human dissection was impossible or forbidden, and in the case of old and limited words which had to be fitted to new concepts.[10–12]

EUSTACHIUS (1500-1574), the only man to whom Fallopius was unjust, was Professor in Rome and made more anatomical discoveries than any of his predecessors. He made countless, and unusually beautiful illustrations, among them the uterus. (He discovered the Eustachian tube of course.) Eustachius and Fallopius quarreled because Fallopius loyally supported Vesalius in opposing Galen, and Eustachius declined to go along.[13]

The only other pupil of Vesalius' who made any noteworthy contributions to anatomy, and it was mainly in anatomy to obstetrics, was Julius Caesar Arantius. He published his *De Humano Fetu Liber* in 1572, and gave the first clear account of pelvic contraction and its influence on labor. He also confirmed the views of Vesalius on the non-separation of the female pelvis.

During the 16th Century, numerous famous physicians abounded, treatises on gynecology, which included physiology of menstruation, sterility, and child bearing in general were very common. Amatus Lusitanus (1511-1568) described large pendulous lipomata or fibromata. Hydatid mole was described by Francois Valleriola.

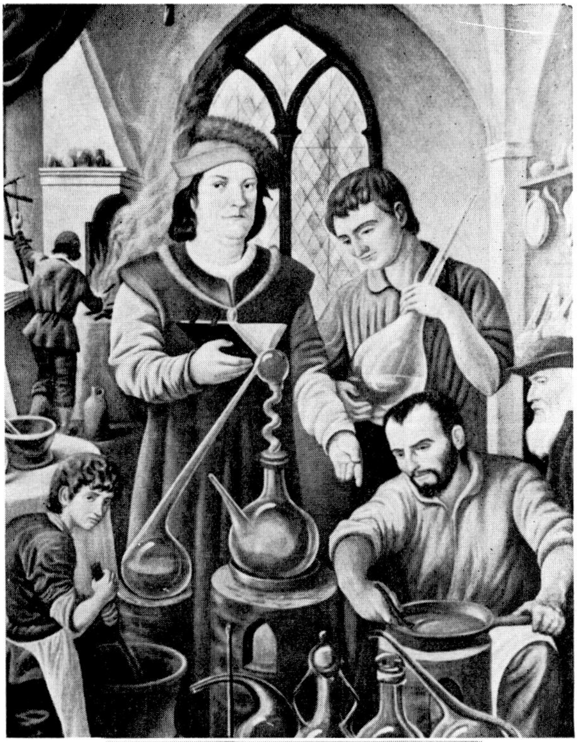

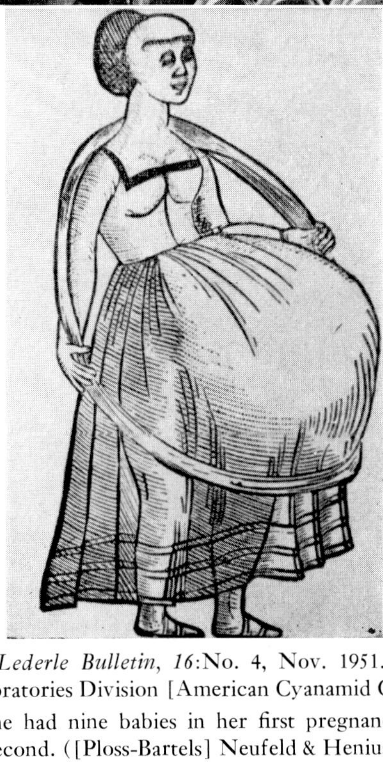

Fig. 55. Paracelsus. (*Lederle Bulletin, 16*:No. 4, Nov. 1951. New York, Lederle Laboratories Division [American Cyanamid Co.].)

Fig. 56. Dorothea. She had nine babies in her first pregnancy and eleven in her second. ([Ploss-Bartels] Neufeld & Henius.)

In 1595, Johann Schenck von Grafenberg (1530-1598) has a case of ovarian tumor adherent to the uterus; he reported deformities of the clitoris, hymen and uterus, including a bicornuate organ. He also described ovarian malignancy, and an ovarian dermoid.

Conrad Gesner (1516-1565) of Zurich, who was called the "German Pliny," graduated from Basel, was a zoologist, botanist, an extremely prolific author, and edited the greatest of the Renaissance anthologies of surgery *De chirurgia scriptores optimi* in 1555. Another contributor from Zurich was Casper Wolff (1532-1601). He published his *Gynaeciorum* in 1566; this was a compilation of all the gynecological knowledge up to that date. In 1586, Caspar Bauhin (1550-1624) enlarged and edited the work of Wolff. Both Wolff and Bauhin's works were later reprinted in one volume by Israel Spach of Strassburg in 1597. This work contained the contributions of twenty-one different authors. It seems unnecessary to quote any of these writers since, in the main, repetition of known practices filled these volumes.

It is an interesting observation that achievements in operative gynecology of the Renaissance era were the result of certain obstetrical surgical performances. It started when a sow gelder named Jacob Nufer did a successful cesarean section of his own wife in 1500. The work of another sow gelder, who contained his experimental furore within "family circles," was Johann Weyer. He did a double ovariotomy on his own daughter for purposes of reforming her sexual ways and keeping her home.

In the early Renaissance, when all forms of medicine showed hopeful signs of advance, obstetrics stood still. As an instance of this advance, we cite Paracelsus, who is considered by many as the initiator of chemical therapy in medicine. He bridged the gap between alchemy and the therapeutic use of drugs. Incidentally, he taught, in the 15th Century, that every wound would heal itself if it were kept clean. In contrast, we have the stasis of obstetrics, in which we see belligerent midwives guarding the lying-in chamber against all medical interference, particularly the male species. According to legend, a physician of Hamburg, Doctor Wirtt, was caught at an accouchement in 1522, disguised in women's clothing, and was promptly burned at the stake. Primitive aspects of Renaissance obstetrics included astrologers keeping a careful and discreet

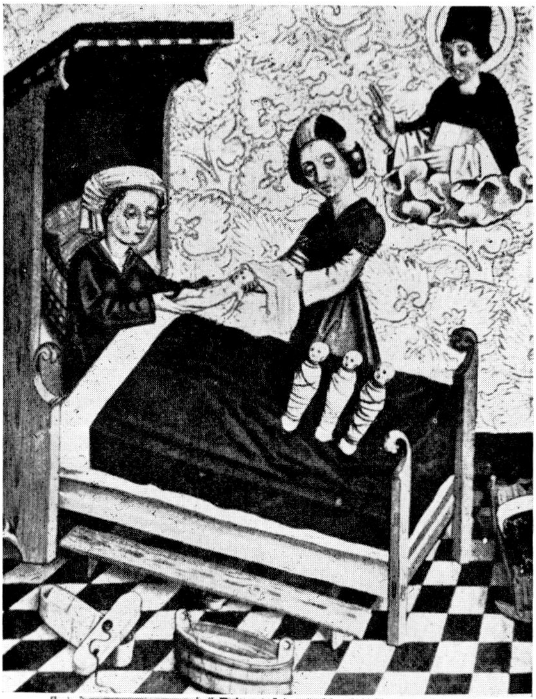

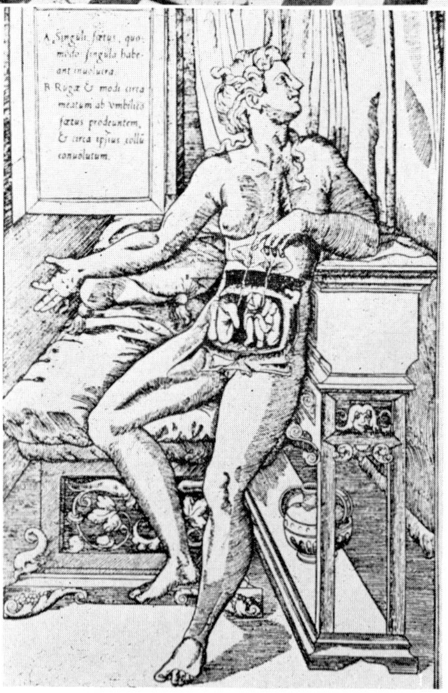

Fig. 57. Quadruplets, about 1450. (Malers, circa 1450.)

Fig. 58. Twin pregnancy, Sixteenth Century conception. (Drawing by Etienne or Stephanie.)

watch on the stars, to determine the child's future. The age-old birth stool was still an implement of labor. One woman eased her burden of multiple embryos with a wooden hoop slung around her neck and under the protruding abdomen to support it; this is one of Paré's stories, for which there is no confirmation.[14] Multiple births were quite as exciting then as now; the numerous references and prints of various multiple births is notable, e.g., print of a 16th Century twin pregnancy, an old primitive painting of quadruplets done in 1450 by a Bavarian painter has had a very wide circulation.

In this illustration (*The Birth of Quadruplets*, Malers, about

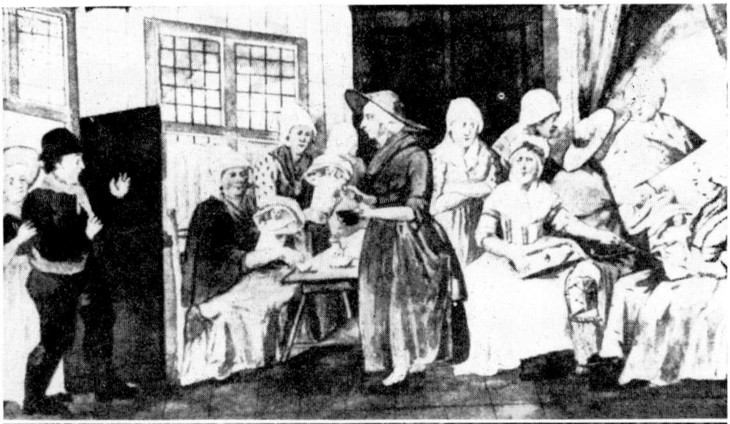

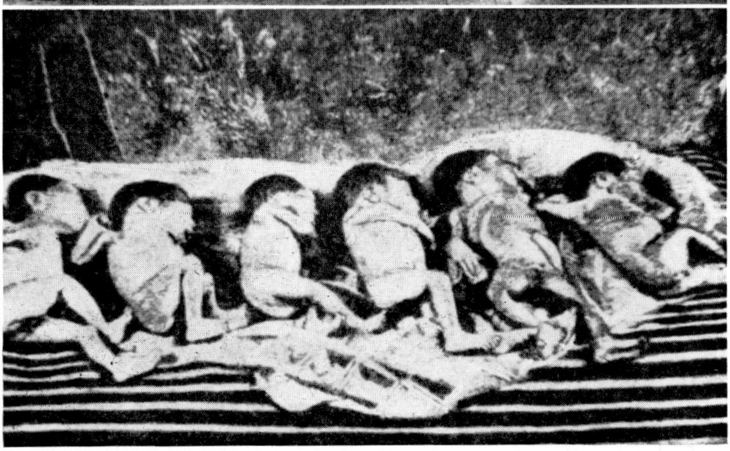

Fig. 59. Quintuplets. Babies were exhibited for a fee, roads were black with carriages. (The Bettmann Archive.)

Fig. 60. Sextuplets. ([Ploss-Bartels] Neufeld & Henius.)

1450) we learn much of multiple births of this period, and not of the medical aspect alone, but of the culture and customs of this era as far as plural births are concerned. First off, we are impressed with the doll-like or papoose-like quadruplets, each wrapped tightly in swaddling bands, just as had been advised by Soranus back in the second century, in order to press the limbs and body into good shape, to remove deformities produced by birth, and to prevent any injury. Each limb is wrapped separately with bandages of seamless clean wool three fingers' breadth wide. Then the longer bandages are used to wrap the whole body into a state of mummification. Boys are wrapped evenly all the way. Girls are wrapped more loosely around the hips. The last swaddling bandage starts round both feet, includes both arms and ends at the neck.

It was generally believed that multiple births were a punishment for adultery, bestiality, or demoniacal intercourse. The Church attempted to correct these beliefs by giving the woman concerned an impeccable married status, and by regarding the wonder birth as a divine manifestation. The importance of clerical approval in these cases was subtly indicated in this picture by Malers. In the upper right hand corner of the picture can be seen a religious personage giving his blessings. There is another well known print of quintuplets. One showing the birth of six babies was also given widespread pulicity during this time. This interest has continued even to this day. Elizabeth Mott, who lived from the latter 18th Century to the early 19th Century, boasts the record of prolificity. She gave birth to forty-two children in forty-two years.

Further evidence of the state of obstetrics of this period are the many weird stories concerning childbearing indicative of the ignorance and superstitions that prevailed. A widespread story of a certain "Maria Tofts giving birth to rabbits" which the famous English artist Hogarth put on copper (etched drawing) is a good example. Word got around that she gave birth to a rabbit. The next week it was a few rabbits. Neighbors were permitted to see her give birth to rabbits every week—for a fee. As Hogarth's print shows, Maria Tofts is sitting on the floor while rabbits are scurrying in all directions from under her skirts. At last the constable investigated this performance and exposed Maria Tofts, who certainly used a most unusual method of making extra money, a not too difficult feat when we appreciate the weird associations that folks had for pregnancy.

In an age marked by such fabulously bizarre beliefs, little that was rational could be expected in the maternity chamber. Peculiar beliefs concerning pregnancy prevail today, but I hope, to a much lesser extent in this enlightened age than in the 1500's. Only recently a maternity patient was told by her friend never to cross her legs on sitting lest she suffocate the baby, and not to step over a rope that lay on the ground, lest the baby's cord would be wound around its neck. Another story of present day vintage is the pregnant woman who was told that if she saw someone with a deformity she should immediately touch her face and carry that hand down to her buttock to touch it so that her baby would not be marked on the face. A southern European superstition that exists today apparently, is one in which a pregnant woman in her puerperium has the power to restore broken marriages and other marital mishaps. I delivered a young Americanized woman of her first baby, at home, some thirty years ago. Her parents were separated, her mother would have nothing to do with her father, who was extremely anxious to be reunited. The delivery took place in the patient's mother's home to which the father had no access. A few days after the delivery he waylaid me and pleaded for a favor. He begged me to obtain a small amount of stool passed by the recent parturient and give it to him. I asked him why he wanted it, and at first he refused to tell me because he said I would not understand, and I would not believe and also I would think him silly, superstitious and simple-minded. He eventually explained that if he were to obtain the specimen of stool, and mix a small quantity of it with food and then eat it, nuptial bliss would be restored to him. It is interesting that when I questioned the veracity of such a procedure, he said he was sure of what he spoke for he knew a number of similar cases that worked *miraculously*. If these are examples of the present time, we can well believe the weird stories of a few centuries ago like the one of Maria Tofts.

Intellectual awakening in obstetrics finally did come, though all the other branches of medicine preceded it by years. Midwifery became molded into a science out of the common play of superstition, ignorance and religious bigotry. For ages, women, denied the serv-

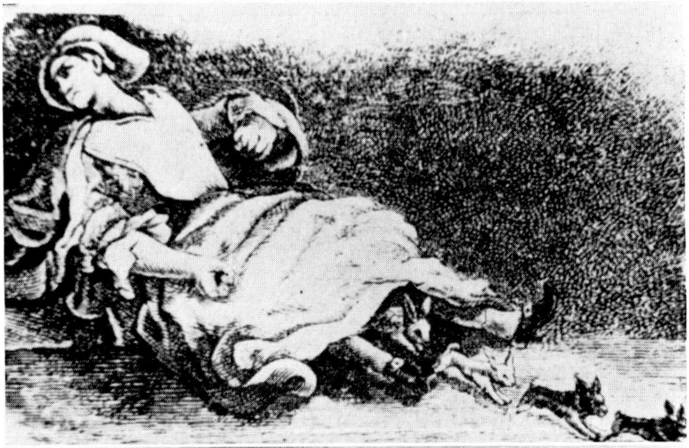

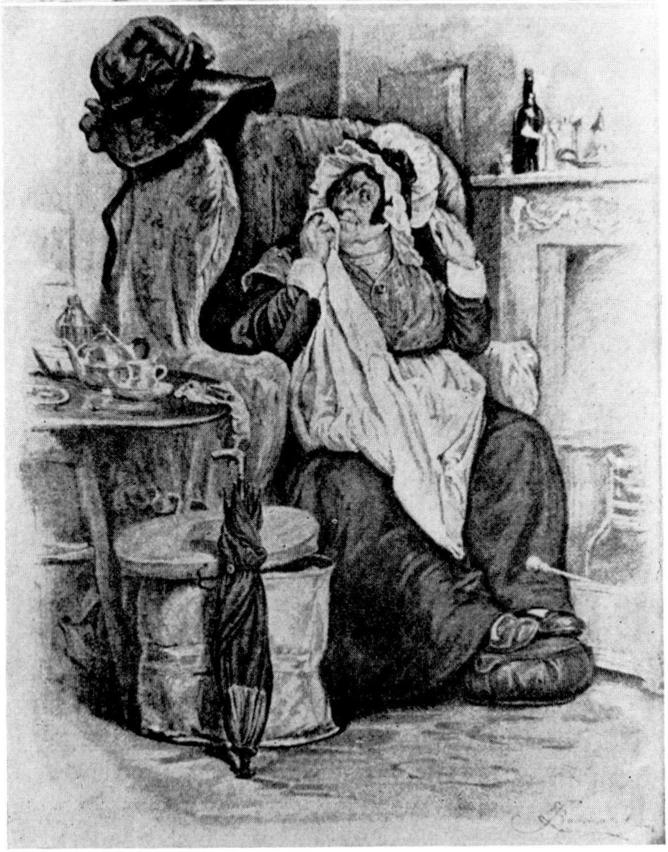

Fig. 61. Maria Tofts giving birth to rabbits. ([Ploss-Bartels] Hogarth.)

Fig. 62. Sairey Gamp, midwife; ignorant, gossipy and uncouth. (Frederick Barnard.)

ices of educated physicians, were compelled to accept the meager assistance of untutored midwives.

The English "Mid-wif" or "with-woman" of the 16th Century (e.g. Sairey Gamp) was a person of inferior education who had borne children herself and watched other women's labors. Relics, charms, and incantations comprised her armamentarium, in the main. The first English midwife on record is Margaret Cobbe, who attended Edward IV's Queen Elizabeth Woodville, when she gave birth to Edward V, on November 1, 1470. By the 16th Century midwives were beginning to receive some instruction, the rejection of the beliefs which had been held for years had not yet come, in spite of the attempt at this time, to inculcate newer and modern methods into these "with-women." But in this period the midwife, the priest physician and the barber surgeons were gradually replaced by men trained in the art of midwifery.

As far as the barber surgeons were concerned, they really were not replaced, instead they merged with the surgeons and were incorporated into one grouping. It was the surgeons themselves who united with the "Barber's Guild" because the politically powerful "Barber's Guild" could thus aid the surgeons' cause in their fight against malpractice and rogues. This was in 1540. The barber-surgeon pact was called the "United Company of Barber Surgeons." Mutilating operations were replaced by more humane and conservative means of delivery, and the foundations of obstetric science were laid in the study of anatomy and physiology of reproduction.

Among the outstanding event of the Renaissance was the development of cesarean section of the living woman, in the major European countries. The death rate of cesarean section at this time, was almost 100 per cent. So it was quite a desperate procedure and attempted only on women who were moribund. However well intentioned the operator, the bereaved relatives always had the feeling that the unfortunate mother might have lived had she been left alone. After Nufer's performance a number of attempts were made to do cesarean, with only the above facts staring them in the face. There were only fifteen successful operations in a period of 100 years, a situation that persisted until the 19th Century.

The performance of the first cesarean by Nufer, initiated the advances in operative obstetrics and gynecology of the Renaissance era. Nufer was followed by Christopher Bain of Italy in 1540. Scipione Mercurio, also in Italy, made his contribution, then came Dirlewang in Germany, in 1549, and later the questionable Francois Rousset of France, in 1580.

Obstetrics of the Renaissance may be prefaced by a number of generalizations applicable to the various countries that were part of this intellectual awakening. In Germany, the Renaissance was marked by the period between Rösslin and Rueff. Midwives were appointed, examined and instructed in the larger municipalities. They delivered the poor and were given charge of sanitary supervision of local brothels. It was the duty of the city physician to examine midwives, and sometimes this duty was left up to the burgomaster's wife. For the first time in centuries poor women became a communal responsibility and were entitled to the care of midwives who should have had some little knowledge of their art. The contribution of France came about in a different manner. While Germany had its passion for organization and regulation, France had a great individualist who achieved in his lifetime more than all the German town councils. This man was Paré, and if Paré was interested in obstetrics then it could no longer be beneath the dignity of his less distinguished brethren. Guillemeau and, to a lesser degree, the name of Rousset may be added. In Italy, Scipione Mercurio was probably the most influential single person to contribute to the advance of obstetrics, and the names of Vesalius, Eustachius, Fallopius, and Arantius may be added, for each one of these great men contributed greatly to the awakening of obstetrics in Italy.

These truly monumental events in the history of obstetrics and gynecology need elaboration in order for the reader to appreciate their importance. Beginning with Germany, the new era in obstetrics was ushered in by the appearance of a series of books especially designed for the instruction of midwives, who were beginning to take on unprecedented responsibilities. Up to then the training of midwives had been handed down from generation to generation, with no intelligent supervision by a medical profession that knew little and cared less. There was real need for authoritative books of instructions for these women, and in a way, these midwives' books provided this much needed information.

Prior to the 16th Century, obstetrical literature (other than that incorporated in works of surgery) consisted of a very few obscure treatises, the earliest being *de Mulierum Passiumbus* by Moschion, in the time of Hadrian (A.D. 117-138).[15] Next to be published was *de secretis mulierum* supposed to have been written by Albertus Magnus in the 13th Century, and about which little is known. In the 15th Century, along came *Das Frauenbuchlein* (Little Book for Women) by Ortolff von Bayerland. Then in 1513, there was published a little book known as the *Rosengarten*, a most widely distributed and translated treatise. Translations of this book endured for two centuries. About twenty-seven years later a book with the title *Byrth of Mankynd* made its appearance in English. (It is supposed to be an English translation of the *Rosengarten*.) Finally we have the *Cheerful Booklet* by Jacob Rueff, published in 1544.

The pre-Renaissance book *Das Frauenbuchlein* antedated the actual Renaissance by a few years, but can readily be considered as the initial publication of this series of books under discussion, for there is no doubt that *Das Frauenbuchlein* was the connecting link between the period of quiescence (primitive) in obstetrics and the flowering of this specialty into an enlightened and intellectual entity embodied with a tinge of science. It may be considered as the seed from which germinated the subsequent Renaissance publications such as the *Rosengarten* and its English translation, *Byrth of Mankynd*. It is therefore included in the series of books dedicated to the intellectual awakening of obstetrics in Germany.

In the *Little Book for Women* there are only thirteen pages, but in this short space the author has given concise instructions for mother and midwife, much of which is sound and eminently practical. Thus:

> The expectant mother must not climb hills, dance, go horseback riding or ride in rough coaches. She should be very careful in order not to fall, not to hurt herself, not to become angry, or give herself up to sadness, and should avoid fright and unchastity. The woman ought to be cleansed first of all, because filth may gather in the lying-in woman and cause many sicknesses. She should receive plenty of sunlight, for women may become blind when kept in a dark room during and after labor. She must regulate her bowels and diet, take proper exercise and baths, though she should avoid hot baths in the last days of her pregnancy, and

should not use any salves, be it oil or fat, on her genitals. She shall wear, on her abdomen and navel, a four to six times folded piece of material or a piece of sheepskin. In the last ten days of her pregnancy she is to anoint the thighs every night with camomile oil to facilitate labor.

In the following quote, the book states the qualifications that should be sought in a midwife, and pertinent instruction to the midwife in the technique that should be employed for the delivery. Thus:

> Every woman who can do it should provide herself with an experienced midwife, one with gentle hands, a fearless and not too talkative one. . . . The midwife ought to pay great attention to the position of the child; for the delivery woman it is best when the head of the child cuts through first and the little hands are to both sides of the hips. But the midwife has to be careful when for instance the hands cut through first, or the hips, a knee or foot. In such cases the midwife must know how to turn the child in order to bring the child into the right position.
>
> Among those above described positions only the first does not undergo any change and so does not the one where the child cuts through with both feet. When everything concerning the child is arranged, the midwife must give her attention to the lying-in woman, help her and advise the woman to do her part, as to draw in her breath, to holler and soon the midwife shall also press the abdomen above the navel; nothing of this kind of help shall be given before the child begins to cut through and parts of it are already seen. By manipulating too early the woman is weakened when her personal help is needed.

The semi-reclining position and the birth stool as used in Italy is recommended. In delayed labor, the midwife is instructed to blow sneezing powder into the nose, to anoint the genitals with oil or fat in which is mixed saphron and barley corn.

> If it happens that the afterbirth is late in coming, make the woman sneeze and close her mouth and nose after having blown into her nose the sneezing powder; she has to suffer it because that is the thing to do in order to call forth the afterbirth. Never shall the afterbirth be drawn out by force; be gentle in order not to tear it or not to leave behind a part in the woman's body. Where a portion of the placenta is retained sneezing powder is again ap-

> plied to the nose, and the navel is anointed. If this fails the midwife is instructed to anoint her hand and insert it into the uterus to remove the placenta. Afterbirth, left in the uterus for awhile, begins to spoil, spreads its rotten vapors to the heart, liver and stomach and makes the woman perish. The uterus should be purged, this power is best obtained from the juice of the rue plant.

In his final instructions, the author commends the midwife to "the mercy of our God, the Lord and his worthy Mother Mary."

To the *Little Book for Women* Ortolff has appended some generalizations which he calls the *Medicine Book.* The following quotation is taken from it:

> The passion of the womb comes to the woman at the age of approximately twelve and lasts till they are forty or fifty years old. Some have it too much and they are yellow and pale, and the urine is red; those who have it too little feel pain in their loins. This is caused by heat and by cold.
>
> A pregnant woman shall not eat anything bitter, shall not undergo any blood letting, shall be careful not to jump nor to beat upon the stomach. . . . The wet nurse must have borne her child at the same time in order that her milk should not be too old or too young. She must have a healthy skin, because the child sucks the sickness from the wet nurse and may become sick. . . . She must be chaste because unchastity spoils the milk. She shall not be fat or meager.

Although the reintroduction of version by Paré was a most impressive event of the Renaissance, a little book known as the *Rosengarten,* published in 1513, had already exerted a mighty influence on midwifery. This book was more widely translated and distributed than any other medical book up to that time, it had no scientific merit, and yet, with its numerous translations it became not only a text book for midwives, but for two centuries served as an authoritative treatise on obstetrics for the medical profession in England and throughout all Europe. The author of this book is supposed to have been a certain Eucharius Rösslin, of Worms. Although the evidence that he was the author is not conclusive, such an authority as Ingerslev, believes him to be. The full title of the book is *Der Swangern Frauen and Hebammen Rosengarten* (*A Rosengarten for*

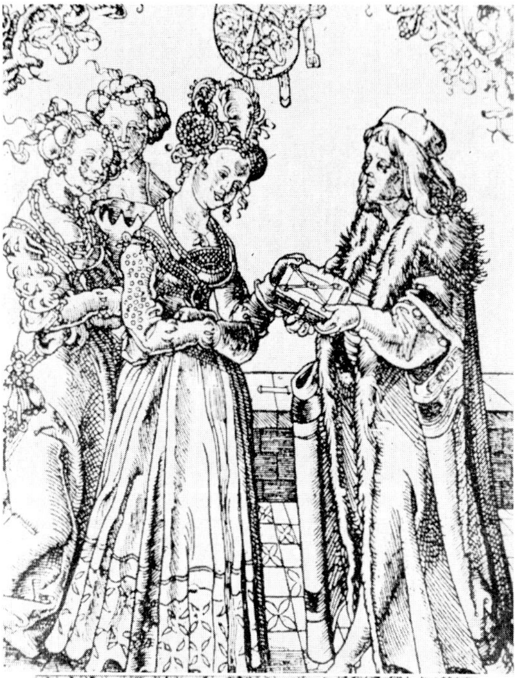

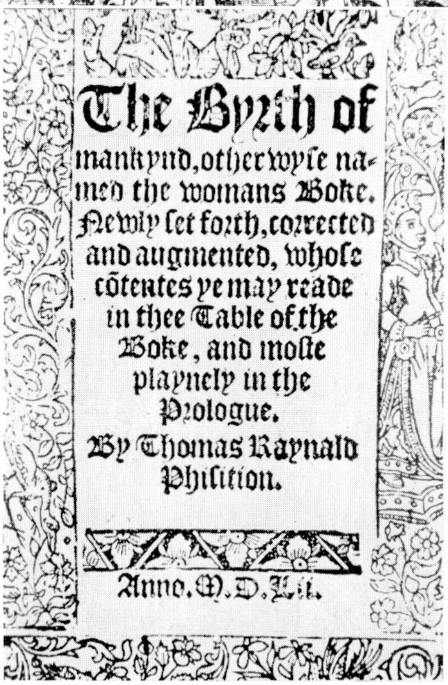

The Byrth of
mankynd, otherwyſe na-
med the womans Boke.
Newly ſet forth, corrected
and augmented, whoſe
cõtentes ye may reade
in thee Table of the
Boke, and moſte
playnely in the
Prologue.
By Thomas Raynald
Phiſition.

Anno. M. D. Lii.

Fig. 63. Eucharius Rösslin presenting his book to the Duchess of Brunswick, 1513.
Fig. 64. Title page of *The Byrth of Mankynd* by Thomas Raynald, 1552. (From *The Byrth of Mankynd* by Thomas Raynald, 1552.)

Pregnant Women and Midwives), and like the authorship, the quaint title is likewise under dispute. The sources of this book are Hippocrates, Galen, Aetius, Magnus and others. It is mostly a compilation and does not represent any marked advance in the science of obstetrics.

The only presentation considered normal was that of the head. Cephalic version (turning by the head) was recommended (as did Soranus) and not podalic version. There are drawings of sixteen positions of the fetus (they look like copies of Soranus' drawings) and also a drawing of a birth stool that goes back to at least the 2nd Century A.D. (also as Soranus). Whereas Soranus made every effort to save the mother at the expense of the child, Rösslin would leave her to her fate when her life was in jeopardy. If the baby was known to be dead, delivery was attempted by medicaments or finally by dismembering operations.

The *Rosengarten* was translated into English by Richard Jones, and published in 1540 by Thomas Raynald, a printer who had a shop in St. Paul's Churchyard. The title of the English translation was *Byrth of Mankynd*.[16] The English midwives and physicians were entirely dependent on this little book for guidance in the practice of obstetrics for over 200 years, when the more scientific works of Smellie and Hunter appeared.

An interesting story by Alfred Brown as to the possible incentive for writing a book of this kind (*Byrth of Mankynd*) is based on the tragedy that befell Jane Seymour, one of the many wives of Henry the Eighth, who rid himself of one wife after another, because they were unable to bear him an heir. When Jane Seymour finally turned the trick, she died of puerperal fever. And according to Brown, it was this event that probably impressed British medical men of the necessity for the study of obstetrics, and three years later *Byrth of Mankynd* was published.

Until now, medieval obstetrics had not emerged from the darkness that had made a martyrdom of childbirth. The anatomy and physiology of the reproductive organs were poorly understood, practice was based entirely upon clinical observations which were handicapped by ignorance, superstition and a goodly amount of religious bigotry. It may have been Paré's version that stimulated obstetric progress toward a more exact science; however, the publication of these books, and the *Byrth of Mankynd* in particular, occurred at the very time when the great transition from the empiric methods of the ancients to the scientific procedures of the moderns was being brought about. The 1560 edition contained lively and expressive figures (drawings?) of all the inward parts of women.

Women of the sixteenth century, while in the throes of labor, would declare that they would never allow themselves to get pregnant again; the same cry we hear in the labor rooms today. Here is Raynald's word picture of this:

> For ye shall heare some women in tyme of theyr trauayle, meued through great payne and intollerable anguyshe, forswere and vowe them selfe, neuer to companye with a man agayne; yet after that the panges be passed, within a short whyle, for entyre loue for theyr husbandes, and singular delyte betwene man and woman, they forget both the sorrow passed and that is to come. Such be the privie works of God, and such be the prickes of nature, which neuer createth no special pleasure unaccompanied with some sorrow.

Raynald considered Pliny's attitude on menstrual blood as nonsense, for Pliny said:

> Menstrual blood is a fatal poison, corrupting and decomposing urine, depriving seeds of their fecundity, destroying insects, blasting garden flowers and grasses, causing fruits to fall from branches, dulling razors, etc.

That a baby "born with a caul" betokens good luck is a fallacy that antedates the time of Raynald, but in this book we find him subscribing to it. The membranes covering the baby's head at the time of birth is called "coyfe," "byggn," "chyldss," and "shert," which "shoulde betoken some great lucke to the child in tyme to come." He makes erroneous references to the afterbirth; while recognizing the fact that the blood vessels convey the mother's blood to the baby through the afterbirth, the author goes far astray when he says that any excess of blood (in the afterbirth) goes to the mother's breast in the form of white blood (milk).

Another fallacy to be noted is that a baby born in the seventh month has a better chance to live than one born in the eighth month. This statement has come down through the ages and is believed by many today. A curious statement is made that the "birth of man is generally easier than the birth of the female." This idea may be based on the fact that in primitive times it was believed that the baby finds its way into the outer world under its own power, and boys being more vigorous than girls, make their exits more quickly; the following sentence bears this out:

> If the child be so faint, weak and tender, that it cannot turn itself or doeth it very slowely. . . . Also if the child be dead in the mother's belly, it is a very perilous thing, for so much as it cannot be easily turned, neither can it move or help itself to come forth, or if the child be sick or weakened so that it cannot for feebleness help itself.

Many reasons are given for the "weakening" of the baby, such as "sore lasked" (purgatives), "daily and unwantened her flowers" (menses). Here, probably, he refers to the hemorrhages of the pregnant uterus due to placenta previa or to premature separation. Drying of the breasts is a sign of death of the fetus.

Normal birth, or as Raynald states: "Natural birth is when the child is born in due season and also in due fashion." He explains that the "due season is about forty weeks after the conception."

The entire book contains truths and absurdities, but is helpful withall. His chapter on the management of difficult labor is similarly laden with half truths and even completely incorrect statements, together with truths and practical hints. Thus premature rupture of the bag of waters is said to prolong labor, but it is difficult to follow the author when he ascribes to delayed labor the eating of certain fruits and vegetables. Certain kinds of baths are thought to retard labor. (No cold baths were allowed after the first month of pregnancy.) If the bag of waters does not break of its own accord (late in labor, presumably), the midwife is instructed to cut it with a pair of shears or a knife. If they rupture too early a dry labor results which requires the oil of lilies, or best of all lubricants, the white of an egg.

Constipation should be relieved because it will hold up the labor, so the woman is advised to eat fresh fruits and wines and abstain from hard eggs. Enemas should be used to relieve constipation. Moderate exercise, "goying or standing, more than otherwise she is wont to doe," is prescribed to strengthen her for labor. To facilitate labor she should use ointments (the grease of hens, ducks, geese, etc.) "where with ye may sople the privie place," and further she is instructed, at the onset of labor pains, to sit still for an hour, then to go up and down the stairs crying "so loude as she can, so to tyre her selfe."

If there are obstructing tumors she is advised to consult a surgeon. Further instruction on complications of labor advises the midwife on a footling presentation, hydrocephalous, twins and retained placenta. With a foot presentation or when the arms are extended alongside the head in a breech, the attempt should be made to turn the baby, bearing in mind that "this is the perylloust manner of birth." A child with a large head, or twins requires of the midwife that "she help all she may be, with her hands first anointed with some oil, opening and enlarging the passageway that the issue may be freer." Oils, ointments, plasters and other medical means may be employed to assist labor when mechanical methods do not avail. Of the plasters to provoke birth, there is "a magic plaster that shall helpe marveylously, made of juyce of Rue and Barlye mixed into a 'meale' with 'wyde Gowarde' (wild gourd, Coeocynth) and placed on the abdomen." When perfumes and vapours fail to facilitate the delivery of the afterbirth, "let her be provoked to sneeze with the powder of Eleborus or pepper put in the nose, holdinge her mouth and noe so close as maybe." If this fails manual removal of the placenta is attempted:

> And if it be so that any part of the secondines (afterbirth) do not appear, let the midwife receive it tenderly, loosing it out well and softly, least it break, then let the midwife tie that part of it which she hath handfast to the womans leg or foot, not very straight, least it break, neither very lax, least it slip in again, and then cause her to sneese. Now if the secondines (afterbirth) tare and stick, so that it come not quickly forewards, then loose it a little and a little tenderly (turn) it from one side to another, till such time it be gotten out, but ever beware of violent and hasty movings of it, least that with the second birth (afterbirth) you remove also.

It can be assumed that he means inversion of the uterus may result from undue pulling of the cord, which he warns against. If the above advice does not result in the delivery of the placenta, the midwife is admonished to let the patient alone with the hope that the afterbirth will "putrifie and corrupt, and dissolve into a watery substance, thick like bryne or other fex myxed with water and so yssue foorth."

Many other suggestions for the complications of labor and pregnancy are given under the title of "how to avoyde, defende, or to remedye the same." For instance, he enumerates countless abominable concoctions devised for the relief of such ailments as "swelling of the body," "fretting and knawing of the guts," "pain in the privie parts," and "outrageous flux of flowres." His picture of exhaustion from prolonged labor is concise and clear:

> Evil signs which betoken a difficult labor are when she sweateth cold sweats, and that her pulse beats and labor are sore, and that she herself in the laboring faints and swoons, these be unlucky and mortal signs.

At one place in the book we find instructions given to the midwife for the performance of a postmortem cesarean operation in the effort to save the life of the unborn child. In another part of this book reference is made to the birth stool:

> Now when a woman perceiveth the Matrix or Mother (womb) to ware lax or loose, and to be dissolved, and that the humors (waters) issue forth in great plenty, then it will be meet for her to sit down leaning backward (in the birth stool) in manner upright. For the which purpose in some regions (as in France and Germany) the midwives have stools for the purpose, which being but low, and not high from the ground be made so round wise and concave or hollow in the middle, that they may be received from underneath which is looked for (the baby) and the back of the stool leaning backward receiveth the back of the woman, the fashion of which the stool, is set in the beginning of the birth figures hereafter. And when the time of labor is come, in the same stool ought to be put many clothes or rags in the back of it, the which the midwife may remove from one side to another according as necessity shall require. The midwife herself shall sit before the laboring woman, and shall diligently observe and wait, how much, and after what means the child stireth itself, also shall with her hands first anointed with the oil of al-

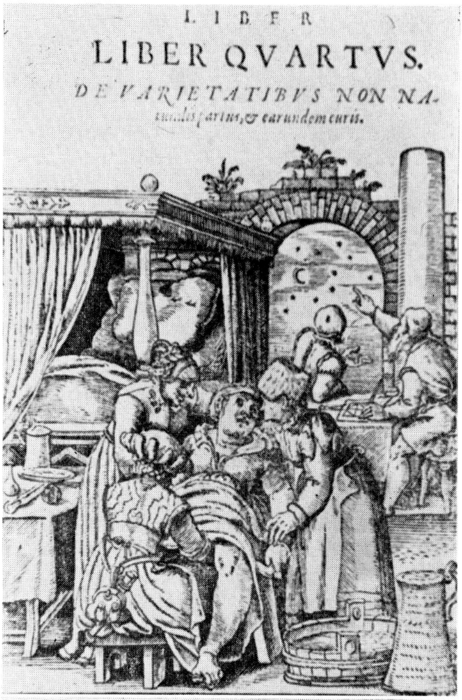

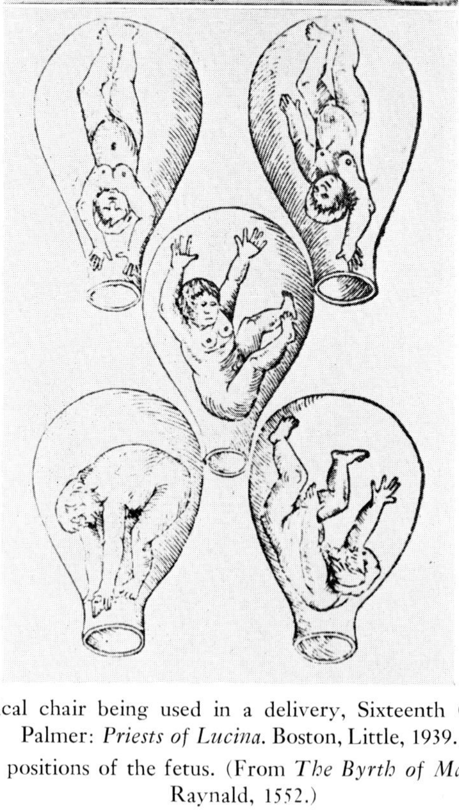

Fig. 65. Obstetrical chair being used in a delivery, Sixteenth Century. (Findley, Palmer: *Priests of Lucina.* Boston, Little, 1939.)

Fig. 66. Various positions of the fetus. (From *The Byrth of Mankynd* by Thomas Raynald, 1552.)

> monds, or the oil of white lillies, rule and direct every thing as shall seem best. Also the midwife must instruct and comfort the party, not only refreshing her with good meat and drink, but also with sweet words, giving her good hope of a speedy deliverance, encouraging and admonishing her to patience and tolerance bidding her to hold in her breath so much as she may, also stroking gently with her hands her belly above the navel, for that helps to depress the birth downward. . . .

Raynald goes on with instructions to the midwife on various complications that she may meet. These we have already mentioned in brief in the preceding paragraphs, the above quote on the birth stool which for ages was the property of the midwife, not only gives a good picture of the birth stool and how used, but also acquaints us with the conduct of labor in the normal parturient.

Of the supposed original illustrations in this book *Byrth of Mankynd,* sixteen came from Soranus in the 2nd Century. In the illustrations the uterus looks like a Florence flask, whose content is a child, twin or monstrous pregnancy stretched out at full length with the arms over the head in almost every attitude of the gymnast. The ages of the fetus might be anywhere from one to ten years, but some look many years older, with the faces of old men. It was 200 years before published illustrations accurately portrayed the positions of the fetus within the uterus; these were by Smellie and Hunter. And yet Leonardo in the 15th Century made a faithful portrayal of the fetus *in utero.* It is difficult to understand why Raynalde chose illustrations from Soranus (2nd Century), when his contemporary Da Vinci did such accurate illustrations.

Nearly all early observers gained their impressions of the structure of the uterus largely from dissections of the hog and other animals and described the organ as having two horns. Many believed that the uterus contained seven chambers or cells. Raynald believed that a cleft in the uterus partially separated the two halves, but the baby developed in only a single cavity. Also he did not differentiate between the vagina, cervix and uterus.

> "The oyaries," by Raynald, "are called woman's stones, wherein are engendered the seed and sperm that cometh from the woman, not so strong, firm and mighty in operation as the seed of man, but rather weak, cold and moist, and of no great

firmness. . . . The stones be nothing so big as the stones of man, but less, flatter, much fashioned after the shape of a large and broad almond."

He called the tube "wormye bodye" which passes from the "stone" (ovary) to the corners of the Matrix (uterus). He taught that the seed of women was for the purpose of moistening the genital passage "as with a dewe." He knew nothing of the physiology of reproduction.*

Another midwife book which appeared in 1544, revised in 1559, was published by JACOB RUEFF (1500-1558). It was perhaps simply an imitation of the *Rosengarten*, but nevertheless, it had a tremendous popularity, though undeserved, by both midwife and doctor. It was called the *Cheerful* Booklet (Trostbuchle); thirty-six years later there appeared a revised edition known as the *Midwives Book*, and even later, a Latin edition entitled *De Conceptu et Generatione hominis, etc.*[18] appeared, so we have a version for the midwives and one for the doctors. Rueff was Professor of Medicine at the University of Zurich; he was an able obstetrician but a mediocre anatomist considering that he was a contemporary of Vesalius. In his writings, he discussed abdominal masses and their differential diagnosis. Etiologically, all uterine growths were the result of degeneration of the seed. He discussed prolapse and its causes, which were internal and external and numbered in the hundreds. He recognized hematoma of the vulva for which he suggested incision; this was about the only really original piece of work he ever produced.

He is known to have used "smoothe" and "toothed" forceps for the delivery of the dead fetus; he was not known ever to use these instruments on the living baby, but he does have the distinction of having first suggested the possibility of delivering the living baby by means of forceps.[19]

About the same time that Vesalius was supreme, there existed a great physician who was proclaimed the father of surgery. His contributions to gynecology and obstetrics were almost equally as

* Dr. J. W. Ballantyne of Edinburgh and Dr. E. Ingerslev of Copenhagen made a critical analysis of the original editions of *Byrth of Mankynd* and the *Rosengarten*. They published a thesis in the *Journal of Obstetrics and Gynecology of the British Empire* in 1906-7-9. This journal has been the source of these quotations.[17]

great as his contributions to surgery. He was largely influenced by Vesalius' *Fabrica;* he even translated an abstract from this work in Latin to his native French.

AMBROISE PARÉ[20] (1510-1590) was this man. He was born in Maine, France. Paré was the first to perform amputation of the cervix (actually Tulpius, in 1652, did the first amputation of the cervix, based on the recommendation of Paré). So it seems that Paré only recommended the amputation of cervix (in cancer). He

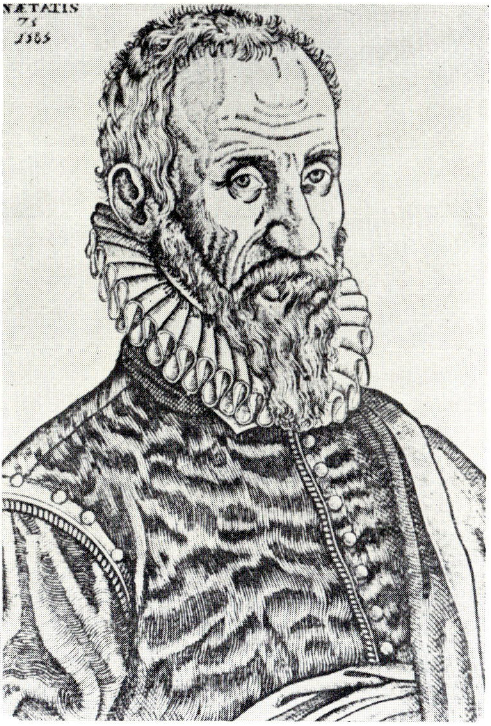

Fig. 67. Ambroise Paré. (Findley, Palmer: *Priests of Lucina.* Boston, Little, 1939.)

is supposed to have used the vaginal speculum in this operation, or at least suggested it. He used to induce premature labor in cases of pregnancy complicated with uterine hemorrhage, a procedure unheard of before his day, and therefore requiring much courage. He was the first to suture a lacerated perineum (the experience no doubt obtained as a result of his attempts at accouchement force). Paré described a fibroid and the differential diagnosis of pregnancy and a fibroid. He reintroduced the ligature to replace the hot iron and boiling oil.

He believed that the slough of apathetic inhumanity into which the practice of obstetrics had been allowed to lapse over the Dark Ages was the unreasonable worship of the Ancients. To prod them out of this lethargy he wrote, "You will have to render account not to the ancients but to God for your humanity and your skill," for with Paré humanity came first and skill second.

He wrote two treatises in obstetrics, *La Maniere de Extraire les enfens tant mors que vivans hors le Ventre de la Mere lorsque Nature de soy ne peult venir a son Effet.* This appeared at the end of his *Briefve Collection Anatomique* and was published in 1551. His second publication was entitled *De la generation de l'homme receuilli des anciens et modernes.* Everything he wrote was in colloquial French. The first publication is the work that contained the description of podalic version, which he reintroduced, after many centuries, from Soranus. He disclaims originality in this procedure, the stimulus for this operation having come after seeing Thierry de Hery and Nicole Lambert do podalic versions in Paris. He failed to popularize it and it remained for Guillemeau, Mauriceau and Portal, who followed him, to do so. The following extract is from the English translation of his thesis on podalic version:

> The woman is first of all to be "aptly placed, that is to say, overthwart the bedside with her buttocks somewhat high." She is then to be trussed as if for a lithotomy operation. The heels are drawn up close to the buttocks and bound there with "broad and soft linnen rowlers." These rolls of linen must "first come about her neck and then crosswise over her shoulders and so to the feet, and there it must cross again and so be rowled about the legs and thighs and then it must be brought up to the neck again and there made fast so that she may not be able to move herself." The midwives or other women are to support her legs and shoulders to prevent fatigue and "that the work may be don with more decencie her privie parts and thighs must be covered." The surgeon is to remove the rings from his fingers and see that his nails are well pared and his hands well anointed with oil.
>
> And supposing that the child presents naturally having the head towards the outlet, to duly deliver it by art you must gently push it back in the contrary direction and seek the feet and draw

> them down. By doing this you will easily turn the child. And when you have drawn the feet into the outlet you must draw one foot outside and tie it above the heel in the manner of a running noose with a moderately long fillet, like that with which women bind their hair. Then you will replace the said foot into the said womb and having found the other foot you will draw it outside and then pull on the fillet. And when you have thus both feet outside the womb you will draw on both equally on one side as on the other, little by little and without violence.
>
> To assist the delivery of the after-coming head the midwives should press the patient's belly with their hands, and the patient must hold her breath and bear down as much as possible. Care should be taken to make sure that there is only one child and not twins. A presentation of the hand or shoulder must be pushed back, for if the arms are pulled down "his head would fall backwards to the great danger of his mother."[21]

Paré's reintroduction of podalic version saved many thousands of mothers who previously had either been left to die or else had been subjected to mutilating operations designed to destroy the child. Paré's own daughter Anne nearly lost her life in childbirth, but was dramatically saved by her father's favorite pupil, Guillemeau, who performed podalic version as he had been taught by Paré twenty years before.

Although Soranus taught midwives to turn the baby under prescribed conditions, and Celsus was the first to demonstrate that the fetus could be delivered with its lower extremities foremost, it remained for Paré to demonstrate the superiority of podalic version; going beyond the indications for version as laid down by Soranus many centuries before by resorting to the procedure in severe hemorrhages and where immediate delivery was indicated.

He adhered to the teachings of Hippocrates, Aristotle, St. Augustine and the Arabian physicians, and though he shared in the superstitions of his time, and believed in magic and witchcraft, he did not subscribe to the belief of the ancients that monstrous babies were begotten by the devil. And yet he proceeded to commit himself to an equally absurd theory when he wrote:

> In times past there have been some who nothing fearing the Deity, neither Law nor themselves, that is their souls have so ob-

> jected and prostrated themselves; that they have thought themselves nothing different from beasts; wherefore Atheists, Sodomites, Outlaws, foregetfull of their own excellency and divinity, and transformed by filthy lusts, have not doubted to have filthy and abominable copulation with beasts . . . for of this various and promiscuous confusion of seedes of different kinde, monsters have been generated and borne, who have beene partly men and partly beasts.

Paré believed the myth of the true hermaphrodite, a theory which has been disproved by embryologists and geneticists of our time. Interestingly, he was ahead of his contemporaries in his views on the correct treatment of the intersexes. He believed, and the modern view is the same, that whatever the external appearances might be, hermaphrodites should be allowed to choose whether they wished to be regarded as males or females, psychosexuality being more important than changes in the external genitalia. This did not apply to mild cases; these were to be treated legally and socially as being of the sex of which the characteristics were dominant.

Paré was uncompromising in his opposition to cesarean operations on the living mother. He did not think it possible to survive so formidable an operation, mainly because of the size of the wound and hemorrhage (he made no mention of infection). One of the errors Paré made in good faith concerned the belief that in childbirth the bones of the mother's pelvis undergo separation. Because of the high esteem and authority with which he was invested, this myth was perpetuated for centuries. Paré was one of the many who shared in the old belief that a baby born in the eighth month would be born dead or die shortly after birth. A very interesting bit of advice from Paré (in view of the present day practice of milking the cord or not tying it until pulsations ceased) was to wait as long as possible before ligating the cord if the baby seemed to be weak.

Paré rose from barber surgeon to surgeon of the King. He suffered from the vanity of self-reverence which accompanies great and even small reputations. He thought that he had left little undone when he said "posterity will not be able to surpass us (be it said without malice or offense) save by additions, such as are easily made to things already discovered." Surely he did not envision the future and its boundless achievements.

Jacques Guillemeau (1550-1613) was a pupil and son-in-law of Paré. He gained a tremendous experience in the large wards of the Hotel Dieu of Paris. He helped to popularize the art of "turning" taught him by Paré. He was not too original, but he did perfect the technique of version in many of its details. In the name of suffering womanhood, he exhorted the medical profession to become better equipped for the practice of midwifery. He lived up to this suggestion by publishing a book in 1609, in Paris, called *L'heureux accouchement des femmes*. Guillemeau was a very practical surgeon and obstetrician, and strangely enough he never assumed the responsibility for determining whether the baby should be sacrificed to save the life of the mother; he left this decision to the clergy. He was very emphatic, however, in deciding whether or not the baby was alive before suggesting any particular method of delivery in a complicated case. In those days most physicians were not overly concerned with the life of the baby and were ever ready to perform mutilating operations. His method of deciding whether the baby was alive or not, was to insert the hand into the uterus and grasp the hand or foot of the baby; if there was no retraction of the limb, he would insert a finger into the mouth of the baby; if living it would suck his finger. His practices and obstetrical thinking ran quite parallel to those of Paré.

Francois Rousset (b. 1535), in 1580, made a far reaching contribution in the form of a report of fifteen cesarean sections, obtained from many different sources. He was like many of his confreres, an intrepid abdominal surgeon from the University of Paris. Like all the other reported cesarean operations, Nufer's included, they were thought to have been abdominal pregnancies. Although his cases were greatly doubted, his interest in this direction had much to do with the progress of obstetrics and gynecology (surgery). He did clear up the question of inversion of the uterus, which, prior to his time, was confused with prolapse. He made a masterful presentation of cause, diagnosis and treatment of inversion. This observation of Rousset's was incorporated in all subsequent treatises on midwifery.

The contributions to Renaissance obstetrics made in Germany and France were bolstered by advances in Italy, in the person of

Scipione Mercurio (1550-1595?)* who was born in Rome in the year in which the *Byrth of Mankynd* was first published. He studied at Bologna, Padua and the Dominican monastery at Milan, where he took the name of Hieronymus. He first studied theology, but did not pursue that road very long, instead turned to obstetrics. He travelled widely through France and Spain where he improved his knowledge of obstetrics greatly, especially from physicians in the city of Toulouse, where he saw two cesarean sections in 1571. He finally settled again in Italy, in a monastery in Venice, where he practiced medicine for sixteen years. He never separated himself from his monastic association; in fact, he was buried in this Venetian monastery. It was his observations on cesarean sections in France that prompted him to study under Arantius at Bologna on his return to Italy. From him, he learned much of obstetrics that bears directly on the problems of cesarean section, such as pelvic contractions.

His writings were the outstanding contributions to Italian obstetrics in the 16th Century (perhaps the seventeenth century can be included). He published *La Commare o Riccoglitrice*[22] in 1596. It was the first work on obstetrics to be published in Italy, and remained an authoritative source in Italy and Germany for 125 years. In this book, he refers to the "hanging legs" position which Albucasis had introduced in the 10th Century and which Walcher popularized in the 19th Century. The hips are elevated on a pillow and the legs hanging over the edge of the bed and resting on a stool, the sacral prominence is elevated and the anterio-posterior diameter of the pelvis is increased thereby. He published also a procedure of bimanual turning of the fetus two and one-half centuries before Braxton Hicks, whose name is appended to the operation. His most important contribution in this book was two chapters devoted to cesarean section. He was, so far as known, the first to suggest the advisability of a cesarean operation on a living mother with a contracted pelvis.

His vanity and superior mental endowment made him many enemies. He respected the old masters, but did not hesitate to take issue with them. He criticized Rueff for his unreasoning devotion

* This date was obtained from the "Index Catalogue of the Library of the Surgeon General of the United States."

to astrology. To him Hippocrates was not infallible; Avicenna sometimes spoke nonsense; and Aristotle was not always the wise philosopher and scientist. He disagreed with Galen that the uterus contained separate compartments, and questioned Galen's assertion that a diagnosis of pregnancy could be made from the examination of the urine. (How does that fit in with today's pregnancy test?) He demonstrated the presence of the hymen that was considered of doubtful existence by Soranus and Paré.

His description of cesarean section is very long and detailed, but a model of clarity. It need not be given here, suffice it to say that they used no anesthesia, made a right rectus incision from the pubis to just above the umbilicus. The patient was held by five men (or strong, courageous women) in a big canopied bed. The incision was outlined in ink first. The uterus was sponged out, as was the abdominal cavity. The abdominal wall was closed by interrupted sutures, the intestines carefully pushed away in the process. The postoperative treatment was the same as for any other form of surgery. He ends his discourse by saying, "This is enough about this new method of aiding difficult deliveries to help miserable patients."[23]

In summarizing the contributions of the Renaissance we start with:

(1) The beginnings of anatomical studies, which may be considered one of the most potent factors responsible for the intellectual awakening of medicine.

(2) The reintroduction of podalic version (Paré).

(3) Cesarean section (Nufer).

(4) Publication of a series of booklets on obstetrics exerted an inestimable influence on its advance; teaching of midwives by physicians became more common, and this indirectly was responsible for improving the maternal mortality and morbidity, a practice which we are stressing in modern times with unbending energy.

First Occurrences and Outstanding Events

Fracastoro was the first to coin the word syphilis, circa 1500.

Recognizable syphilis was first mentioned by Emperor Maximilian I, and shortly afterwards by Theodoricus Ulsenius in his "*Vaticinium* (1500).

Bartolomeo da Montagnana, in 1460, gave the clearest ideas on female anatomy by dissection.

Alessandro Benedetti da Legnano (1460-1525) was the first to use the words perineum, cervix and procedentia.

J. Berengario da Carpi (1460-1530) was the first to state that the fundus contained only one cavity (this was long after DaVinci's pronouncement). He was the first to do vaginal hysterectomy. Was first (after Leonardo) to make anatomical drawings from nature. He was the first to describe the appendix.

Nicolaus Massa (1499-1569) was the first to describe the three layers of the uterus.

Leonardo was the first to show that the uterus had only one cavity, and he also described fetal membranes for the first time.

Vesalius, by his *Fabrica*, founded modern anatomy. He was the first to show that the uterus was not round. He was the first to show that cartilage united bone joints, and that the pubic arch does not separate.

Fallopius was the first to describe precisely the clitoris. He gave the first accurate description of the tubes and ovaries. (Rufus and Soranus and Vesalius described them, but less accurately.)

Fallopius named the vagina and the placenta.

Eustachius discovered the Eustachian tube; made countless other anatomical discoveries; also made beautiful drawings of the uterus.

Arantius gave the first clear cut account of pelvic contractions.

First cesarean by Nufer.

First English midwife with recognition was Margaret Cobbe who delivered Edward V in 1470.

Scipione Mercurio was the most influential single person to contribute to the advance of obstetrics.

The *Rosengarten* exerted a mighty influence on midwifery for 200 years.

Reuff was the first to "suggest" forceps delivery of the living baby.

Paré was the first to amputate the cervix (actually Tulpius in 1652 did it on Paré's recommendation). First to suture perinei. First to make differential diagnosis between pregnancy and a fibroid. He reintroduced the ligature to replace the cautery and boiling oil. He reintroduced podalic version since the time of Soranus.

Celsus was the first to demonstrate a delivery with the lower extremities foremost.

Rousset, in 1580, was the first to make differential diagnosis between inversion and prolapse of uterus.

Scipione Mercurio was the first to publish obstetrical work in Italy. He was first to do a Braxton Hicks version (Braxton Hicks did it 250 years later). He was the first to advise cesarean on a living mother for contracted pelvis.

References

1. Riesman, David: *The Story of Medicine in the Middle Ages.* New York, Hoeber, 1935.
2. Sarton, G.: *Science in the Renaissance; the Civilization of the Renaissance.* Chicago, Univ. Chicago Press, 1929.
3. Graham, Harvey: *Eternal Eve.* London, Heinemann, 1950.
4. Ricci, J. V.: *Genealogy of Gynecology.* Philadelphia, Blakiston, 1950, p. 243.
5. *Ibid.*, p. 242.
6. *Ibid.*, p. 246.
7. *Ibid.*, p. 246.
8. Spielmann, M. H.: *The Iconography of Andreas Vesalius.* London, J. Bale, 1925.
9. Libby, W.: *The History of Medicine, in Its Salient Features.* Boston, Mifflin, 1922.
10. Favaro, G.: *Gabriello Falloppia, Modenese.* Modena, Studio Biografico, 1928.
11. Speert, Harold: Obstetrical-gynecological eponyms; Gabriele Fallopio and fallopian tubes. *Obst. & Gynec.*, *6*:467-470.
12. Castiglioni, Arturo: *A History of Medicine.* New York, Knopf, 1941.
13. Baas, J. H.: *Outlines of the History of Medicine and the Medical Profession*, transl. by H. E. Handerson, New York, Vail, 1889.
14. Bettmann, O. L.: *A Pictorial History of Medicine.* Springfield, Thomas, 1956.
15. Findley, Palmer: *Priests of Lucina.* Boston, Little, 1939.
16. Roesslin, Eucharius: *The Byrth of Mankynd*, transl. by Raynald. London, Raynald, 1545.
17. Ballantyne, J. W. (Edinburgh) and Ingerslev, E. (Copenhagen): Critical analysis of the original editions of *The Byrth of Mankynd* and the *Rosengarten; J. Obst. & Gynec. Brit. Emp.* 1906-7-9.
18. Rueffus, Jacobus: *De Conceptu et Generation Hominis et iis quae circa ihaes, potissimum considerantur*, 6 books. Tiguri, C. Froschoverus, 1554.
19. Brown, Alfred: *Old Masterpieces in Surgery.* Omaha, privately printed, 1928.

20. Packard, F. R.: *Life and Times of Ambroise Paré* (1510-1590). New York, Hoeber, 1921.
21. Findley, Palmer: *Priests of Lucina*. Boston, Little, 1939.
22. Mercurio, Scipione: *La Commare o Riccoglitrice*. Venetia, Ciotti, 1601.
23. Thoms, Herbert: *Classical Contributions to Obstetrics and Gynecology*. Springfield, Thomas, 1935.

Chapter XI

PHYSIOLOGY AND MICROSCOPY (A.D. 1600-1700)

THE 17TH CENTURY was an era of great names such as Thomas Hobbs, Sir Isaac Newton, Francis Bacon, Pepys, Burton, Dryden, John Locke, Sir Thomas Browne, the Chamberlens and greatest of all, William Harvey. These great men managed to remain aloof from the civil, political and religious strife that prevailed in England, and, as a result, England witnessed a superb literary and scientific outburst. France, on the other hand, had emerged from a devastated, disorganized, bankrupt country on the verge of collapse in the beginning of the century, to become a leading continental power. She extended her frontiers to the Rhine, built colonies in the four corners of the world, greatly improved her national finances and civil administration, excelled in war, and her art and literature were unmatched, as were certain phases of the sciences. In spite of the fact that France was up and coming, as a country, and England was enmeshed in almost total disaster as an Empire, it was from England (London) that progress emanated mostly, in the 17th Century, while the rest of continental Europe continued to involve itself in almost fifty years of uninterrupted warfare to gain economic supremacy. All this had its influence on medicine because at no time in its history has medicine been entirely independent of the prevailing trends of thought.

Physiology

The seventeenth century has often been called the "age of physiology" because of the discovery of the circulation of the blood by

Harvey in 1616 in England, an event that has been considered the greatest physiological discovery of all time. The physiology of Galen, which contained practically nothing but simple notions, plus some theoretical abstractions from Aristotle and the Scotists, was the sort of physiology known up to the middle of the 16th Century. The first glimpse of a change was noted when the Greek doctrine of the four elements was severely shaken by the speculations of the alchemists. Then came an attempt at creation of a new system of physiology and pathology by Fernel (1497-1558);[1] in other words a science guided by metaphysical speculation prevailed up to the close of the 16th Century. With the introduction of higher mathematics, of astronomy, physics and chemistry in the Seventeenth Century came a change. It was through these sciences that they explained all physiological conduct as a response to physical laws. Ideas on the circulation, respiration, nervous system and generation were changed completely. Pulse taking and the thermometer resulted from these newer concepts. Malpighi had demonstrated microscopically the pulmonary flow in 1661; Maurocordato had experimented on the course of the blood through the lungs; Stensen had described the true structure of the heart in 1664 (this description was improved upon by Lower in 1669); Leeuwenhoek had demonstrated capillary anastomosis and the corpuscles.

Anatomy

While the 17th Century was devoted primarily to advances in physiology, some very notable discoveries in anatomy took place, a sort of continuation of the great advances in anatomy that laid the foundations of modern surgery in the 16th Century. As a basis for this new anatomical knowledge, stands Leeuwenhoek's microscope, which helped to found the sciences of histology and embryology.

There were some very valuable contributions in anatomy by the English. They were the antrum of Highmore in 1651, Glisson's capsule in 1654, the circle of Willis in 1664, the Haversian canals in 1691, and Cowper's glands in 1694. Robert Hooke (1635-1703) was the first to depict the biological cell. Then we have Wharton's duct in 1656. It was to him, Thomas Wharton, that we are indebted for the description of the jelly of the cord. He was born in Winston on

Fig. 68. Thomas Wharton. (*Obstetrics and Gynecology*, *8*:No. 3, p. 380, Sept. 1956. New York, Hoeber.)

Tees, England, attended Cambridge and Oxford. Primarily an anatomist, his greatest contribution was the "*adenographia*."[2]

Mauriceau introduced the terms "fourchette" and "fosse naviculaire." Guillaume des Noues, a French surgeon teaching anatomy in Genoa, described the Nabothian cysts of the cervix. In 1692, Nuck described the peritoneal prolongation of the round ligaments (the canal of Nuck). Anatomical advances and discoveries and correction of erroneous concepts of earlier years were the result of more frequent dissections on diseased patients instead of criminals. Also, numerous changes in anatomy resulted from the science of injecting specimens through the vessels, instead of by the scalpel and mere exposure of the organs.

Rapid progress was made after Vesalius threw off the shackles which had, since the days of Galen, hemmed in the study of human anatomy. Johann van Horne (1621-1670) of Leyden was among

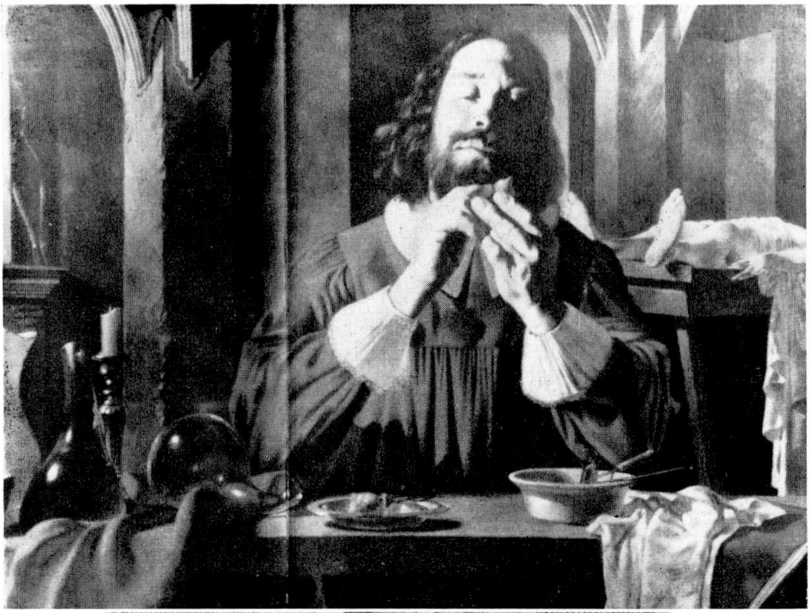

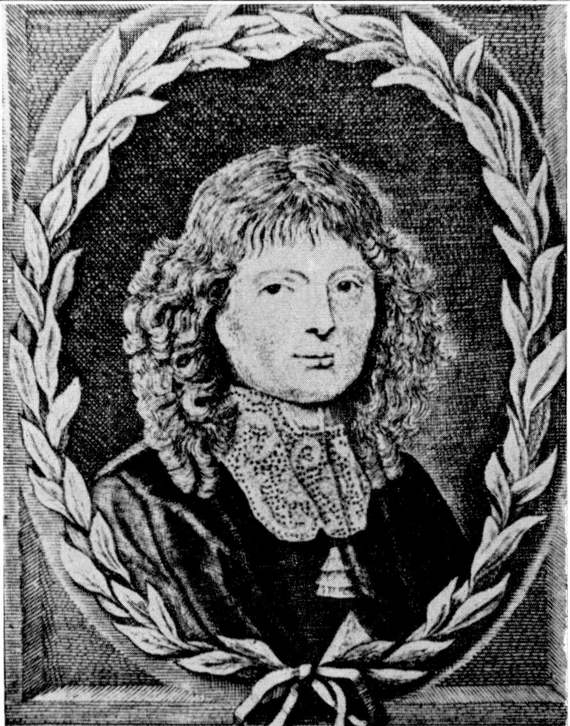

Fig. 69. Johann van Horne. (*Lederle Bulletin, 18*:No. 2 (cover), May 1953. New York, Lederle Laboratories Division [American Cyanamid Co.].)

Fig. 70. Regner de Graaf. (*Obstetrics and Gynecology, 1*:No. 5, p. 582, May 1956. New York, Hoeber.)

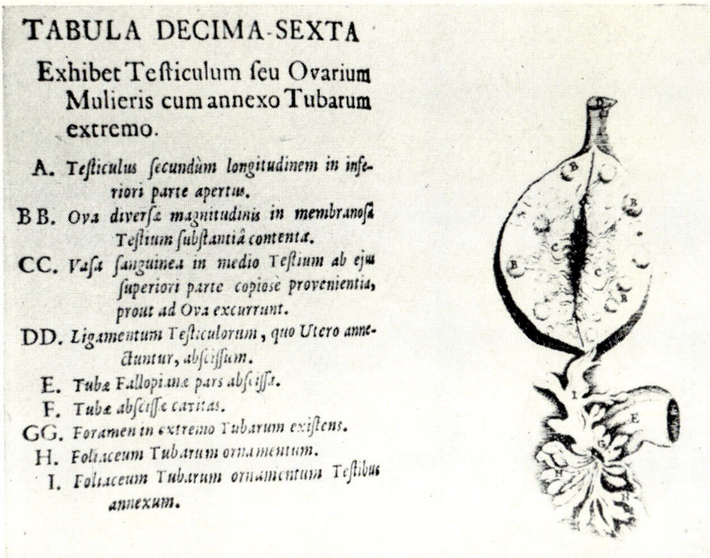

TABULA DECIMA-SEXTA

Exhibet Teſticulum ſeu Ovarium Mulieris cum annexo Tubarum extremo.

A. *Teſticulus ſecundùm longitudinem in inferiori parte apertus.*

BB. *Ova diverſæ magnitudinis in membranoſâ Teſtium ſubſtantiâ contentæ.*

CC. *Vaſa ſanguinea in medio Teſtium ab ejus ſuperiori parte copioſè provenientia, prout ad Ova excurrunt.*

DD. *Ligamentum Teſticulorum, quo Utero annectuntur, abſciſſum.*

E. *Tubæ Fallopianæ pars abſciſſa.*

F. *Tubæ abſciſſæ cavitas.*

GG. *Foramen in extremo Tubarum exiſtens.*

H. *Foliaceum Tubarum ornamentum.*

I. *Foliaceum Tubarum ornamentum Teſtibus annexum.*

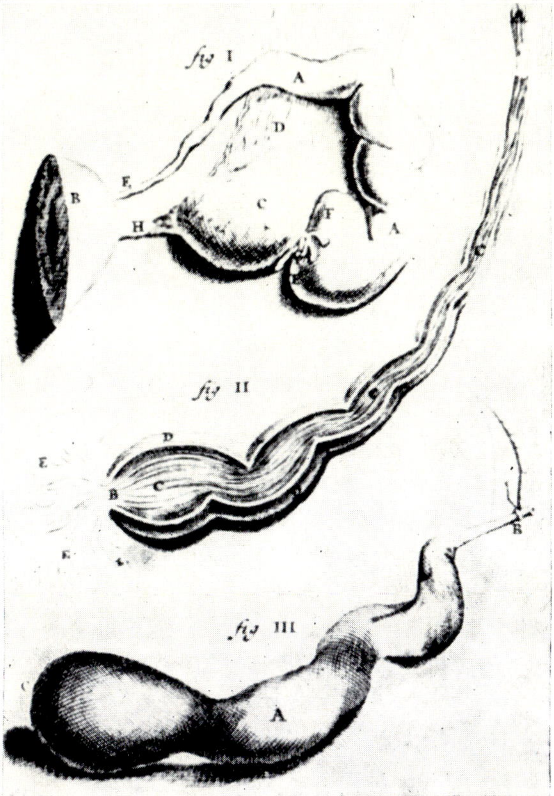

Fig. 71. Exhibit Testiculum feu Ovarium Mulieris cum annexo Tubarum extremo, by Regner de Graaf. (*Obstetrics and Gynecology*, *1*:No. 5, p. 584, May 1956. New York, Hoeber.)

Fig. 72. First illustration of a closed Fallopian tube (from *De Mulierum Organis*). (*Obstetrics and Gynecology*, *1*:No. 5, p. 587, May 1956. New York, Hoeber.)

the greatest of these early post-Vesalian anatomists. He was the first to call the ovary by that name; before this time it was designated as the "female testicle." He was also the first to name and describe the round ligament accurately, and to attempt to differentiate a true corpus luteum from a simple small ovarian cyst. The most important contributions to the study of the ovary, appeared in 1672 by de Graaf, a pupil of Johann van Horne.

REGNER DE GRAFF (1641-1673) of Schoonover, Holland, studied at Delft and later in France. He opposed the Aristotelian doctrine of the egg being formed in the uterus as a result of activation of the menstrual blood by the male semen, but held that generation takes place from the ovum pre-existent in the ovary. He believed that each ovum was surrounded by a glandular substance and ripens as it moves toward the periphery of the ovary. He discovered the ovarian follicles as they exist within the ovary, and the outer coating of which, after rupture, forms the corpus luteum.[3] To these Haller gave the name "Graafian follicles." He described the corpus luteum minutely, which already had been discussed by Fallopius in 1561 and his pupil Coiter in 1566. He did work in digestive juices and the pancreas. He also made many ingenious inventions such as an enema for self-administration. Before this, quasi-physicians travelled to many places, and did nothing but give enemata. His great literary contribution was his *De Mulierum Organis Generationi Inservientibus* in 1672, which embodies the best contemporary knowledge of the genitalia of women. Among his many reports on various gynecological entities, he distinguished between gonorrhea and leucorrhea by the presence of purulent discharges in the para-urethral ducts. He claimed that these para-urethral ducts secreted a thin fluid which stimulated the parts and augmented sexual desire.[4]

NIKOLAAS TULPIUS (1593-1674) of Amsterdam, made the first accurate notations on hydatid mole and he also described cervical polyps. He is the central figure in Rembrandt's painting *The Lesson in Anatomy*. Mauriceau in 1664 gave a detailed account of the removal of a mole by intrauterine finger manipulation, and it was Mauriceau who believed that too frequent intercourse was the cause of mole formation. It remained for Marcello Malpighi and Antonio Vallisnieri to advance the view that hydatidiform mole developed from placental tissue.

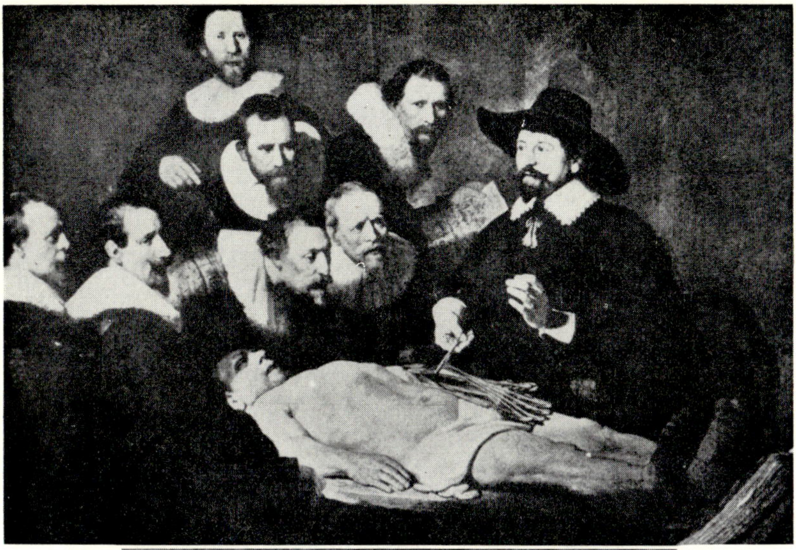

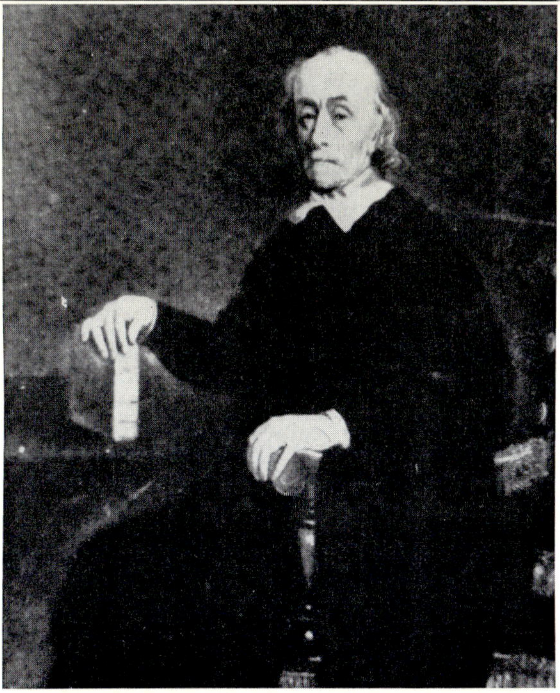

Fig. 73. Doctor Nikolaas Tulpius in *The Anatomy Lesson* by Rembrandt. (*MD Medical News* Magazine, Aug. 1958. New York, MD Publications, Inc.)

Fig. 74. William Harvey. (Herbert Spencer)

Adrian Spigelius (1578-1625) was the author of the first and finest anatomical atlas of the century. It contained a series of superb plates executed by his master Giulio Casserio. His descriptions began with the external genitalia; this was contrary to the accepted custom of beginning with a description of the uterus.

Caspar Bartholin (1655-1738) described the vaginal glands which now bear his name and which had previously been discovered by Duverney in the cow. The discovery of these glands was a partial solution to the problem of the origin of the feminine semen of which so many scientists had written since the time of Aristotle and which was believed to be a necessary concomitant to fecundation. He should not be confused with Thomas Bartholinus (1616-1680) who published an interesting dissertation on uncommon deliveries.

During the 17th Century approximately 150 authors published well over 200 different treatises on anatomy, mostly on female genitals. Most of these authors repeated the views of earlier or contemporary anatomists, but a few made original contributions.

William Harvey (1578-1657) was born at Folkestone. He graduated from Cambridge in 1597, then studied at Padua for the next five years under Fabricius of Aquapendente, the anatomist and successor of Fallopius and Vesalius. During the same years, he came under the influence of the great mathematician Galileo, who gave Harvey his first lessons in exact observations. Galileo, who studied medicine, was observed counting his pulse as he watched the swinging lamps in Pisa, an observation that led to the pendulum law and the invention of the astronomical clock. From Aquapendente, Harvey received his first lessons in embryology, a subject that played such a big part in his life afterwards.

While Harvey studied in Padua, Bacon, his friend and later his patient, published in 1605 his *Advancement of Learning*, which stressed particularly the inductive method on which all modern scientific work is based. Harvey was as greatly influenced by this work as by Bacon himself; so like Bacon, he appealed for the accumulation and systematic analysis of facts obtained by observation and experiment, and not to rely upon other men's experience but on their own.

In 1600, while in his third year of study at Padua, he returned to Cambridge to receive his degree in medicine. In 1607 he was admitted to the College of Physicians of London and to the staff of St. Bartholomew Hospital. He became physician extraordinary to the King, Charles I, had a large private practice and, withall, found time to conduct experiments on animal generation. He was not wealthy as were his seven brothers; his wealth was in his destined greatness. Although his King, Charles I, was in sympathy with Harvey's work and experimentation, his colleagues were envious and not so charitable. It got around that he was a crackbrain and that all physicians were against him. As a result his practice declined, and his income suffered. However, it does not seem that he suffered too great a pecuniary loss, for he later gave to the College of Physicians a building equipped with a library and a collection of instruments.[5]

His great publication *De Motu Cordis* in 1628, a 72-page book, is a landmark in medical history, and will ever be associated with the name of Harvey. It is considered to have revolutionized medicine. We, in gynecology and obstetrics, are probably more concerned with his other great contribution *De Generatione Animalium* in 1651 with the famous chapter "De Partu." The great merit of Harvey's work lies in the careful and methodical observation and record of the embryo and of the fetus at all stages. Prior to this time, we find the records barren concerning embryology. The primitive races had no conception of animal creation. The ancient civilizations of Egypt, Babylon, Assyria, India and China produced nothing in their writings to indicate that they had given the subject any serious thought. They were more concerned with the religious aspects of the embryo; the point at issue was when the soul entered the body of the embryo. The philosophers of the ancients gave no consideration to the soul, but the Christian Church was vitally concerned with this problem and vigorously denounced the practice of destroying the life of the unborn child. Pythagoras gave us the first written record relative to conception; he said, in the 6th Century, that from the brain and nerves of the male a moist vapour descends in the act of coition and from this vapour the embryo is born. He taught that the soul resided in the brain and in the nerves and imagined that all the "grosser parts" were made from the blood and humors of the womb. Hippocrates wrote on the development of the fetus, and not too many years later Aristotle laid the foundation for the science of embryology. Aristotle dissected animals, both warm- and cold-blooded, and studied the human embryo, which he thought was the product of male semen mixed with menstrual blood.

Harvey spent many years in the study of the development of the chick in the egg and making many dissections of the human embryo. While he was Warden of Merton College at Oxford, he spent much of his time there with the Reverend George Bathurst, in whose rooms a hen was kept to hatch successive batches of eggs. Each day an egg was opened so that they could watch the development of the chick embryo. His observations of the minute changes in the developing embryo were made through a simple lens for Leeuwenhoek had not yet invented the microscope. From these studies Harvey eventually evolved his book on generation. His chapter "De Partu," on labor, approaches the subject from a scientific and practical point of view. There is detailed criticism of earlier opinions on the anatomy and physiology of the fetus and of parturition, based on Harvey's own observations. Briefly, he recommended patience, watchfulness, and gentleness in all things. In the ordinary case nature was to be imitated and encouraged, but never subjected to unnecessary interference. The difficult case was subjected to podalic version.

Harvey's work produced many new approaches to the studies of generation, but unfortunately he never reached a conclusion as far as conception was concerned. He admitted he was at a loss to explain this phenomena; it remained for the discovery of the microscope to show us the sperm and the ovum. His method of attack is well illustrated in his description of the varying sizes of the uterus. He does not refer to misty authority; instead the record is one of personal observation: "as I have found" or "as I have seen" recur repeatedly.

> Various, then, is the constitution of the uterus, and not only in its diseased but also in its natural state, that is, at the period of fecundity and barrenness. In young girls, as I said, and in women past childbearing, it is without blood and about the size of a bean. In the marriageable virgin it has the magnitude and form of a pear. In women who have borne children, and are still fruitful,

> it equals in bulk a small gourd or a goose's egg; at the same time, together with the breasts, it swells and softens, becomes more fleshy, and its heat is increased.
>
> Wherefore women are most prone to conceive either just before or just subsequent to the menstrual flux, for at these periods there is a greater degree of heat and moisture, two conditions necessary to generation. In the same manner, when other animals are in heat the genital organs are moist and turgid. Such is the state of the uterus as I have found it before birth.
>
> In pregnant women, as I have before stated, the uterus increases in proportion to the fetus and attains a great size. Immediately after birth I have seen it as large as a man's head, more than a thumb's breadth in thickness, and loaded with vessels of blood. It is, indeed, most wonderful, and, as Fabricius says, quite beyond human reason how such a mass can diminish to so vast an extent in the space of fifteen or twenty days. . . .[6]

It is remarkable that so much of Harvey's work was confirmed rather than upset by the new precision which the microscope gave to experimental work. He was correct when he maintained, as pure theory, the doctrine of epigenesis, that is, that the organism does not exist preformed or encased in the ovum but is evolved from it by a gradual building up and aggregation of its different parts and layers. But he was quite wrong about fecundation. He believed the fertilization of the ovum to be "incorporeal, as iron touched by the magnet is endowed with its own powers." Twenty years after his death, Antonj van Leeuwenhoek of Delft through one of the microscopes he had devised saw the highly corporeal spermatozoa, which Hamen, one of his students, had first pointed out to him in 1674. So because Harvey was mightily handicapped by the lack of the proper tool, the microscope, it fell to the lot of Malpighi, Spallanzani, de Graaf, von Baer, and Wolff to formulate definitive principles in this matter of conception and generation.

Harvey's work on the circulation covered a period of many years of research, study and experimentation. Yet his work on the heart and circulation began on a more sure footing than his work on generation, for the way had been prepared by many investigators and it was left to him to bring to conclusion the work that had been in the making since the days of Hippocrates. And yet, even under these circumstances, the lack of the microscope did have its retarding effect on Harvey's work on the circulation, even if not seriously so. It was Huxley who pointed out that Harvey's demonstration of the circulation was a chain of observations lacking only one link. Because he did not have a microscope, he could not see the capillary anastomosis between the arteries and veins. This fact was later confirmed by the microscope, though Harvey did not live to know this. Harvey presented his views on circulation many years before his publication; he deplored the foolish rush into print until he had confirmed his facts in every possible way. In one of his lectures he said:

> On account of the structure of the heart, the blood is constantly passed through the lungs into the aorta, as by two clacks of a water bellows to raise water. Moreover, on account of the action of a bandage on the vessels of the arm, there is a transit of blood from the arteries to the veins. It is thus demonstrated that a perpetual motion of the blood in a circle is brought about by the beat of the heart.[7]

Though much of Harvey's teaching was to be superseded with the coming of the microscope, particularly his embryology, much remains valid to this day as do his observations of the lungs in the newborn. He noted that a child, immediately after being born, stretched its lungs in taking the first breath of life. This changed the color of the lung tissue so that it became possible to say with certainty whether a child was born dead or alive (the lungs are whiter when filled with air). These findings were confirmed in 1667 by Jan Swammerdam of Amsterdam, who added that once the child has breathed the fetal lungs will float. If the child had not breathed the lungs sink. This is an important criterion in determining whether a child is stillborn or not.

Harvey did not enjoy the esteem of his colleagues or the distinction of being the greatest anatomist and physician of the age. It was Aveling who designated Harvey as the "Father of British Midwifery," because it was Harvey who published in 1651, the first original English book on obstetrics. It was the publication of his book that started the Renaissance of Midwifery in England; Germany, France and Italy having embarked on their Renaissance at an earlier date. Prior to Harvey's obstetric work, England had used the translation of an original publication from Germany that became known, in England, as *The Byrth of Mankynd.* Also, they had been using a number of translations of the works of Ambroise Paré of France. Harvey's book *De Generatione Animalium*, with its chapter "De Partu," was a brilliant replacement of the German and French books. He was considered the founder of modern physiology because of his discovery of the circulation and his work on generation. Yet, we might be misled if we fail to understand that much that he taught and did was not too far removed from the metaphysical speculations of the 16th Century in spite of his great bulk of work that was based on the newer concepts of mathematics, astronomy, physics, and chemistry, and his new approach of explaining all physiological conduct as a response to physical laws. For instance when Harvey tried to explain the cause of birth he could not do so. He held to the theory that labor comes when the waters fail to provide sufficient nourishment for the baby. He used this simile:

> Oranges in this country usually remain on the trees two years before they arrive at maturity; and figs, which in Italy ripen two or three times annually, scarcely come to perfection in our climate; the same thing happens to the fruit of the womb; it depends on the abundance or deficiency of nutriment, on the strength or weakness of body, and on the right or wrong ordering of life . . . whether the child arrives sooner or later at maturity.[8]

He clung to the age-old belief that the baby makes its own way through the narrow passage to the outer world. He contended that the head of the baby "attacked the portals of the womb, opened them by its own energies and thus struggled into day"; he cited birds which break through their shells on their own volition, and all kinds of flies and buterflies that pierce the delicate membranes in which they are encased. He also likened the opening of the womb to permit the escape of the baby to ripened fruit that softens when coming to maturity, to the little point of a sprouting almond germ breaking the shell that could scarcely be crushed by a hammer, and the tender fibers of an ivy root penetrating the narrow chinks of the stone and causing rents in mighty walls. He believed that moisture and heat are necessary to generation, and therefore the most favorable time for conception is just before or immediately after menstruation.

During the 17th Century, it was customary to treat prolapse of the uterus by conservative means, and only in extreme cases, such as carcinoma complicating the prolapse, was surgery advisable. The quacks on the other hand always resorted to surgery for the cure of this condition and in most instances with fatal results. It seems that the guillotine method of amputation was in vogue, and numerous instances are recorded where part of the sigmoid or large arteries were included in the amputation; death was usually rapid. Harvey was an exponent of the conservative school which treated prolapse with pessaries, replacement and other such means unless carcinoma was present, when surgery was occasionally suggested. A very interesting case of "prolapse," that turned out to be a pregnancy with a dead fetus in a prolapsed uterus, is found in Harvey's *Anatomical Exercitations Concerning the Generation of Living Creatures* in 1653. A quotation from it follows:

> And now at this time, it (the prolapsed uterus) was as large as a Bulls cod dangling between her leggs. . . . It grew at last bigger than a man's head, being then a hard tumour, and hanging downe to her knees did much pain her so that she could not goe, (but upon all foure). . . . I did suspect it to be a Cancer of the wombe, and therefore did bethink my selfe of a Ligature, and cutting it off. . . . But the following night an Infant perfectly shaped, of a span long, was cast out of that Tumour, but it was dead.[9]

Harvey died in his eightieth year and maintained his mental vigor to the end. He was buried in Hempsted, Essex.

Marcello Malpighi (1628-1694) whose name stands highest in the field of microscopy in the 17th Century was the father of tissue studies of descriptive embryology. His discovery of the capillaries and their circulation in the lung completed Harvey's discovery of the circulation of the blood. He was professor of medicine at Messina and Bologna. In 1681, at the age of fifty-three, he published *De Utero Epistola* in which he described the mucous glands in the uterus of the calf, the muscular fibers of the uterine wall, and corpora lutea of the ovary. Before this, in 1668, he contributed his masterly treatise on the incubation of the egg. When Antonio

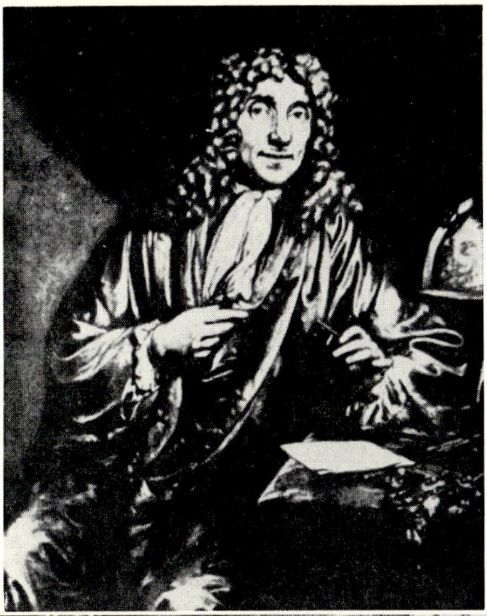

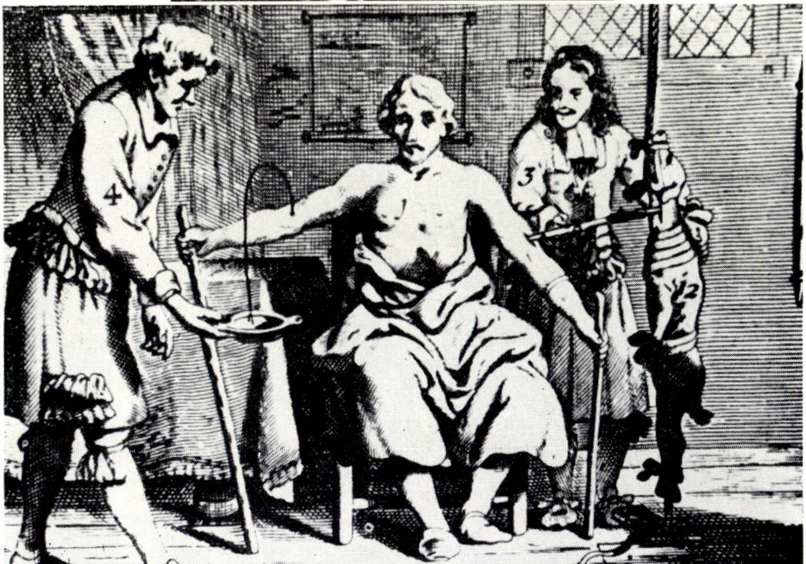

Fig. 75. Anton Van Leeuwenhoek. (Findley, Palmer: *Priests of Lucina*. Boston, Little, 1939.)

Fig. 76. Transfusion from lamb to man. (The Bettmann Archive.)

Vallisnieri advanced the view that hydatidiform mole developed from placental tissue in 1690, Malpighi had already spoken of chorionic degeneration. He described the structure now known as Gartner's duct as seen in the cow. Gartner, in 1822, redescribed it in the sow.

ANTONJ VAN LEEUWENHOEK of Delft (1632-1723) is considered the inventor of the microscope. He demonstrated capillary anastomosis and the corpuscles, and gave the first description of the spermatozoa which, however, had been pointed out to him by Hamen in 1674.[10]

JOHANN SCULTETUS of Ulm (1594-1645) was graduated from Padua. His name is associated with the many tailed bandage. He wrote about the vaginal speculum, a bivalve and a quadrivalve speculum resembling those of the late 19th Century. He was thirty years old when he devised a crude but effective method for amputation of the breast. Thin rope-like cords inserted with a thick needle held the breast up and away from the thoracic wall. A single sweep of the large amputation knife completed the operation.

FABRICIUS HILDANUS (1560-1634) was known as the father of German surgery, but made a few gynecological contributions. He began to do breast amputations after the method of Scultetus. Later he followed the method of Vesalius making a wide excision for cancer of the breast, and still later removed the axillary nodes in such cases, which is recorded as the first such attempt. He described three cases of imperforate hymen. He recognized that bleeding long after the cessation of menses probably meant cancer. He had a clear conception of a blighted ovum, stating that the size of the fetus did not correspond to the length of the period of amenorrhea. He spoke of pregnancy in a prolapsed uterus, and a prolapse occurring in virgins. One such case was only 16 years of age. In agreement with most of the surgeons of the 17th Century, he advised against operation in prolapse, especially if fibroids or polyps are present in the fundus, unless absolutely necessary; he noted that these cases do not prove serious if left alone even over a long period of time. He cured a case of vesico-vaginal fistula by using frequent vaginal injections of barley water and a decoction of fenugreek mixed with the mucilage of quince seeds, administered for eight months.

HENDRIK VAN ROONHUYSE was born in 1622. He lived and practiced general surgery in Amsterdam; he was a contemporary of Rembrandt. He was particularly interested in the diseases of women and made a remarkable contribution to 17th Century gynecology when in 1663 he published his *Heelkonstige Aanmerkkingen Betreffende de Grebrecken der Vrouwen.* This book has often been referred to as the first textbook on operative gynecology. His two major contributions to female surgery were the revival of the cesarean operation and the cure of vesico-vaginal fistula. His book contains detailed accounts of the cesarean operation and its technique; it cites a case history of a delivery per rectum in which the baby survived and the mother lived and was cured of the extensive rent to her perineum. He discusses the etiology and treatment of prolapse. An accepted procedure for the treatment of prolapse was the use of cork with a hole in it for discharges plus wax pessaries or the cork dipped in wax. He describes a case which he delivered that had been so treated. Quote:

> The like example I have met with in a woman living upon the "Herengracht," whose womb, as she thought, had also been replacing by such wax balles; but this prov'd also unhappy. For I was at last sent for, to deliver her of her misery, which I also did, though with no small trouble. For this piece as big as a man's fist, and having obstructed her lochia, caused great pain, a fever, stench and putrefaction; though by God's blessing, she was delivered of this child of wax. . . .[11]

He wrote on atresia of the vagina, congenital and acquired (from gangrene), and on stenosis of the cervix which he treated by dilating and keeping it dilated by the use of intracervical pessaries. He also discussed deformities of the urinary tract, and imperforate hymen. His operation for vesico-vaginal fistula is extremely interesting, not for his technic alone but because of some of the basic principles involved, such as the use of sharp instruments for cutting so as not to devitalize the tissues that they may heal better. He evidently was aware that a dull instrument compresses and contuses tissue thus making it more susceptible to infection. He advocated exposure of the fistula with a retracting speculum, the patient being placed in the lithotomy position, marginal denudation of the tract is performed, exclusion of the bladder wall is sought when making approximation of the denuded edges of the fistula by means of quills fastened with silk threads. He is aware of the importance of the fitness of the patient to undergo such an operation; in other words her general health must be good, and her lochia must have ceased (this assumes the etiology is childbirth). He talks of bladder irrigations to promote healing, and there is some suggestion of a procedure like the use of our indwelling catheter.

It was van Roonhuyse to whom the elder Hugh Chamberlen is said to have sold the secret of the obstetric forceps about 1693. He was supposed to have discovered the Vectis.

Richard Lower (1631-1691) was the first person to show interest in the subject of transfusions. He was an Oxfordian. He used sheep's blood for transfusion, eight to sixteen ounces at a time, and with success usually. The first transfusion was attempted in 1665, but was not described by him until 1669. Jean Denis of Paris also performed transfusions in the same manner as Lower, but because of the numerous fatal outcomes, the Paris medical faculty forbade transfusions. As a result, nothing further was done in the way of transfusions. until the 19th century, when it was revived but only as a life-saving measure.[12]

It seems that everybody is a father or founder in medicine's various branches. In keeping with this tradition of medical history, we now come to the founders of modern obstetrics and gynecology—Francois Mauriceau and Van Deventer.

Francois Mauriceau (1637-1709) of Paris was the most able accoucheur of his time. His clinical ability was the result of an intimate knowledge of anatomy and physiology, however it would seem that in some respects his information of these subjects was not always accurate. He was at loggerheads with de Graaf concerning the ovum and its fertilization, and he thought ligaments were ejaculatory ducts. He thought that conception could occur at any time of the month and therefore unrelated to the menstrual period. He believed that the uterus distended like a full bladder and that its walls did not thicken. He denied the possibility of fertilization of the ovum in the Fallopian tube, and yet he was the first to report a tubal pregnancy.

Mauriceau gave detailed descriptions of the mechanism of labor and was the first to describe brow presentation. He described the

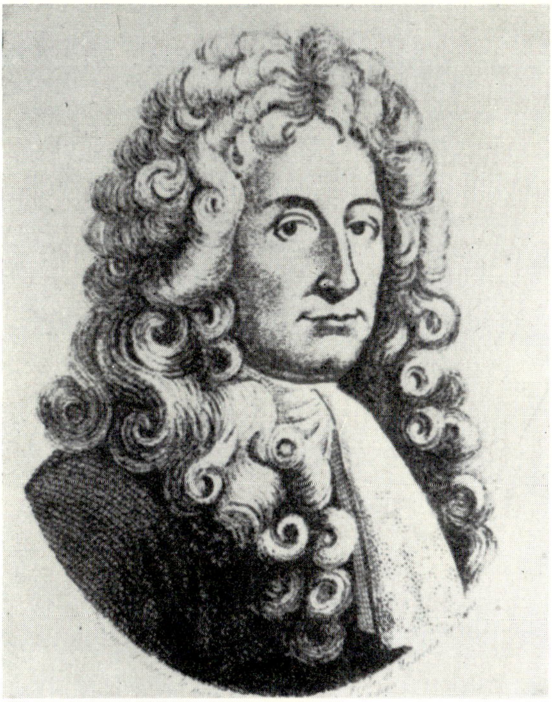

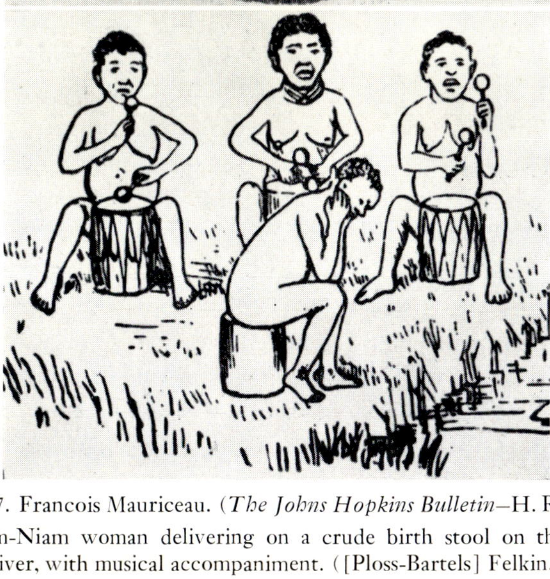

Fig. 77. Francois Mauriceau. (*The Johns Hopkins Bulletin*—H. Robb.)

Fig. 78. Niam-Niam woman delivering on a crude birth stool on the bank of a river, with musical accompaniment. ([Ploss-Bartels] Felkin.)

management of the after-coming head and considered the lochia as a wound secretion. He was the first to rupture the membranes to induce labor and control hemorrhage in placenta previa. He was one of the first to describe in detail an epidemic of puerperal fever, seeing many cases in the wards of the Hotel Dieu in Paris. He ascribed it to humors which flowed into the womb and decayed there. He was acquainted with toxemia and hyperemesis, stating that convulsions occurred more often in first births; his treatment was bloodletting. He wrote on fertility and sterility, abortions, leucorrhea and menstrual irregularities. He did not agree with Hippocrates that the male child is developed earlier than the female since they both come to term at the same time. He wrote that there are too many poor women who have been caused to miscarry by medicines and bleeding because they were not aware of their pregnancy. He charged doctors and midwives with being guilty of murders, either through ignorance or rashness, for besides the death of the innocent baby, they often put the mother into great danger.

Mauriceau was far from a doctor of science; indeed, he was not immune to the vagaries of his time. He held that the baby at birth had its face turned toward the earth because it felt itself guilty of the sin of Adam; that its first cry was "O-A" meaning "Oh Adam, why had you sinned?" The cry of the mother in her final pains he interpreted as "O-E" meaning "Oh Eve, why did you lead our first father into sin?" Referring to twins of opposite sex and occupying separate chambers in the uterus, he likened them to boys and girls in a church where the boys sit on one side and girls on the other side of the church. This segregation of the sex in the uterus, he said, is for the purpose of breathing into men, from the first moment of their formation, the laws of chastity.

In difficult labors when it seemed impossible to deliver a living baby, he resorted to the crotchet, saying that he at least could preserve the life of the mother. He did not countenance the cruel and barbarous cesarean section, in which " 'tis absolutely impossible (though many imposters whom Rousset favors, assure the contrary) that a woman should ever escape." When one or both hands protruded, he replaced them and turned the baby and preferred to deliver it by its feet rather than as a vertex.

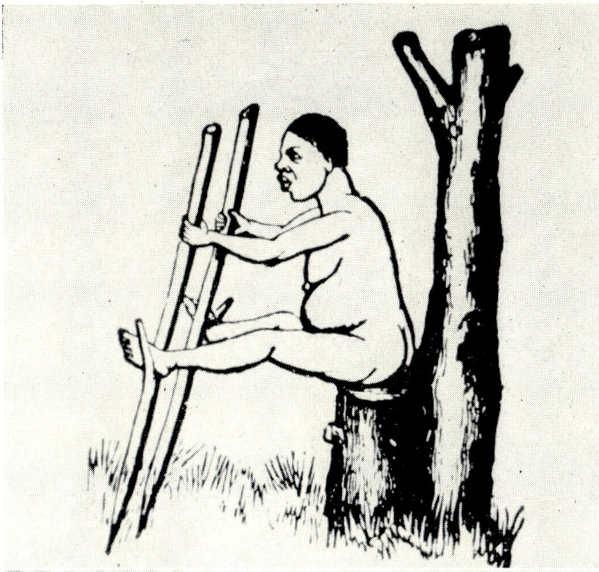

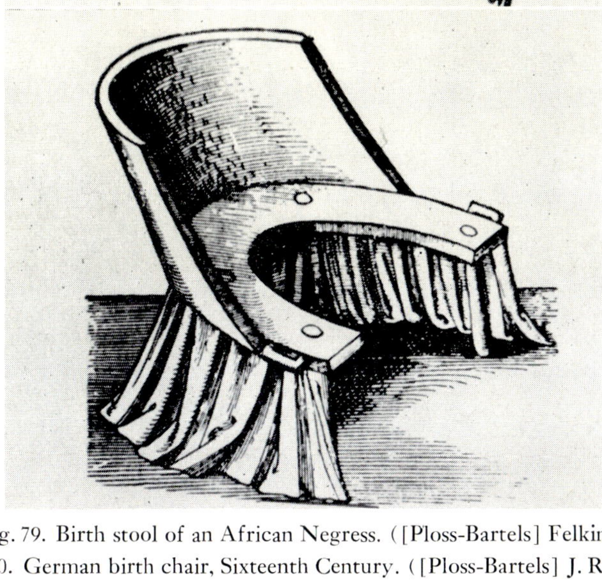

Fig. 79. Birth stool of an African Negress. ([Ploss-Bartels] Felkin.)
Fig. 80. German birth chair, Sixteenth Century. ([Ploss-Bartels] J. Reuff.)

"Whensoever the infant comes wrong, in what posture soever, from the shoulders to the feet, it is the best way, and soonest done, to draw it forth by the feet; searching for them, if they do not present themselves, rather than to try to put it in a natural posture, and place the head foremost. For the great endeavors

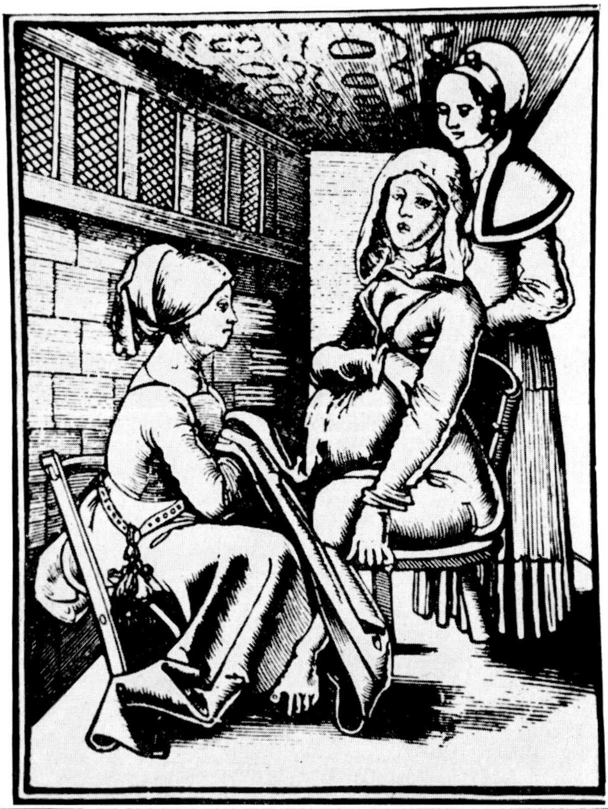

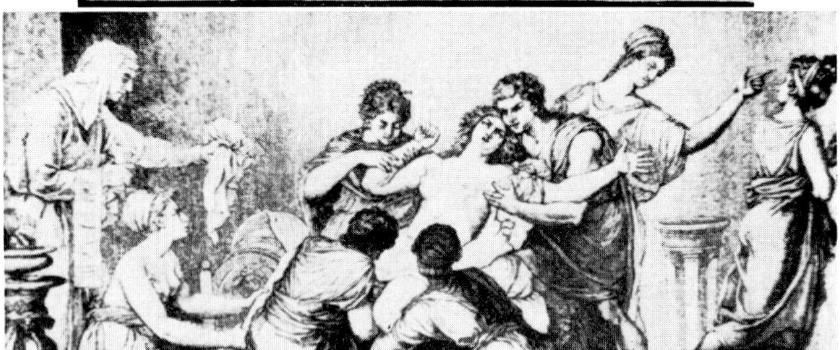

Fig. 81. Delivery of a German woman in a birth chair, 1513. ([Ploss-Bartels] Neufeld & Henius.)

Fig. 82. Childbirth in a Roman house. Soranus, circa A.D. 100, recommended obstetric chair with two women standing in back, one kneeling in front. (The Bettmann Archive.)

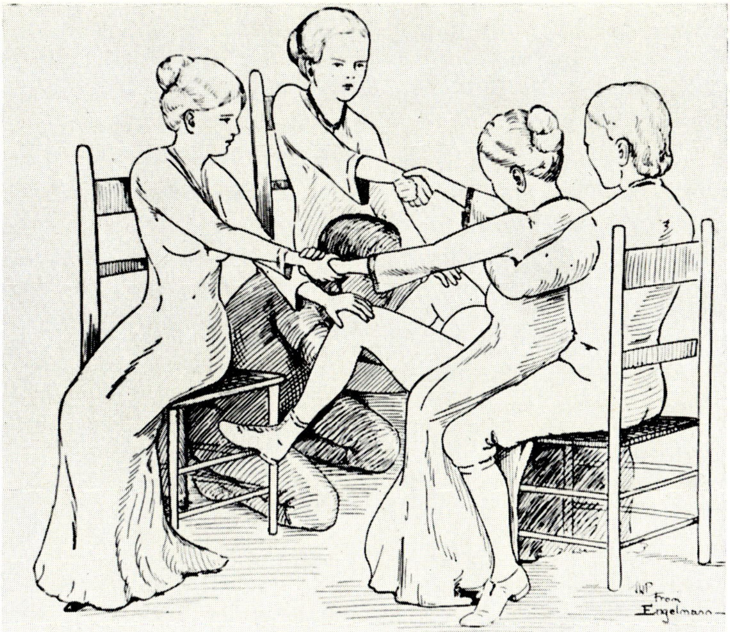

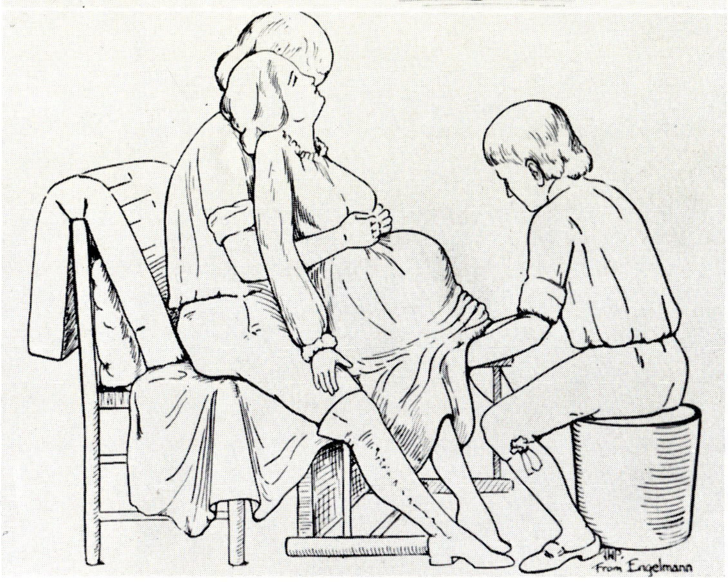

Fig. 83. Delivery scene in Virginia in early Nineteenth Century. (Englemann)
Fig. 84. Delivery scene in Ohio in early Nineteenth Century. (Englemann)

> often necessary to be used in turning the infant in the womb (which is a little harder than to turn a pancake in a frying pan), does so weaken both mother and child, that there remains not afterwards strength enough to commit the operation to the work of nature, and usually the woman hath no more throws nor pains fit for labor after she has been so wrought upon . . . the infant would certainly perish in the passage, without being able to be born.[13]

Mauriceau was the first to substitute the bed for the birth stool and we know that toward the end of the 19th Century the delivery table followed the use of the bed. The birth stool was used for centuries: crude birth stools were used by primitive people and right along the various periods of history a similar contraption has been in use, e.g., the Germans in the 16th Century used a birth stool; the Romans in A.D. 100 (recommended by Soranus) used the birth stool not unlike the stool seen in a delivery of the 16th Century by the Germans. However, primitive methods used by aborigines, e.g., strapping a woman to a table and shaking it to hasten delivery, instead of using the birth stool, was still often used in this period. The early Pennsylvania settlers, in the 18th Century used a modified birth stool or chair. In fact many peoples used similar methods of delivery until Mauriceau delivered patients in bed. Yet, in the United States, in rural areas, the same method of delivery continued, e.g. in Virginia and Ohio, the chair and the usual assortment of assistants officiated.

It is interesting that the position assumed by the patient, accoucheur and assistants has remained similar from ancient times, e.g., the centuries old "Ancient Peruvian Urn" (illustrated) shows the same disposition of patient, accoucheur and assistants as noted in deliveries centuries later, up to the 19th Century in fact, when Mauriceau instituted the bed for the birth stool.

Mauriceau belonged to the school of Paré in obstetrics and to the time when the science of obstetrics was in the making. He was on the threshold of a new era in midwifery. The Chamberlens had not yet revealed the secret of the forceps, antisepsis and anesthesia had not yet arrived, so Mauriceau and his contemporaries could not help but carry on a practice by which they were responsible for the mutilation of countless living babies.

His outstanding literary contributions were *Traite des Maladies des Femmes Grosses, etc.*, published in Paris in 1668. He also wrote *Observations sur la Grossesse et L'accouchement des Femmes et surs maladies et celle(s) des enfens nouveaunes, etc.* in 1709; this was later, in 1752, translated into English by Hugh Chamberlen.[14]

Two contemporaries of Mauriceau but of lesser stature were PAUL PORTAL (1630-1703) was born in Montpellier, and studied at the Hotel Dieu (as did Mauriceau). He was a great obstetrician and urged that the dilatation of the cervix be left to nature, a fact that J. A. Dührssen and many of his followers have long since disregarded.[15]

PHILIPPE PEU (1623-1707) also a pupil of Mauriceau and practiced in the Hotel Dieu was known mostly for his meritorious work on the management of the third stage of labor. He tried to change a practice that had been in vogue for ages. He countenanced against undue haste in delivery of the placenta. While Mauriceau would leave placental remains to decay and pass with the lochia, Peu contended that retained particles of placenta would interfere with the flow of the lochia and advised their removal without delay.

HENDRIK VAN DEVENTER (1651-1724) was the co-founder of modern obstetrics and possibly of gynecology. He was born in the Hague. He studied medicine at Groningen, practiced midwifery chiefly, but was acutely interested in orthopedics and problems that were vexing the practitioners of his day. His bent towards orthopedics was the basis for his contributions in pelvic anatomy; he was the first to make a study of the bony pelvis and its deformities. Until the time of Deventer, the anatomists, except for Arantius, confined themselved mainly to the soft parts of the pelvis. The importance of the bony pelvis as a factor in delay and difficulty in labor was almost universally neglected, so much so that when Deventer focused his attention in this direction he did so almost apologetically. He described the pelvis with inlet contraction, and pelvis with general contraction. He noted elongation of the fetal head in cases of general contraction, and in these cases as well as those with a flat pelvis, he considered the possibility of brain injury to the baby, aside from a delay in its passage. He was aware of the importance of the axis of the birth canal and described it accurately. He dismissed pubic separation as rare and as unimportant, and yet he

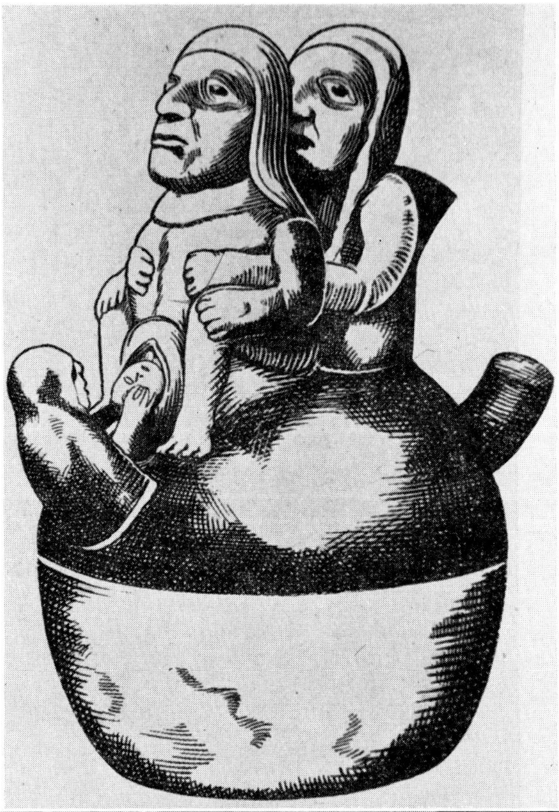

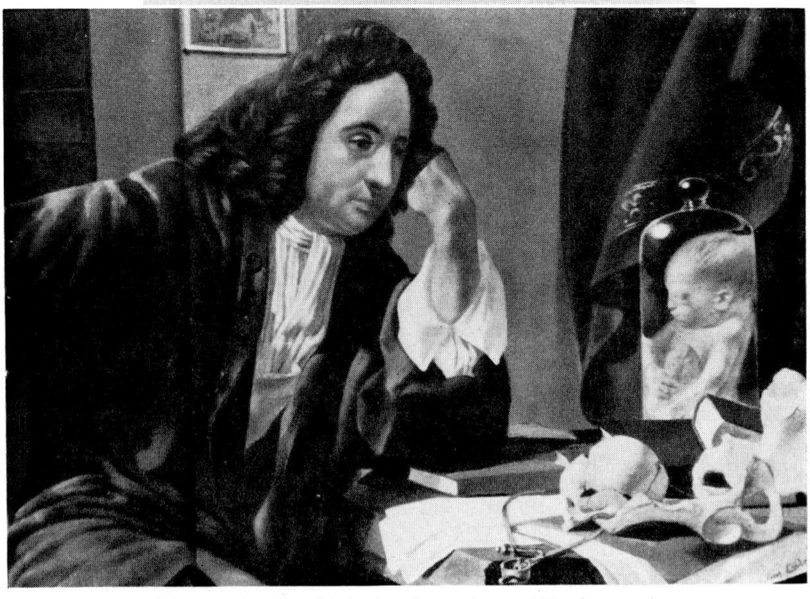

Fig. 85. Ancient Peruvian funeral urn. (Englemann)

Fig. 86. Hendrik Van Deventer. (*Lederle Bulletin 17*:No. 3 (cover), Aug. 1952. New York, Lederle Laboratories Division [American Cyanamid Co.].)

attached great importance to the movement of the sacrum and coccyx, which he believed both swung backwards to make room for the passage of the child's head. He was unwilling to undertake the hazardous procedure of cesarean operations on the living mother. He did the best he could with delivery by both hands for he also abhorred the use of hooks and such. He had only two indications for the use of instruments, one where:

> by Reason of the monstrous Bigness of the whole Body, or any Part, cannot pass through the Pelvis whole.

and the other where:

> by Reason of the Neglect or Ignorance of the Midwife, the Head of a well turned Infant, in a Womb oblique to the highest Degree, falls down in the narrow Cavity of the Pelvis, and is there so straightened along with the Shoulders, that the least Descent is not perceived upon the Force of the Strongest Pains, and all remedies have been tried in Vain; for the Safety of the Mother, the Infant is to be handled and drawn out, as a dead one.[16]

In face and in transverse presentations he preferred version to "the turning of the head into the Passage." He decried the stretching and tearing of the soft parts to hasten labor, a procedure common to the midwives; they should be taught the bony anatomy so that they might realize the retardation came from that source and not the soft parts, and would be better able, therefore, to direct the parts more properly in relation to the bony parts.

In the opening chapter of his *The Art of Midwifery Improved*, Van Deventer defined the qualifications required to make a woman fit for practice of midwifery. He excluded all malformed, diseased and consumptive persons and all fat and gross women:

> whose hands and arms are quite unfit to be made use of . . . the maimed with crooked fingers, hands and arms; those with a stupid and dull sense and incapable of perceiving things distinctly; the illiterate, slothful persons who are neither willing, nor know how to handle anything; those of wilfule disposition and obstinate as well as vagabonds, or tattlers and tiplers. The men midwives should possess the virtues of chastity, bashfulness and modesty, nor should they be rash swearers, drinkers or company keepers.[17]

This book (*Art of Midwifery Improved*) was published in 1728. He also published *Dageraat* in Leyden in 1696, *Novum Lumen* in

1701, and a thesis *Diseases of the Bones.* Van Deventer was the accepted authority for a century and a half until Michaelis wrote *Das Enge Becken* from the foundations laid down by Van Deventer.

Up to the 17th Century, the problem of difficult labor was solved by the use of small doses of ergot to increase the contractions, podalic version which was reintroduced by Paré, and cesarean section which was commenced by the sow gelder Nufer and later made safer by Mercurio. To these procedures was added the obstetric forceps, discovered in 1598 by Peter Chamberlen I, the Elder.[18]

Contributions in gynecology during the 17th Century can be enumerated by a terse account of the accomplishments of the following men:

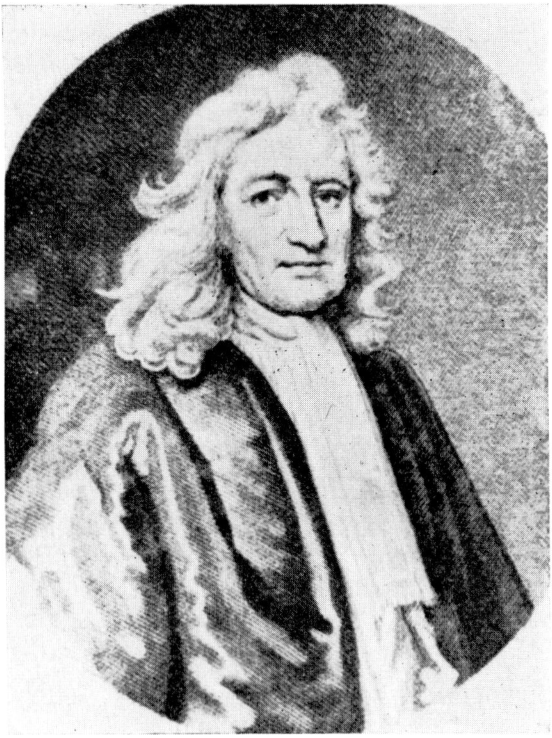

Fig. 87. Peter Chamberlen. (Findley, Palmer: *Priests of Lucina.* Boston, Little, 1939.)

Johannes P. Lotichius (1598-1652) of Frankfort, wrote a dissertation entitled *Gynaicologia.* This was the first time that the term "gynecology" made its appearance in medical literature. It was a hundred years later before this term was seen again; it was spelled "Gynaecologia" this time, 1730, and the author was Martin Schurig of Dresden.

J. B. de Lamzweerde in 1686 was the first to write on fibroids and on ovarian cysts. His text was a remarkable contribution of a mixture of judicious observations and wildest speculations; this may be noted in his adherence to the ancient idea that fibroid growths were the result of degeneration of the semen. He wrote "neither virgins nor married women could generate uterine tumor masses merely by entertaining sexual thoughts. The development of fibroids in widows was not possible without the 'auxilium' of a new husband."

Justice Theodorus Schorkopff in 1685 wrote the earliest work, a thesis for his degree at the University of Bale, devoted entirely to ovarian cysts. He is the first to use the term annexa (adnexa), the first to mention ovarian abscess, and the first to suggest extirpation as a cure for ovarian cysts.

Jean Riolan (1580-1657) of Paris reported the first authentic case of ectopic pregnancy with rupture. This occurred in the fourth month of the patient's eighth pregnancy in 1604 and another case in 1638. Both patients died the next day after the onset of symptoms and they were both found to have ruptured ectopic (tubal) pregnancies at post-mortem examination.

de Saint Maurice of Perigod in 1682 observed a case of ovarian pregnancy, the first such case ever to be reported. This report is in the *Philosophical Transactions* and was abstracted by Smellie in his *Theory and Practice of Midwifery*, Vol. II (p. 51, ed. 1877). This patient had safely delivered eight children; five years later she became pregnant again. She went along thinking she was normally pregnant when she became seized with severe pain, bleeding and fainting. She called in her physician and died upon his arrival. Clinically she had all the symptoms of a ruptured ectopic pregnancy. After her death, her abdomen was opened, with these findings:

> On opening the integuments of the belly, all the entrails of the epigastric region were seen floating in blood, which was taken out with a spoon to the quantity of two pounds. To avoid changing the situation of the parts, a large quantity, which was coagulated, still remained in the right flank; and trying to take this out with the hand, a little fetus was found in the first clots, about the bigness of a man's thumb, and a third less in length, all very distinctly formed, and in which was manifestly discovered the sex of a boy, but naked and without covering. The right cornu of the womb was found near this place; the testicle or ovary was torn long ways, and through the middle on the side, that it did not much touch the tube. This testicle was near the bigness of a hen's egg, and seemed to be the place where the fetus was contained and which had burst through the same, for the left testicle" was no bigger than a little chestnut; the tube was not dilated, neither was there any wrent of the uterus, which appeared to be in its natural state. . . .[19]

Laurentius Strauss (1603-1687) and H. Eyssonius of Groningen (1620-1690) both published cases of long standing lithopedia, the latter reporting a case of twenty years standing in 1661.

During the 17th Century, certainly in its early part, the old concept of hysteria, also known as hysterical or uterine suffocation, remained unchanged since the time of Hippocrates, 2,000 years before. This condition was supposed to be due to a diseased condition of the uterus. The ancients believed that hysterical attacks resulted from a wandering uterus, which lodged temporarily in the upper abdomen. Rhazes, the Arabian clinician, and Mondinus de Luzzi, in 1316, stated that such a phenomenon was impossible, that the uterus was a fixed organ. The idea was finally completely discarded when in 1618, Charles Le Pois, physician to King Henry II, published his treatise showing that hysteria occurred in both men and women. (de Luzzi signifies Mondinus' coat of arms)

During the 17th Century procedentia was discussed very often, as it had been in the past. In this century some attempts at surgery were made, but even so, the consensus of opinion was that it was not a surgical condition. Much of the medical literature of this period contained gynecological material in conjunction with other specialized phases of medicine. In proportion to the large number of books on anatomy, on generation, on the ovary and on medicine in general, the texts devoted solely to gynecology were strangely few. And the bulk of these merely reflected the views prevalent in the preceding century. Although great strides and advances were made during the preceding century and shortly before, gynecology and obstetrics were still extremely crude when compared to present day standards. To illustrate this, a few quotations from LAZARUS RIVERIUS (1589-1655) are interesting and revealing. They are taken from an English translation of his *Practice of Physick*.

> From p. 403 "Of the stoppage of the Terms": The Terms are said to be stopped, when in a Woman ripe of Age which gives not suck, and is not with Child. . . . Divers Diseases of the Womb may cause this Disease; namely, a cold Distemper and dry, which thickeneth and bindeth the Body of the Womb; or a hot and dry distemper by drying the part, or burning up the nourishment thereof, from whence come evil humors, which being fastened in the part, hinder the Terms from flowing. . . . The Vessels of the Womb do often suffer Obstruction, which is the chief cause of stopping of the Terms, and they come from and thick humors. . . . The blood offending either in quantity, quality or motion, may be a cause of the obstruction of the Courses. . . . The blood offends in motion, when it passeth otherways, as by the Nose, vomiting, spittle, Urine, Hemorrhoids, and many other parts. I saw a Maid who had a sore in her Head, which opened every month, and bled plentifully, and we have many that have sent forth blood at fixed times by their Lungs; and this evacuation was instead of a Menstrual flux. . . . The External Causes are cold and dry Air, Northern Winds, often going into cold water especially in the time of their flux, etc., etc.
>
> From p. 413 "Of the Whites": a Woman is said to have the Whites, the Woman's Flux, the Flux of the Womb, or the white menstruals, when Excrementitious Humors do flow from the Womb, either continually, or at least without any certain order or course of time observed in their flowing.[20]

In the same chapter is this interesting paragraph:

> In the Gonorrhea, the matter which comes away is not so much in quantity, is thicker, of a more shining whiteness, holds up longer from flowing, and seldom or never stinks. But if it be a virulent or venemous Gonorrhea (such as accompanies the Letch-

ers pox) it is known by sharpness of Urine, Ulcers of the privy parts, and other signs that argue Malignity.

As a result of Harvey's work on the circulation and physiology of fetal respiration, the invention of the microscope by Leeuwenhoek, the histology and embryology of Malpighi, and the work of de Graaf, all of whom gave us new data on gross and minute anatomy and physiology, we come to a period in the 17th Century when glandular therapy begins to emerge as an entity. Organotherapy was a very ancient form of therapy. The Egyptians were known to eat the penis of the ass for impotence. The Greeks and Romans prescribed the testicles of the ass for this purpose. Galen, Dioscorides and Pliny referred to hepatic juices for the treatment of maladies referrable to the liver. Lusitanus recommended the testicles of a rooster as a means of regaining lost sexual vigor in 1551. The blood of animals in "heat" (deer) was thought to increase sex desire. In 1663, Sylvius de la Boe (1614-1672) vaguely began to mention internal secretions of the organs. Thomas Willis (1621-1675) suggested that puberty occurred as a result of ferments generated in the gonads and passed into the blood stream; M.F.X. Bichat (1771-1802) was the first to lend experimental proof to Willis' theory. Many of their concepts were incorrect as far as ova and ovulation went, such as the speculations of Theodorus Kerckringius (1640-1693) of Amsterdam, who said he had found ova, at autopsy, the size of large peas, and therefore urged married women to look for ova in the menstrual blood, for he believed they were expelled with it, and in the coitional issue.

By the close of the 17th Century the subject of generation was being discussed vociferously. But these discussions were no longer being guided by metaphysical speculation as in the past, but by a basically sound scientific approach from which also arose the creation of physiology and pathology, and these in turn formed the basis of a newer and sounder practice of obstetrics and gynecology. This clinical improvement owes its emergence to two men of the 17th Century, primarily, William Harvey and Peter Chamberlen and his forceps.

First Occurrences and Outstanding Events

Seventeenth century was called the "age of physiology" because of the discovery of the circulation by Harvey in 1616.

Robert Hooke was the first to depict the biological cell.

Mauriceau introduced the terms fourchette and fossa naviculaire.

Johann Van Horne was first to call the ovary by that name, and first to accurately describe the round ligament, and first to differentiate between a true corpus luteum and a simple ovarian cyst.

Regner de Graaf discovered the ovarian follicle, and was among the first to differentiate leucorrhea from gonorrhea.

Nikolaas Tulpius gave the first accurate notation of mole and cervical polyps.

Caspar Bartholin discovered the gland bearing his name.

Pythagoras gave us the first written record relative to conception.

Aristotle laid down the foundations for the science of embryology.

First microscopic vision of a spermatozoa by Hamen, 1674.

Harvey was called "the Father of British Midwifery" by Aveling, besides being considered the founder of modern physiology.

Malpighi was the father of tissue studies on descriptive embryology. He discovered the capillary circulation (of the lungs).

Leeuwenhoek discovered the microscope.

Scultetus discovered the many-tailed bandage.

Fabricius Hildanus was the father of German surgery.

Henrik van Roonhuyse wrote the first text book on operative gynecology.

Henrik van Roonhuyse has often been credited with being the inventor of the "lever."

Richard Lower did the first blood transfusion in 1665.

Mauriceau was the founder of modern obstetrics and gynecology, among the first to report tubal pregnancy, the first to describe brow presentation, the first to rupture membranes to induce labor to control hemorrhage in placenta previa, one of the first to describe puerperal fever (epidemic), the first to substitute the bed for the birth stool.

Deventer was the co-founder with Mauriceau of modern obstetrics and gynecology. He was the first to make a study of the bony pelvis and its deformities.

Peter Chamberlen I the Elder discovered the forceps, circa 1598.

J. P. Lotichius was the first to use the term gynecology in literature.

J. B. de Lamzweerde was the first to write on fibroids and ovarian cysts.

Schorkopff in 1685 was the first to use the term annexa (adnexa); ovarian abscess; and first to suggest extirpation as a cure for ovarian cysts.

Riolan in 1604 was the first to report a ruptured ectopic pregnancy. de Saint Maurice was first to report a case of ovarian pregnancy. Strauss and Eyssonius were the first to report lithopedia, 1661.

References

1. Capitaine, A.: *Un Grande Medecin du XVI Siecle.* Jean Fernel, These, Paris, 1925.
2. Speert, Harold: Thomas Wharton and the Jelly of the Umbilical Cord. *Obst. & Gynec., 8*:No. 3, Sept. 1956.
3. Leonardo, R. A.: *History of Gynecology.* New York, Froben, 1944, p. 207.
4. Speert, Harold: Regner de Graaf and the Graafian Follicles, *Obst. & Gynec.*, 7:No. 5, May 1956.
5. Aveling, J. H.: Biographical Sketch of Harvey. *Obst. J. Brit. Emp., 1*:23-31, 1873 (London).
6. Graham, Harvey: *Eternal Eve.* London, Heinemann, 1950, p. 244.
7. *Ibid.*, p. 249.
8. Findley, Palmer: *Priests of Lucina.* Boston, Little, 1939, p. 121.
9. Ricci, J. V.: *Genealogy of Gynecology.* Philadelphia and Toronto, Blakiston, 1950, p. 303.
10. Leonardo, R. A.: *History of Gynecology.* New York, Froben, 1944, p. 202.
11. Ricci, J. V.: *Genealogy of Gynecology.* Philadelphia and Toronto, Blakiston, 1950, p. 313.
12. Bettmann, O. L.: *A Pictorial History of Medicine.* Springfield, Thomas, 1956.
13. Findley, Palmer: *Priests of Lucina.* Boston, Little, 1939, p. 134.
14. Robb, H.: The Writings of Mauriceau. *Bull. Johns Hopkins Hosp., 6*:51-7, 1895.
15. Gaul, P.: L'ostetricia di Paul Portal. *Rev. distoria sc. med. e nat., 16*: 1925 (Siena).
16. Findley, Palmer: *Priests of Lucina.* Boston, Little, 1939, p. 142.
17. *Ibid.*, p. 139.
18. Aveling, J. H.: *The Chamberlens and the Midwifery Forceps.* London, Churchill, 1882.
19. Ricci, J. V.: *Genealogy of Gynecology.* Philadelphia and Toronto, Blakiston, 1950, p. 302.
20. *Ibid.*, p. 289.

Chapter XII

HISTORY OF THE FORCEPS

In ancient literature there are numerous allusions to instruments used in delivering dead babies. Records go back as far as 400 B.C., during the time of Hippocrates. Mention of the hook, compressor and machaire is made by Soranus and Celsus, in A.D. 50, and Aetius in the 6th Century A.D. Paulus, in the 7th Century, used two hooks to grasp the baby's head; these hooks were the nearest thing to the Palfyn and Chamberlen forceps, even though they were used for extracting dead babies only. Then came a period when forceps with teeth were used; it began with Avicenna, in the 10th Century, Albucasis, in the 12th Century, and from descriptions and woodcuts by Paré, and Rösslin, in the 16th Century. Extractions of the living child, up to this time, were done by version or unaided hands. In the 16th Century, Jacob Rueff, stated that he could deliver a living baby with forceps if the teeth were omitted. He left no evidence that he succeeded in this.

In Hodge's book of 1864,[1] there is a very clear picture of forceps and other instruments employed "for the preservation of the child." They are described under four heads; these varied considerably in their forms, and the demand for their use depended usually upon different circumstances. They are the "fillet or bandage"; the "blunt hook," the "vectis or lever," and the "forceps."

"Fillet is a bandage, which may be cast around the limbs, or the head of the child, and is doubtless not only the most simple, but the most ancient instrument employed in obstetrics. Formerly [this is now 1864] when the science of midwifery had not been cultivat-

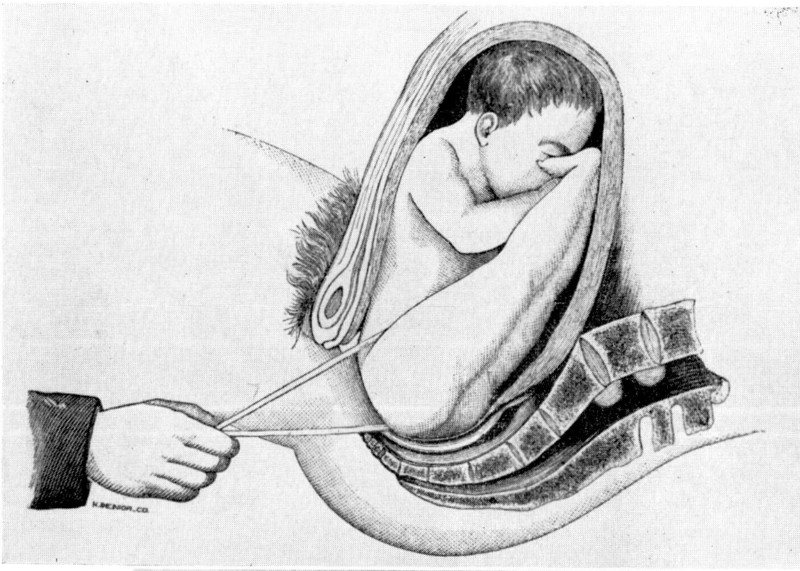

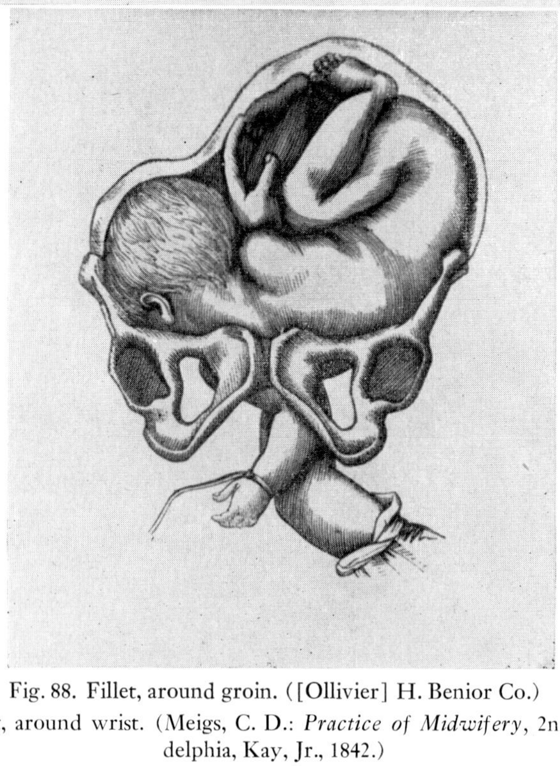

Fig. 88. Fillet, around groin. ([Ollivier] H. Benior Co.)
Fig. 89. Fillet, around wrist. (Meigs, C. D.: *Practice of Midwifery*, 2nd Ed. Philadelphia, Kay, Jr., 1842.)

ed, this mode of operation was often injudiciously and injuriously resorted to. Of late it has been almost entirely restricted to breech presentations; but, doubtless, it might be extended very advantageously to some other cases. . . . A strong band or fillet may be in-

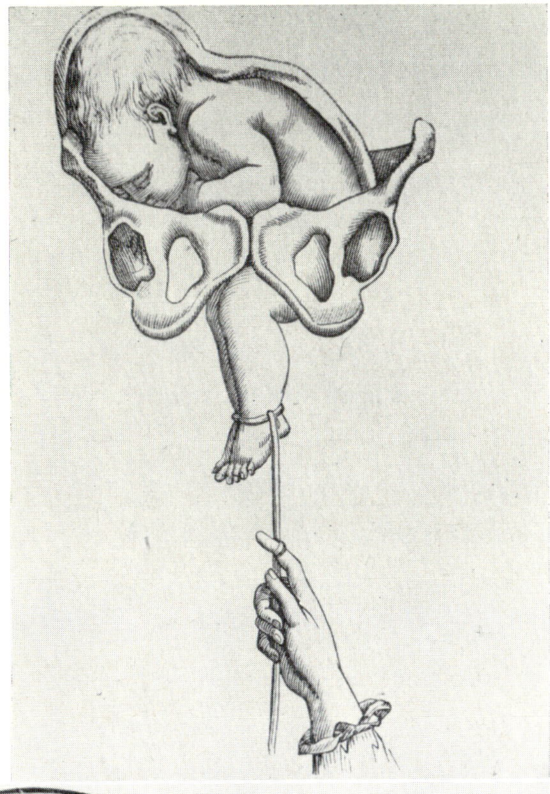

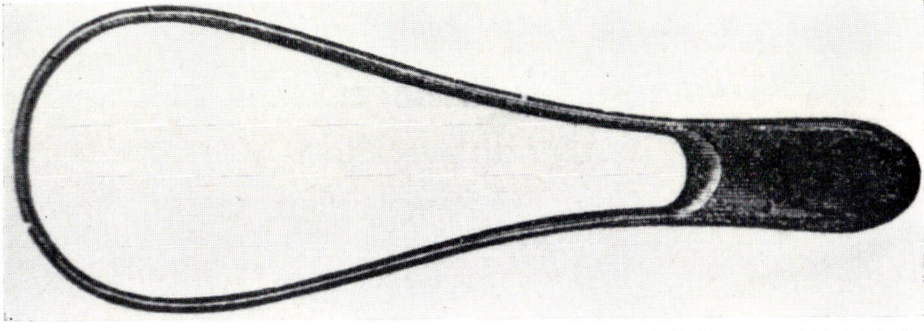

Fig. 90. Fillet, around ankle. (Meigs, C. D.: *Practice of Midwifery*, 2nd Ed. Philadelphia, Kay, Jr., 1842.)

Fig. 91. Whalebone fillet. (Hodge, H. L.: *Principles and Practice of Obstetrics*. Philadelphia, Lea, 1864.)

troduced between the thigh and body of the child over the groin, so that, by this means, traction effort can be made to cause the descent of the fetus until its breech be expelled at the vulva, and the limbs unfolded; after this, of course, the fillet is useless, and delivery must be perfected by manual means.

"The character of the fillet is of importance. It should be strong, and at the same time, a very soft, pliant material, so as not to injure the skin by its roughness or stiffness, or lacerate the tissues, when traction is made. Muslin, linen, or soft leather is often employed. A fillet of thin whalebone has also been recommended, especially in cephalic presentations. The mode of application of the fillet is often a difficult operation, so that another mode of application of the fillet, perhaps more easily executed, is by means of a curved spring canula, this canula contains a stilette which is pushed out after proper placing of the instrument. A thread is attached to the stilette, which is grasped and to which a fillet is then attached. As the stilette is pulled into the canula the fillet takes the place of the thread around the thigh. The instrument is then removed and the fillet is in place. The modus operandi of the fillet is simple traction. In modern practice the fillet is occasionally employed in cases of prolapsed arm or leg, not for the purpose of traction, but merely to prevent the retraction of the protruded extremity too far within the maternal organs.

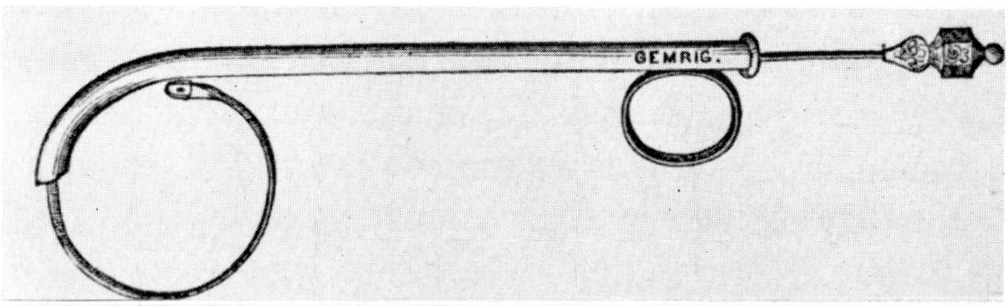

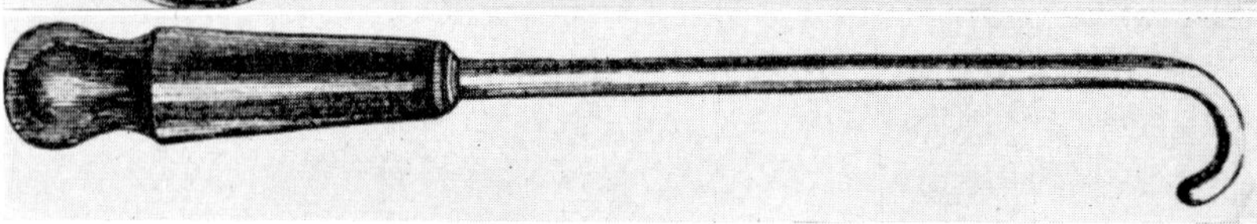

Fig. 92. Spring canula, type of fillet. (Hodge, H. L.: *Principles and Practice of Obstetrics*. Philadelphia, Lea, 1864.)

Fig. 93. Blunt hook. (Hodge, H. L.: *Principles and Practice of Obstetrics*. Philadelphia, Lea, 1864.)

"Although the use of the fillet is thus greatly restricted at the present time, there are cases of cephalic presentations in which a bandage may be safely and advantageously employed to facilitate delivery, when properly applied by one well acquainted with the mechanism of labor, and who has clear ideas of the indications to be fulfilled. This instrument, however, must in such instances, be regarded as a mere substitute for the lever or forceps, when such agents should, unfortunately, be not at command."

"Blunt Hook. This, like the fillet, was much employed in ancient times in conjunction with sharp hooks or crotchets; constituted the chief agents of the practitioner. Its use, however, is now greatly restricted, . . . it is limited almost exclusively to breech presentations, under the circumstances to which the fillet is applicable. Indeed, it depends upon the convenience or judgment of the operator, whether the blunt hook or the fillet should be resorted to; the former, perhaps, has the advantage of being more easily applied, but it is not, by any means, more efficient, and is more liable, from its hard, unyielding character, to injure the tissues of the groin, than a fillet, especially when this last is 'stuffed' with soft materials." Hodge's text goes on with a description of the actual application of the hook; he precedes this description with the following admonition, "the usual preparations for delivery being arranged, and the friends of the patient being advertised of the necessity of the operation, etc., etc." He concludes the section on the blunt hook by saying that the blunt hook, therefore, should be generally restricted to embryotomic operations."

"Vectis, Tractor, or Lever. This is a long, narrow steel instrument, having usually a wooden handle at one extremity, and at the other it is enlarged to a triangular shape, and curved, so as to be adapted to the convexities of the cranium; the curve is termed, therefore, cephalic . . . It is thin, so as not to occupy more space than is requisite; . . . it is also fenestrated, not only for lightness, but that it may slip less readily over the scalp. The degree of curvature varies. . . . the greater the curve the more difficult may be the introduction, but the greater will be its efficiency. The instrument which the author has been in the habit of using is somewhat of the form of the letter S, about nine and a half inches in length, and a blade with a cephalic curve at either extremity, one

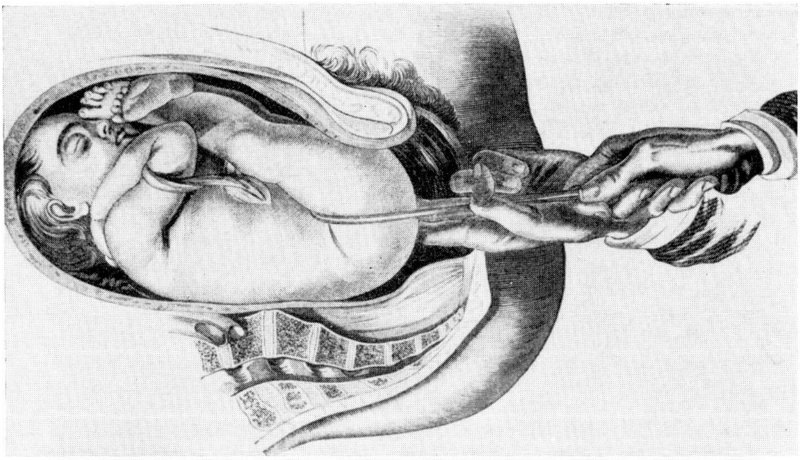

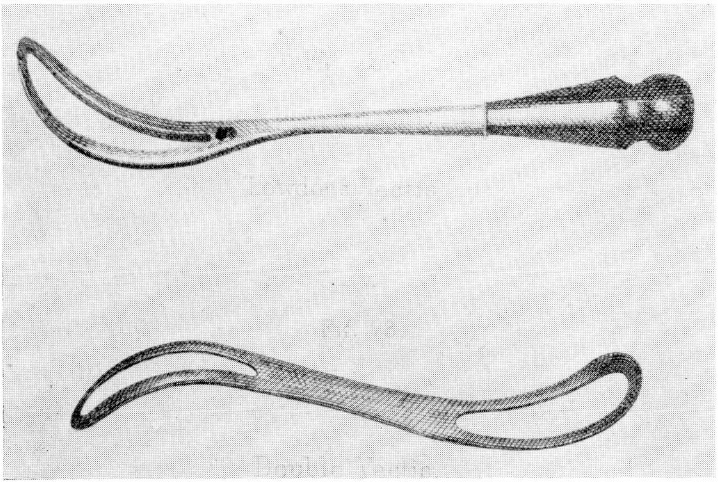

Fig. 94. Blunt hook in breech presentation. (Hodge, H. L.: *Principles and Practice of Obstetrics*. Philadelphia, Lea, 1864.)

Fig. 95. Single and double vectis. (Hodge, H. L.: *Principles and Practice of Obstetrics*. Philadelphia, Lea, 1864.)

end larger and adapted to the form of the head, the other smaller for the extraction of globular pessaries or other foreign bodies from the vagina.

"The question as to who was the original inventor of the vectis has excited great discussion, and the whole original history of this instrument is still veiled in obscurity. It is most probable that the Chamberlens of England, to whom the credit is now universally

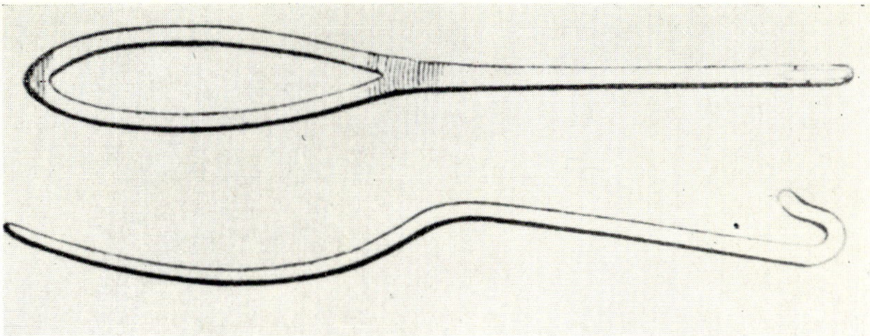

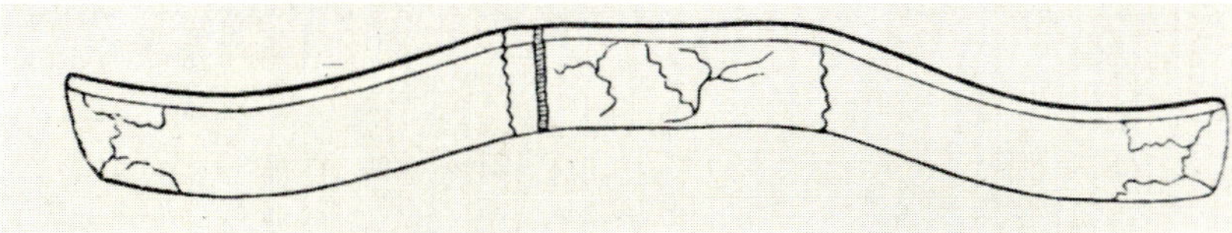

Fig. 96. Chamberlen's lever, front and side views. (Hodge, H. L.: *Principles and Practice of Obstetrics.* Philadelphia, Lea, 1864.)

Fig. 97. van Roonhuyse's lever. (Hodge, H. L.: *Principles and Practice of Obstetrics.* Philadelphia, Lea, 1864.)

given of devising the modern obstetric forceps, were also the inventors of the lever. This has been rendered the more probable of late by the discovery in 1813 of a box of obstetric instruments, concealed in a vault in a house in Essex, England, originally the property of Peter Chamberlen, in which was a small lever, in addition to several modifications of the forceps. This lever has a curve and a fenestra, similar to those of the modern vectis, with a comparatively short handle. Moreover, it is asserted that Hugh Chamberlen fled to Holland in 1687, and became intimate with van Roonhuyse and other distinguished obstetricians at Amsterdam, to whom, it is reported, he confided his secret. Years, however, elapsed, during which the knowledge of this instrument was confined to a few practitioners in Holland; and when the secret was published, in 1753, the whole credit of its invention was given to van Roonhuyse. His lever . . . was a thin piece of iron, curved at either extremity, and without the fenestra; certainly therefore, different in many respects, from the vectis of Chamberlen, although possessing the curve, which constituted the essential part of the instrument.

"The reputation of the vectis has fluctuated greatly. Its early advocates in Holland and England were numerous, and insisted that it was far superior even to the forceps. It is still recommended by Bodaext, of Belgium, as very efficient even in cases of deformed pelvis, where the forceps has failed. In France and Germany it has received less attention. . . . The vectis eventually has fallen into comparative disuse in Europe and America. . . . This neglect has, we think, been very unfortunate. It has arisen partly from ignorance of the mechanism of labor in the various presentations and positions of the child, and partly from the want of a due appreciation of the respective value of the vectis and forceps, and the peculiar circumstances under which the one may be preferable to the other. Although one may be frequently substituted for the other, they have each their respective spheres, and hence are applicable to different cases of labor, or even to different periods of the same labor; the lever altering the presentation or position of the head preparatory to the employment of the forceps. They should not, therefore, be considered as rivals, but as co-ordinate agents. Their relative advantages can be better understood after proper consideration of the application and *modus operandi* of each of these most valuable instruments.

"The modus operandi of this instrument, as its name indicates, is two-fold: First, as a Tractor or Vectis, by which portions of the head may be made to advance, by simply drawing the instrument more or less directly downward; and second, on the principle of a Lever, so that an additional force may thus be given to its tractile power. . . . Flexion and rotation, or even extension, may be advantageously facilitated by this tractile power of the instrument. Accoucheurs accustomed to the lever can safely and powerfully facilitate the flexion and descent of the head; and some have given it preference to the forceps, as but one blade is to be introduced, and there is no difficulty in its adaptation to the head of the child. Although the lever may be used in some cases as a substitute for the forceps, yet nearly all practitioners, at the present day, consider it far less efficient than the forceps, not only as being more liable to slip and thus injure the tissues of the mother or child, but as being much less powerful, as Dr. James, in his edition of Merriman, quaintly observes, he cannot conceive how one lever can act more powerfully than two. We shall hereafter demonstrate that the lever is a very important and invaluable instrument in cases of defective rotation, where it should often be employed as a substitute for the forceps.

"The disadvantages of the vectis are its instability, and the danger of bruising or otherwise injuring the tissues of the child and the parent. For these reasons, as well as for its comparative inefficiency as a tractor, it has fallen relatively into disuse; but, nevertheless, in special cases, it must be regarded as a most valuable agent in many complicated labors."

FORCEPS. The possibility of delivering the living baby by forceps was first suggested by Jacob Rueff, in 1554, when he first described his instrument. It had a poor cephalic curve and shanks that could not be disengaged; it would seem therefore impossible of application and devoid of necessary traction. He used a forceps

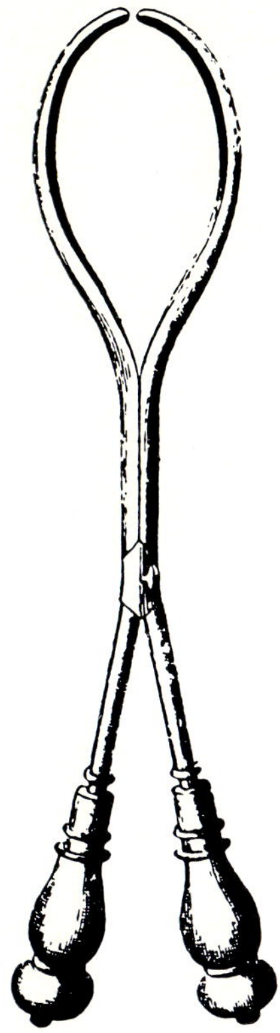

Fig. 98. Rueff's forceps. (Dill, L. V.: *The Obstetrical Forceps*. Springfield, Thomas, 1953.)

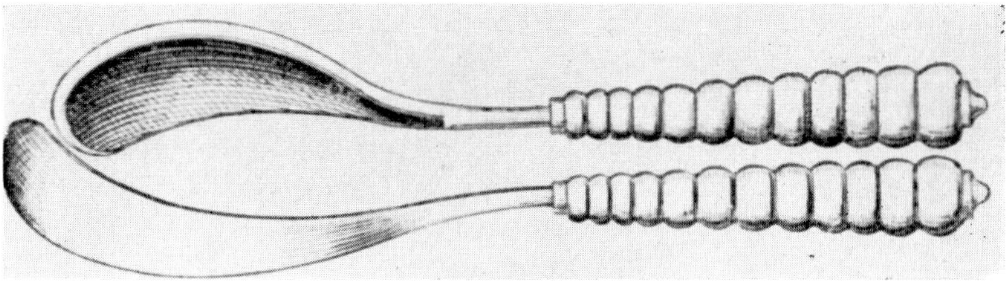

Fig. 99. Palfyn's forceps or "hands." (Hirst, B. C.: *Text Book of Obstetrics.* Philadelphia, Saunders, 1918.)

similarly constructed, with the addition of teeth on the blades, for delivery of the dead baby. For such a purpose his forceps with teeth would be feasible, but practically impossible for the extraction of a living child. Actually he was not known to ever use the forceps for the delivery of a living child.

It was approximately forty-four years later, shortly before 1598, that a practical midwifery forceps for the extraction of the living child was invented. This honor went to Peter Chamberlen, the Elder.

The literature is not in agreement with the fact that Peter Chamberlen, the Elder, invented the forceps, however the preponderance of evidence favors him. Igerslev[2] expressed the conviction that JEAN PALFYN (1650-1730) of Ghent was the first to exhibit "safe" forceps for the delivery of a living baby, but questioned his claim as the inventor. Known as the Palfyn forceps in France and the Douglas forceps in England, these forceps had been in secret use for a century. He believes that Palfyn must have seen the Chamberlen forceps. The story goes that Palfyn had a glimpse of one blade of the Chamberlen forceps that was owned by van Roonhuyse, having bought it from Hugh Chamberlen, Sr. Some say that Hugh fleeced van Roonhuyse by selling him only one blade, which amounted to a vectis, an instrument that van Roonhuyse had already invented; others say that van Roonhuyse fooled the public, and Palfyn, by showing only one of the blades of the forceps that he had bought from Hugh.[3]

Palfyn exhibited his forceps before the Academie Royale des Sciences in 1723 (or 1720 according to some sources). The next year, 1724, a description appeared in print, published by Heister of Helmstadt, but unfortunately this write-up was derogatory and showed not the least appreciation of the worth of these forceps. Six years later Palfyn died and was soon forgotten.

Confusion and secrecy pervades the history of the forceps. The Chamberlens were supposed to have a secret method of delivery of the complicated cases, and it was said that other physicians were let in on the secret at a price. At any rate, there are certain names that stand out during this era because of their interest in the forceps;

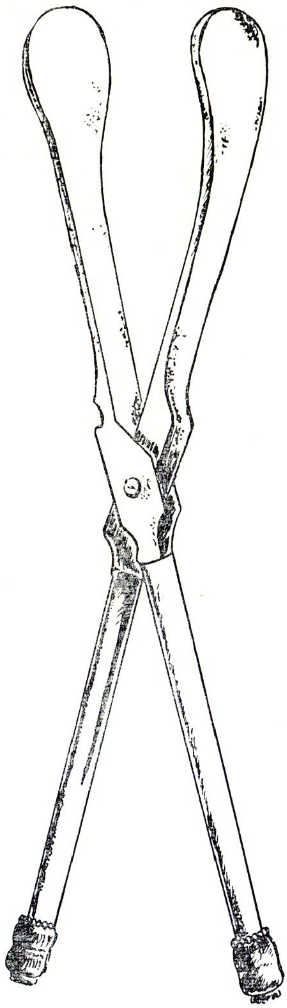

Fig. 100. Dusée's modification of the Palfyn forceps. (Dill, L. V.: *The Obstetrical Forceps.* Springfield, Thomas, 1953.)

many of them were reputed to have in use a forceps somewhat similar to the "secret forceps."

William Giffard (d. 1731), an English obstetrician best known for his forceps in an era when most physicians were kept in ignorance of this instrument. Like Palfyn he eventually published an account of his forceps in 1734, one year after Chapman did the same with his forceps.

Dusée (d. circa 1733) was using a forceps made of steel and solid curved blades about the time that Palfyn was laying claim to his forceps. Sometime later, in 1733, Dusée modified the Palfyn forceps by providing an articulation of the branches which prevented the longitudinal displacements of the blades, and by increasing the curvature of the branches, prevented compression of the fetal head. The characteristic features of the perfected Dusée forceps were the very broad blades, exaggerated cephalic curves and the double lock arrangement. He never published anything about this forceps. The Dusée instrument was unknown to anyone except Paul de Windt, Gregoire, J. Boswell and Alexander Butter, all of whom were shown the forceps by Dusée himself while visiting him socially.

Alexander Butter (fl. 1733) went to Paris to study, became acquainted with Dusée, saw his forceps, but never saw him use it for Dusée died shortly thereafter. Butter bought the forceps from Dusée's heirs and brought it to Edinburgh where he placed it on display. This was in 1733, the same year that Chapman described his forceps. He and Chapman were practically using the same instrument, for they both liked the same characteristics that were required in a forceps.

About the same time that Butter had placed his forceps, which he obtained from Dusée's heirs, on exhibition in Edinburgh, he wrote a letter for public consumption. This letter was the trigger that set off the exposé of the secret of the forceps. Among other things, it stated:

> that the forceps for taking hold of a Child's head, when it seems to make no Advances to the Birth by the Throws of the Mother, is scarce known in this country, though Mr. Chapman tells us, it was long made use of by Dr. Chamberlaine who kept the form of it a secret, as Mr. Chapman also does. I believe therefore that

> a sight of such an instrument which I had from Mr. Dusée who practices Midwifery in Paris, and who believes it to be his own Invention, would not be unacceptable to you, and the publication of a Picture of it may be of Use to some of your Readers . . . etc.[4]

EDMUND CHAPMAN (1680-1756) settled in London and became the second public teacher of midwifery. His fame rests on the publication of a book in which he illustrates and describes the forceps. Palfyn, Drinkwater, Butter, Dusée, Giffard and Chapman himself had been using the forceps, either the Chamberlen or one which was slightly modified, for quite a few years. In 1733, the same year that Butter displayed his (Dusée) forceps, he published the first edition of a book entitled *An Essay for the Improvement of Midwifery*[5] in which he gave a detailed description and praised its usefulness, and urged everyone to use them; this was five years after the death of Hugh Chamberlen, Jr. He states in the preface of his book that the use of the forceps had been going on for at least twenty-five years, but was rarely discussed openly. In 1735, one year after Giffard's publication of the forceps, Chapman published the second edition of his *Essay* in which he illustrated his forceps with unusually beautiful engravings, and stated that it was not very different from that of Giffard, and that both of them were better than Dusée's forceps, because it takes better hold of the child's head. In the beginning, Chapman used the forceps only occasionally, because it was made of soft metal and slipped from the baby's head too often, and also because he had modified the instrument with a replaceable screw to hold the blades together, and this got lost so often, that he was unable to use them when needed. Later, he found that he could work them to a greater advantage without the screw at all, and then began to apply them often.

So it is to Chapman that we are indebted for the publication of the "Chamberlen secret;" this was accomplished when he published his book which described in detail and illustrated beautifully the Chamberlen forceps.

PETER CHAMBERLEN I, the Elder (1560-1631), was born in Paris, and went to England in 1569. He is credited with the invention of the forceps sometime before 1598, and was one of a large family of physicians who shared the secret use of the forceps. He, the first born, and his brother PETER CHAMBERLEN II, the Younger (1575-1628)[6] or (1572-1628)[7], the fifth born, were the sons of WILLIAM CHAMBERLEN (circa 1540-1596—some say he died before 1596). Both were secretly practicing a method of delivery of difficult cases unknown to anyone else, a secret which they would not divulge; in fact, it was more than a hundred years before the secret became known. They were both members of the Barber Surgeons' Company. They were in frequent conflict with the College of Physicians for practicing medicine. They did not have the qualifications necessary to become members of the College; a Doctorate of either Oxford or Cambridge was necessary. Nevertheless, the Elder was physician to King James I and Anne, his Queen. When Peter II, the Younger, died, he left a son PETER CHAMBERLEN III (1601-1683) to whom he passed on the secret of the forceps; he had the qualifications for the College, and was so elected. Then Peter I died, and his nephew Peter III took over his royal appointment to Charles. Like the other two Chamberlens, Peter III also did not divulge the secrets of their deliveries when all others failed.

The Chamberlens went to great ends to preserve their secret. They arrived at the patient's house in a carriage of special design, with a huge wooden box with beautiful carvings. This box was carried into the room of the patient, all others were excluded, and the patient blindfolded. All sorts of ideas circulated, and it was generally thought that the box contained a huge complicated piece of machinery.

HUGH CHAMBERLEN, SR. (1630 fl. 1702) was the fourth member of this family to be associated with the forceps. He was the fourth son of Peter III. He was born in Holland. Hugh, Sr., is the Chamberlen who "in the early part of the year 1670 went to Paris in the hope of finding a purchaser for the family secret. Here he met Mauriceau, who to test the value of Chamberlen's pretenses, suggested that the latter should attempt the delivery of a woman with extreme contraction of the pelvis, upon whom he (Mauriceau) had previously decided to perform a cesarean section. Hugh declared that nothing could be easier, and at once, in a private room, set about the task. After three hours of vain effort he was obliged to acknowledge his defeat. The woman died. The negotiations for the sale were dropped, and Chamberlen returned, with his secret unrevealed, to England."

In 1672, Chamberlen published a translation of Mauriceau's work upon midwifery, and in the preface stated:

> My Father, Brothers, and myself (though none other else in Europe, as I know) have, by God's Blessing and our own Industry, attained to, and long practised a way to deliver Women in this Case without any Prejudice to them or their Infants; tho all others (being obliged, for want of such an expedient, to use the common way) do or must endanger, if not destroy, one or both with hooks.[8]

Hugh Chamberlen, having failed to sell "his forceps" in Paris in 1670, tried again in 1688, this time to van Roonhuyse in Amsterdam, for a large sum. A number of other Hollanders were admitted to the exclusive group that knew the secret, for which they were supposed to have paid a price. The graduates of the Medico-Pharmaceutical College at Amsterdam were not allowed to practice midwifery without first obtaining the secret, also for a price. In 1753, it was learned that the "secret" was simply one blade, a vectis that Roonhuyse himself invented.

Hugh Chamberlen, Sr., had two brothers, PAUL CHAMBERLEN, and JOHN CHAMBERLEN, who lived in Essex, England. Except for the fact that they practiced and shared the secret of the forceps, very little else is known about them.

HUGH CHAMBERLEN, JR. (1664-1728), the eldest son of Hugh, Sr., was the last of the Chamberlens. Except that he was modest and retiring, he followed the exact pattern of the other members of the family before him, having served as physician to the royal family, as did his father, uncles and grandfather. Like them, he, too, kept the secret of the forceps.

As already mentioned in this chapter (section on the lever), the whole matter of the secrecy of the forceps was set to rest in 1813, by the discovery of a chest containing a variety of patterns of the vectis and a number of pairs of forceps.

Dr. Aveling, a recognized authority, states that Peter Chamberlen I, the Elder, was the inventor of the obstetric forceps. Lusk, in his book of 1892, so quotes Aveling. Lusk obtained his information from an essay by Dr. J. H. Aveling,[9] in 1882, and from a treatise upon midwifery by Chapman,[10] in 1735.

Since Chapman's publication in 1733, and a second in 1735, with engravings, the modifications made of the forceps by obstetric practitioners have been exceedingly numerous. About the middle of the 18th century, Levret of France, and Smellie of England came up with the same idea, that the efficiency of the forceps depended on the addition of a pelvic curve, so that the forceps would be accommodated to the direction and form of the pelvis. To this end they devised instruments with a curve in the direction of the long axis; this made it possible to make an application to a head lying in the mid-plane of the pelvis. They worked independently, but published a description of their respective forceps in the same year, 1751. Since then, nearly every prominent obstetrician has developed a modification of the Levret and Smellie forceps.

Lusk,[11] in his book, further states that in selecting forceps, a distinction between the long and short forceps must be made. He discusses each type thusly: "Short forceps: The original instrument of the Chamberlens furnishes the type of the short variety. The Chamberlen forceps consisted of two levers, made to cross each other like a pair of scissors, with short fenestrated blades, diverging just

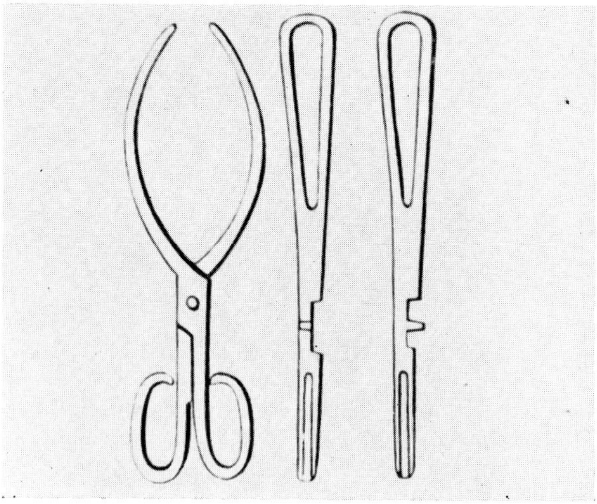

Fig. 101. Forceps of Chamberlen. (Lusk, W. T.: *The Science and Art of Midwifery*. New York, Appleton, 1892.)

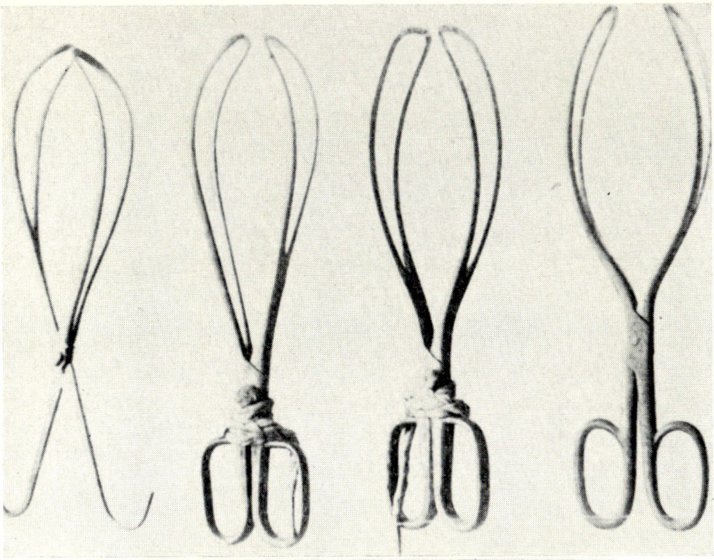

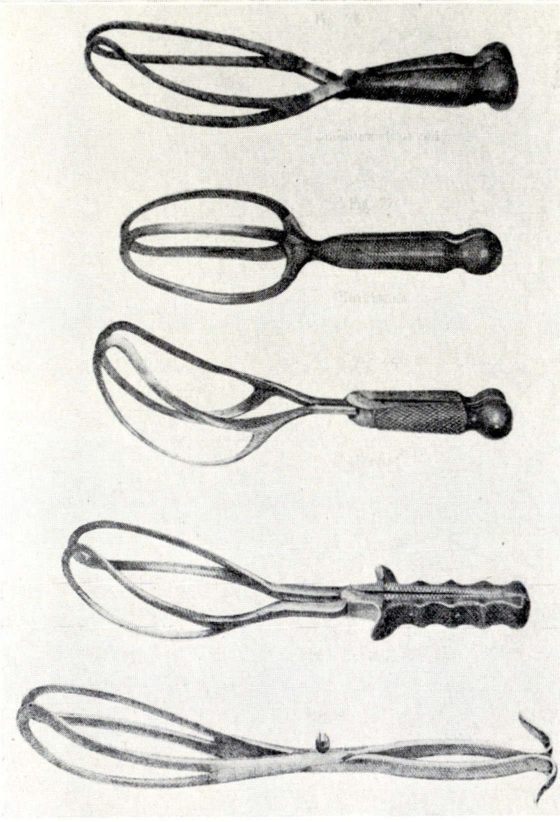

Fig. 102. The four forceps found in the Chamberlen chest. (Hirst, B. C.: *Text Book of Obstetrics*. Philadelphia, Saunders, 1918.)

Fig. 103. Early forceps, from above downward they are Smellie's (curved), Haighton's, Davis', long English forceps, Levret's. (Hodge, H. L.: *Principles and Practice of Obstetrics*, Philadelphia, Lea, 1864.)

beyond the point of articulation. The fenestration helped to lighten the instrument and to enable them to seize the head with greater security. They were furnished with a cranial curve, as has been stated, but they were straight when viewed in profile. Though somewhat crude in appearance, they were capable of rendering good service when the head had once entered the pelvic cavity. Smellie, in place of the mortise lock of the Chamberlen forceps, which required to be secured by tape or cord, invented the easily adjusted English lock, and covered the handles with wood and a durable coat of leather. The handles were five and one-half inches in length, and the blades six inches. Short forceps, slightly modified, are used by some still. It has been thought an advantage because they can be concealed in the pocket, and slipped over the child's head without

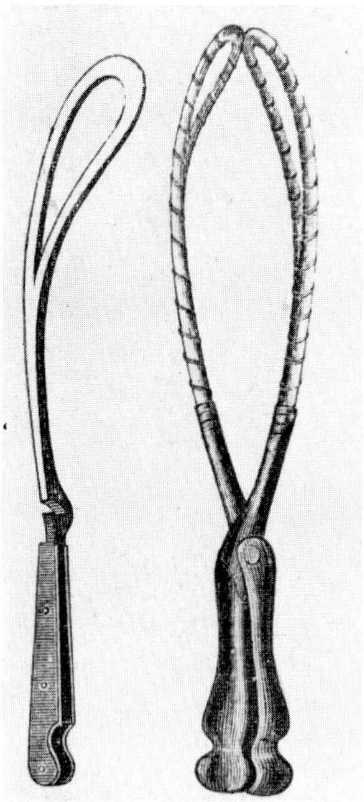

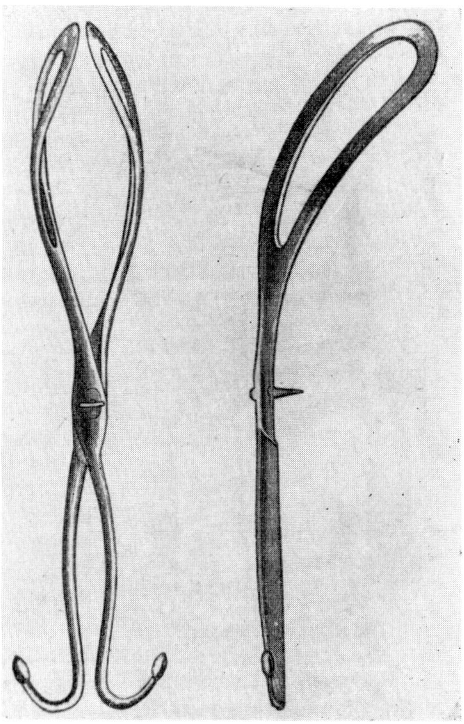

Fig. 104. Smellie forceps. (Lusk, W. T.: *The Science and Art of Midwifery*. New York, Appleton, 1892.)

Fig. 105. Levret's forceps. (Lusk, W. T.: *The Science and Art of Midwifery*. New York, Appleton, 1892.)

the knowledge of the patient or of the assistants. Smellie laid great stress upon this point, and says: "As women are commonly frightened at the very name of an instrument, it is advisable to conceal them as much as possible until the character of the operator is fully established." In these enlightened days, however, secrecy is no longer advisable.

"Long forceps: Smellie states that in pelves with jutting-in of the sacrum, he could not push the handles far enough backward to include, between the blades, the bulky part of the head which lay above the pubes. To remedy this inconvenience, he contrived a longer pair, curved on one side and convex on the other. Although "Smellie was deeply impressed" with the dangers of high forceps operations, and sought to diminish the risks incidental to them by making the handles short, to free himself, as he said, "from the temptation of using too great force"; he nevertheless applied the curved forceps to the head when not engaged in the inlet.[12]

"Levret, on the contrary, contemporaneously with Smellie, converted the forceps of Chapman, into a powerful tractor and compressor; and yet he forbade the use of his forceps "when the head lay within the uterus." He retained the iron handles, but roughened the surfaces, and made them slightly convex, to adapt them to the palms of the hand. The chief peculiarities, however, consisted in the weight and length of the instrument and in the extent of the pelvic curve. The articulation was effected by means of a pivot and a mortise. So far from these features proving objectionable, they have been substantially retained in modern French instruments. The forceps of Smellie and Levret are the two type-forms from which are derived the great number of the models in vogue at the present day.[13]

"The Naegele forceps is a modification of the Smellie instrument which it resembles closely.[14]

"The Simpson forceps possesses a relatively short handle, with transverse shoulders, and indentations for the fingers of the under hand. The English lock is improved by the addition of knees or projections to diminish its mobility. The cephalic curve, in place of starting at the lock, is carried away two and three eighths inches by straight, parallel shanks, an arrangement which makes it possible to lock the instrument outside the vulva even when applied to the head at the brim, and which enables the operator to bring the head to the floor of the pelvis without placing the vulva upon the stretch. The pelvic curve does not exceed one and one half inches. I have

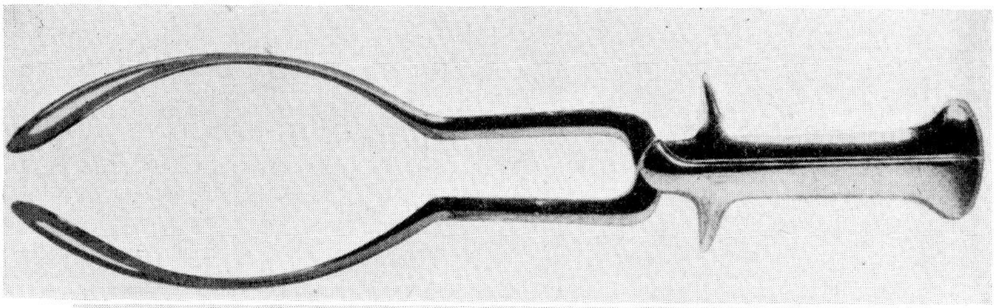

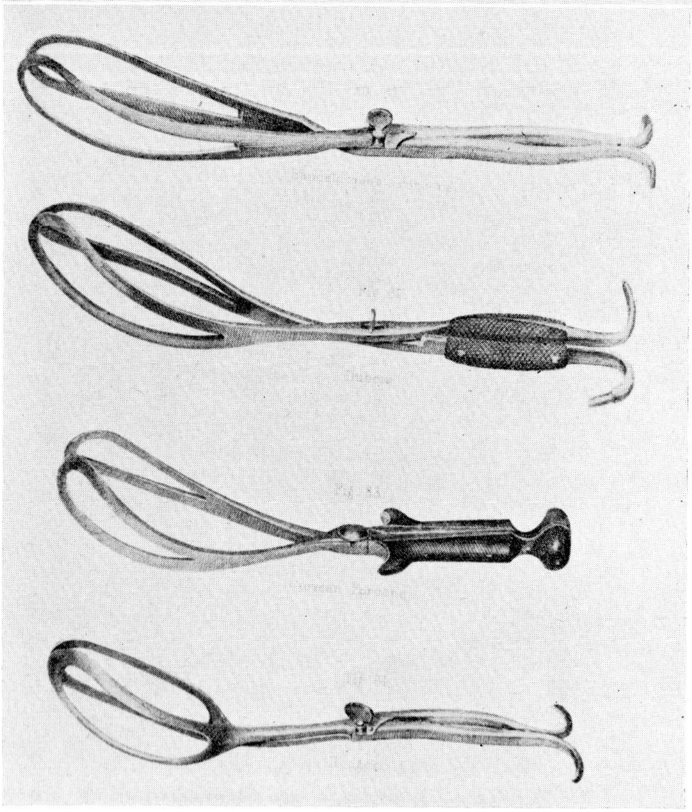

Fig. 106. Simpson's forceps. (DeLee, J. B.: *Principles and Practice of Obstetrics*, 5th Ed. Philadelphia, Saunders, 1929.)

Fig. 107. Other early forceps, from above downward are Baudelocque's, Dubois', German forceps, and Hodge's forceps. (Hodge, H. L.: *Principles and Practice of Obstetrics*. Philadelphia, Lea, 1864.)

been in the habit of recommending this forceps to my classes of medical students, on account of the ease with which it can be applied, its solidity, and the slight markings it leaves, under ordinary circumstances, upon the child's head. It is, however, defective in compressive power, when such action is necessary."[15]

In Simpson's *Obstetrical Memoirs and Contributions*, published in 1855, the following information is to be found:

"The blades (of Simpson's forceps) are the same as Dr. Ramsbotham's, but scarcely so much curved. The lock is Smellie's, but with knees or projections above it of such size as to prevent the blades readily unlocking in the intervals between the pains, thus giving it the character of the locks of Levret and Brünninghausen's instruments, without their complexity. The joints are made so loose as to allow of their lateral motion and overlapping to a very considerable degree, thus facilitating their introduction and application. And, lastly, the handle is that used by Naegele and other German accoucheurs, viz., with transverse knees or rests below the lock for one or two of the first fingers of the right hand to drag by, the long forceps being only properly used as an instrument of traction, not of compression. In addition, the handles are grooved and marked on the anterior side, to distinguish that from the other side when the blades are within the pelvis."

Simpson used his forceps almost exclusively for rotations as well as ordinary difficult deliveries. At this time there was still much controversy as to the necessity of forceps in most instances; for example, the vectis (single uncurved blade) was still the most common method of delivering a posterior position. Simpson further discusses this in his book, and seems to know all about it despite the fact that he never used it. He said, as did most obstetricians of his time, that "posterior positions would deliver themselves without forceps, and at any rate it was perfectly proper to use the vectis if so desired. It was a matter of flexing the head, and then assisting in the rotation, by hand or with the vectis, and then allowing the patient to deliver herself." If inertia were the cause, then the problem took on a somewhat different aspect. He used his forceps to rotate only after the proper treatment for inertia failed.

He also discussed the proper mode of application of the forceps. He states that "the long forceps differ from the short in their modes of application. The short forceps are applied always to the lateral surfaces of the child's head, in whatever position the head may be. This is generally in the right diameter, so the forceps are usually applied in the left diameter."

"If the long forceps are ever, for inertia, hemorrhage, or other such complications, in any case applied while the head is passing through the brim, and the brim and head are natural in size, the instrument may be perhaps applied, like the short forceps, directly to the lateral surfaces of the child's head. But the common reason for the employment of the long forceps is morbid contraction of the brim of the pelvis in its most general form, and from its most general cause, viz., in the conjugate or antero-posterior diameter, from the projection forward of the promontory of the sacrum. . . . In this state the child's head is usually in the transverse diameter, and not in the right diagonal. If the forceps are applied to the short diameter of the head, one blade would be under the symphysis, and other in front of the promontory of the sacrum. Firstly the application is almost impossible, and secondly considerable damage is done to the mother, such as injuries to the bladder. If the application is made with one blade over the face and other over the occiput (transversely), you end by really applying them obliquely. And it is only so after much waste of time and damage. So (Simpson deduced) that the proper mode of application in the transverse head is to directly apply the blades obliquely; one, the posterior, over the side of the occiput, and the other, the anterior, over the side of the brow or temple; and consequently they should be generally situated somewhat in the oblique diameter of the brim."[16]

The Hodge, Wallace and White forceps were the instruments most commonly used in the United States in 1892. Interesting innovations in forceps were made by David D. Davis[17] (1777-1841) who was professor of midwifery in the University of London produced five varieties of forceps. There were those with symmetrical blades, those with assymetrical blades, those with blades of unequal length, blades covered with leather and padded with flannel so as not to injure the face.

The introduction of the forceps was not accepted cordially and unequivocally. Many approved, and very many disapproved. Among those who endorsed it wholeheartedly was Frederich Ben-

JAMIN OSIANDER (1759-1822) who, born in Zell, Württemberg, and "professor of midwifery in Göttingen, was an ardent advocate of the forceps." He urged everyone to qualify in the forceps and use them unsparingly. He proclaimed the forceps as an instrument well qualified to shorten labor. With a record of 175 forcep deliveries without injury to mother or child, he boasted of its value in obstructed labor, and had no time for craniotomy. When he performed cesarean section, he preferred the lower uterine segment because he could thus push the head against the symphysis and then make the incision through the abdominal wall.[18]

Among those who bitterly disapproved was THOMAS DENMAN (1733-1815) to whom mankind is indebted for fostering a conservatism in obstetrics and thereby saving many lives before obstetrical powers were understood. He was born in Bakewell and graduated from Aberdeen. Like William Hunter, he opposed symphysiotomy. He never performed a cesarean operation, but concurred in its performance if an absolute indication were present and the outcome was quite assured to be successful. He practiced watchful waiting in cases of postpartum bleeding instead of going in and performing a manual removal of the placenta. He was among the first to suggest the contagious nature of puerperal fever and blamed the physician for its spread. He wrote about this in 1768; his *Essay on Puerperal Fever* was published in London.

As usual, his conservative approach to version permitted him to point out the limitations in the indications for the procedure, a condition greatly ignored by many of his colleagues. He cited as a contraindication the woman with pains which were strong but not progressing, with a head low in the pelvis, and more important with the uterus tightly wrapped around the baby.

He declared that the fillet was too often ineffectual. He believed, like Mariceau, that the forceps were capable of more harm than good. Quoting him in this regard:

> If we compare the general good done with instruments, however cautiously used, with the evils arising from their unnecessary and improper use, we might doubt whether it would not have been happy for the world if no instrument of any kind had ever been contrived for, or recommended in, the practice of midwifery.

He maintained that the vectis was as efficient as the forceps.

Other important objectors to the use of the forceps were William Hunter and Osborn.

In the history of the forceps, we begin with the original instrument of Chamberlen and the few men who used a forceps similar to Chamberlen's, with minor modifications. In its evolution we note the first really important addition when Smellie and Levret added the pelvic curve. With every change that came subsequently, and

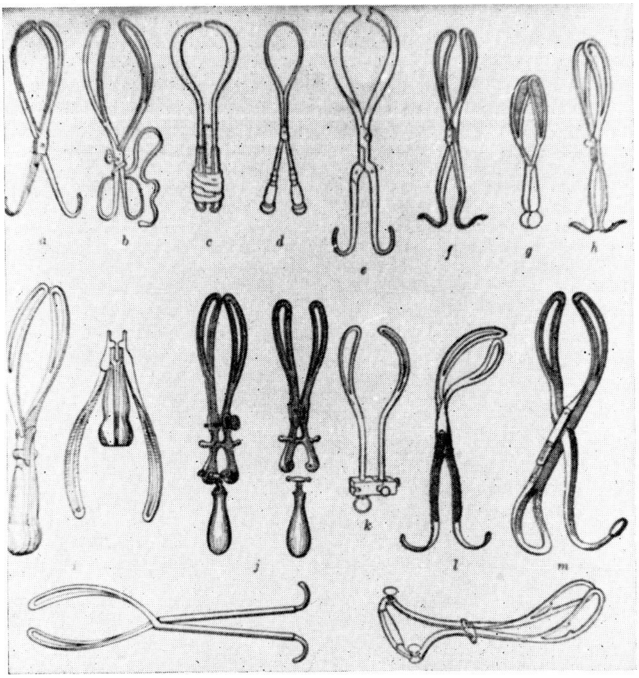

Fig. 108. A few of the hundreds of forceps models; a. Chamberlen No. 1; b. Chamberlen No. 2; c. Palfyn; d. Palfyn, 1721; e. Dusee, 1733; f. Gregoire, 1746; g. Smellie, 1752; h. Levret, 1747; i. Mathias Saxtorph, 1791; j. Coutouly; k. Hamon, 1867; l. Baumers of Lyon, 1849; m. Santarelli, 1794; n. Japanese forceps; o. Chassagny. (DeLee, J. B.: *Principles and Practice of Obstetrics,* 5th Ed. Philadelphia, Saunders, 1929.)

there were many hundreds (600 according to Dill), there was nothing radically different in the fundamental design to improve it. Dill,[19] in his book on the obstetrical forceps, has aptly, if briefly, discussed some of the more important modifications of the forceps, from which some of the following information has been obtained:

Different forms of blades were evolved and perhaps thus improved; there is the Simpson forceps with the fenestrated type of blade originated by Chamberlen. A radical departure from the fenestration of blades came in 1799 by Osiander to provide a solid blade with a large surface area; its counterpart today is the McLean Tucker type of forceps. A still further modification is

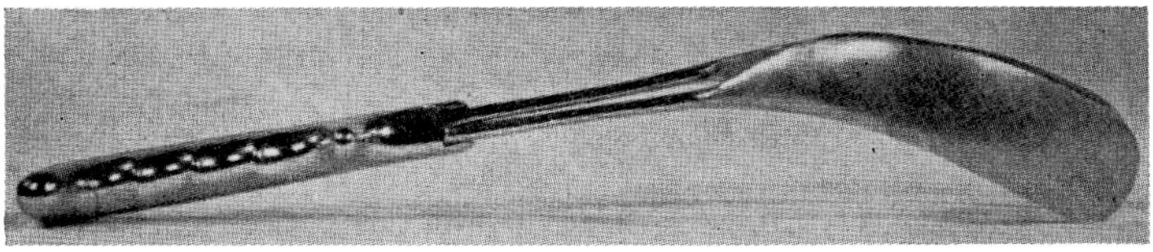

Fig. 109. The McLean Tucker forceps with solid blades. (This fig. 7, p. 11 of Dill's book.) (Dill, L. V.: *The Obstetrical Forceps.* Springfield, Thomas, 1953.)

seen in the very much used blade of the Luikhart McLean type of forceps which retains the fenestration on the fetal side of the blade, but solid on the pelvic surface. This idea was originated by Hohl of Halle in 1850.

All sorts of modifications of the pelvic curve have occurred, all based on Levret in 1747 and Smellie almost simultaneously. We have forceps with extremely acute pelvic curves down to

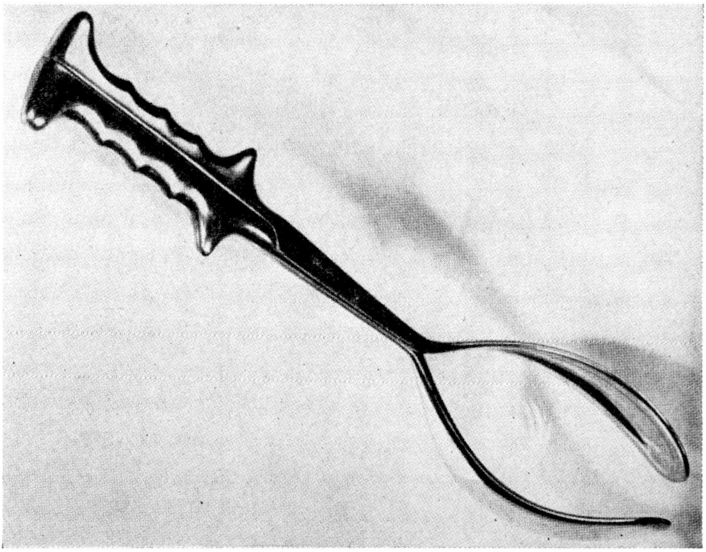

Fig. 110. The Luikart McLean forceps with fenestration of blade on fetal surface, but solid on pelvic surface. (This fig. 8, p. 12 of Dill's book.) (See new note in text.) (Dill, L. V.: *The Obstetrical Forceps.* Springfield, Thomas, 1953.)

those with only a slight curve; one modification actually reversed itself and practically omitted the pelvic curve in order to be able to do rotations, this is the Kjelland forceps.

Cephalic curves changed, some have little curvature such as Tarnier's forceps, and others were extremely curved such as the Davis forceps, or the Hodge forceps.

Changes in the shank took place so that we have the closed type such as the Luikhart McLean type; the Chamberlen forceps had this sort of shank. The Simpson type of shank is open; the Palfyn forceps was the original example of the open type shank.

Locks were varied. There was the "English lock" seen in the Simpson forceps, described by Smellie originally; the "French lock" as in Tarnier's forceps, which is practically the same lock used by Chamberlen; and the "sliding lock" as in the Kjelland forceps. The sliding lock was first made by Boerma in 1907.

Handles have changed little. Forceps were made in which the ends of the two shanks curved outward to produce a traction surface; this idea originated in the Chamberlen forceps. Palfyn's forceps with large and bulbous grip handles was the basis of many of the subsequent models introduced; all sorts of notches and indentations for the grasping fingers have been devised, but basically it is the Palfyn idea.

However, in 1860 a new principle to the forceps appeared. This occurred when Hubert constructed a forceps with the ends of the handles bent backward at a right angle, to which he later attached a bar near the lock. By this ingenious device he could make traction in direct line with the pelvic curve of the instrument. By so doing the head could be drawn in the proper axis of the pelvic inlet with more certainty and less force. This invention of Hubert of Louvain, which was known as the "Compensation Curve" was suggested to him by a forceps designed by Wallace Johnson, in 1769, a forceps that was designed with a perineal curve with the idea that its handles would not make pressure on the perineum. Hubert's forceps aroused no interest, but it is very important because it served later as a model for the Tarnier axis-traction forceps, an invention that was truly another milestone in the improvement of the forceps.

ETIENNE STÉPHENE TARNIER[20] (1828-1897) born in Aisery, studied in Paris and interned in the Maternite Hospital when puerperal

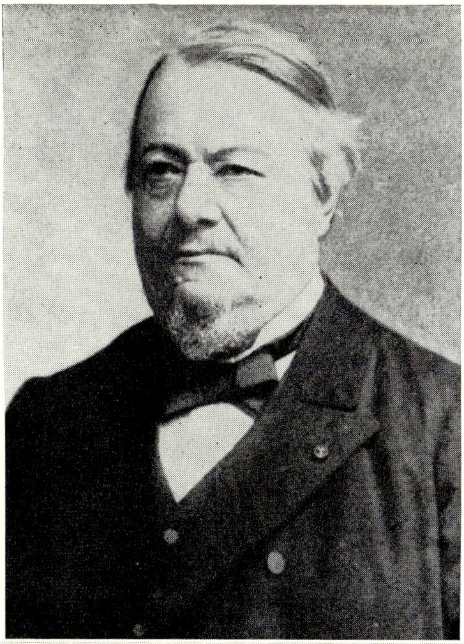

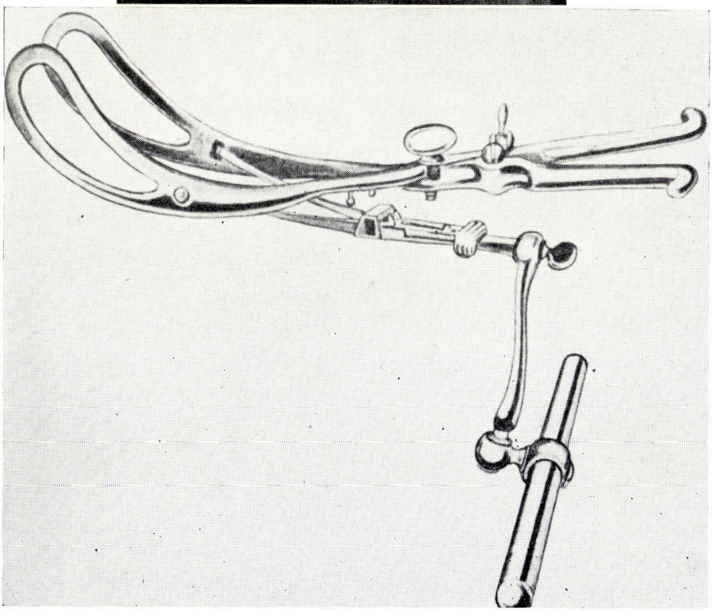

Fig. 111. E. Stéphene Tarnier. (Findley, Palmer: *Priests of Lucina*. Boston, Little, 1939.)

Fig. 112. Tarnier axis-traction forceps. (DeLee, J. B.: *Principles and Practice of Obstetrics*, 5th Ed. Philadelphia, Saunders, 1929.)

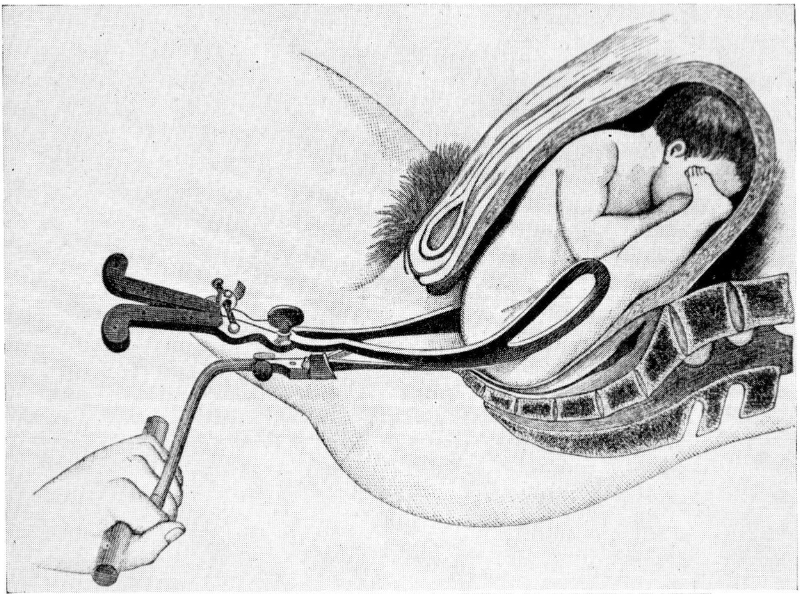

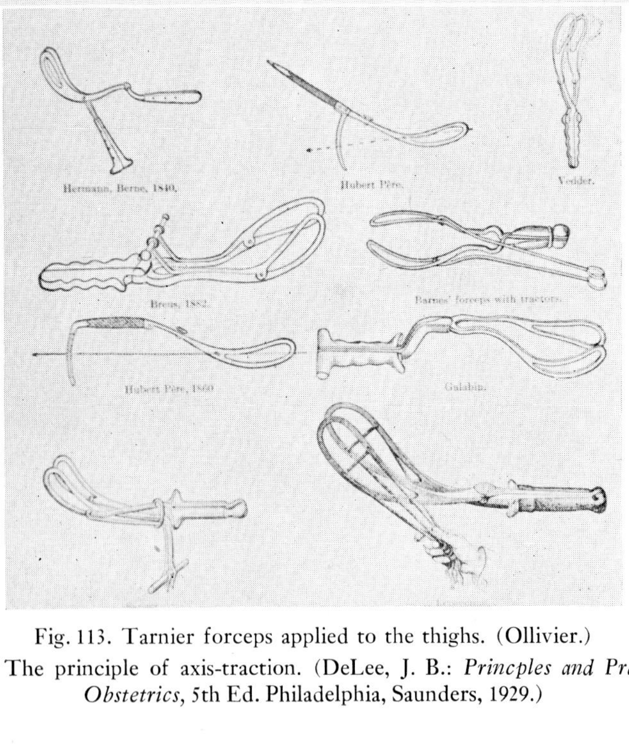

Fig. 113. Tarnier forceps applied to the thighs. (Ollivier.)
Fig. 114. The principle of axis-traction. (DeLee, J. B.: *Princples and Practice of Obstetrics*, 5th Ed. Philadelphia, Saunders, 1929.)

fever was rampant; this, plus numerous other obstetrical problems with which he had to deal, aroused his interest in obstetrics. By the addition of traction rods attached to the handles of the forceps, he was able to direct the head in line with the axis of the inlet with the least amount of force. Intelligent traction replaced blind force, a force that was otherwise misdirected and ineffective. There were adverse critics of his newly invented axis-traction forceps, and a few who maintained faith in its greatness. Matthews Duncan was one of the critics who denounced its worth, expressing his disapproval on the grounds of too much pressure exerted on the baby's head by Tarnier's forceps.

Numerous modifications of this invention, all bearing the same principle, were made by Lusk of New York, Burge of Germany, Sänger of Prague, and even Simpson. Farrior,[21] a student of Dr. B. C. Hirst somewhere around 1900, devised an excellent handle that may be attached to any forceps, by which one utilizes the axis traction principle perfectly.

The problem of delivering the aftercoming head was solved by Smellie originally. Levret, who worked pretty much hand in hand with Smellie, was noncommital in this aspect of the use of the forceps. Karl Schroeder was very actively opposed to the application of the forceps on the aftercoming head. Michaelis, Naegele and Veit and also Credé concurred with Smellie in its efficacy.

Smellie failed whenever he attempted such an application with the short forceps, but he always succeeded with his long instrument. Apparently the longer the handles the more efficient was the forcepts for delivering the aftercoming head, for one of the most successful and most universally used forceps for this purpose was invented in America at the University of Pennsylvania about 1924 by Edmund Piper.

If the Chamberlen forceps were still available today it would find its use in the same cases for which the Kjelland forceps is used, and the Kjelland forceps is used almost exclusively for rotation; for a minimal pelvic curve is required for this maneuver.

Another forceps used only in the transverse position was developed by Barton in 1926 in the United States. The same principle was utilized by Baumers of Lyon in 1849 (see Fig. 108 l) and described but never manufactured by Uyterhoven in 1805.

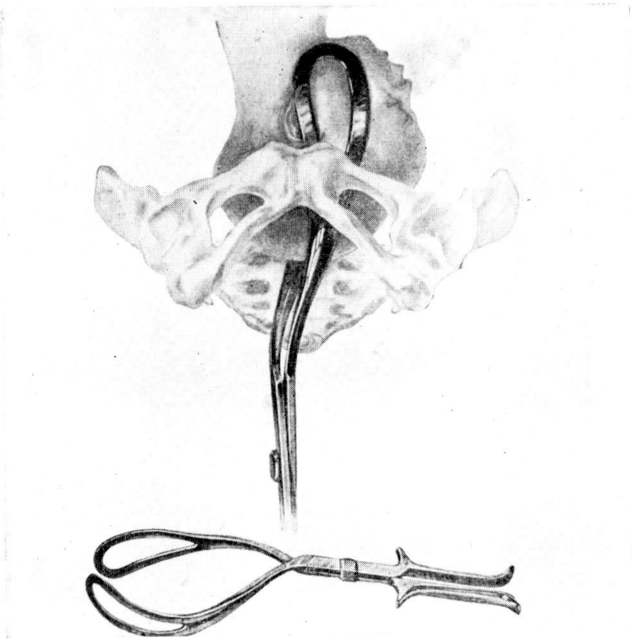

Fig. 115. Kjelland's forceps. (DeLee, J. B.: *Principles and Practice of Obstetrics*, 5th Ed. Philadelphia, Saunders, 1929.)

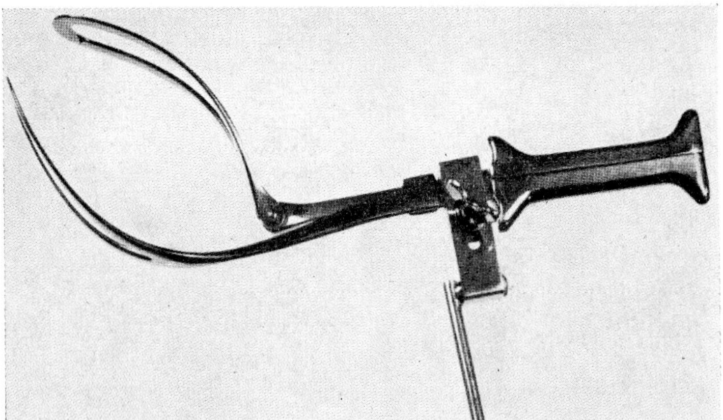

Fig. 116. The Barton forceps. (Dill, L. V.: *The Obstetrical Forceps*. Springfield, Thomas, 1953.)

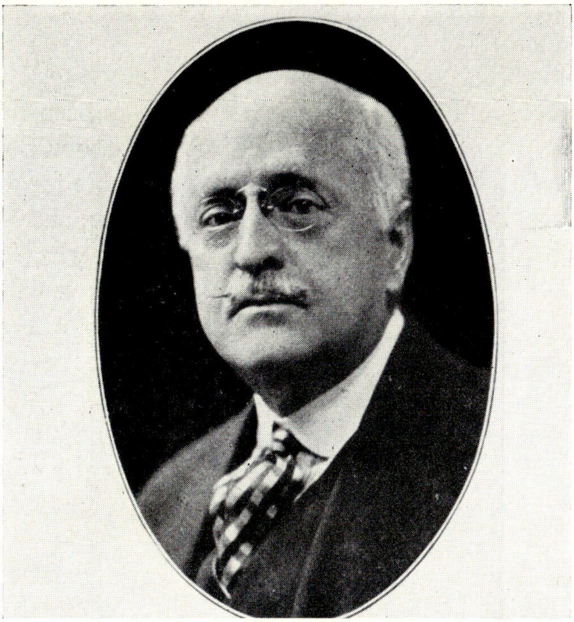

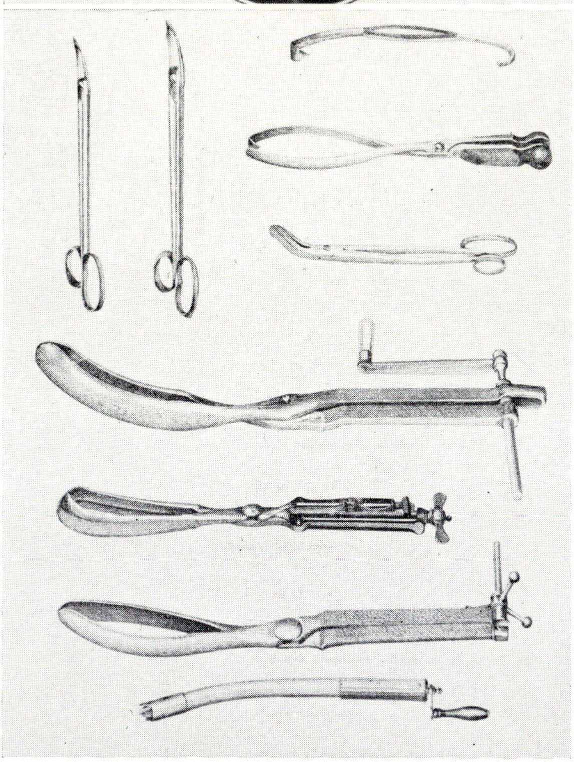

Fig. 117. Barton Cooke Hirst.

Fig. 118. Embryotomy instruments. (Hodge, H. L.: *Principles and Practice of Obstetrics*. Philadelphia, Lea, 1864.)

The basic requirements of a good forceps has been summed up by Hodge,[22] who remarked that the obstetrician would do well to become accustomed to a good long forceps suitable for application at any portion of the pelvis, he will need no other; and by the late Professor of Obstetrics at the University of Pennsylvania, Barton C. Hirst (1861-1935) who said, "That device is best which is simplest and which is most perfectly under the control of the skill and intelligence of the operator." "The essential features of any instrument," he further stated "whether long or short, are that they be made of strong, well tempered steel, devoid of rough edges, nickel or chrome plated (rustless steel), smooth handles of hard rubber or steel, approved pelvic and cephalic curves and a readily adjustable lock."

The embryotomy group of instruments, those formidable instruments, long the stock in trade of physicians, continued as such for many years before the forceps were accepted and cesarean section attained its great stature; yet even to this day these instruments of destruction are included in the armamentarium of some maternity hospitals for occasional use, if anyone around knows how.

First Occurrences and Outstanding Events

Fillet, the most ancient instrument employed in obstetrics.

Jacques Rueff was first to suggest the possibility of using forceps for delivery of living child, in 1554.

Peter Chamberlen I, the Elder invented the forceps circa 1598.

Palfyn was the first to exhibit forceps (his own) in 1720 (or 1723) at the French Academy of Sciences.

Chapman in 1733 was the first to publish an account of the Chamberlen forceps.

The Chamberlen instruments, five of them in a box, were found in his home in 1813.

Levret in 1749 and Smelie in 1753 made the first basic contribution to forceps by the addition of a pelvic curve.

Another new principle was added in 1860 by Tarnier, the axis traction. The idea actually originated with Hubert.

Other major innovations were the forceps for the aftercoming head by Piper in 1924. However this was first attempted by Smellie.

Then we have the Kjelland forceps in 1915, and later in 1926 we have the Barton forceps for transverse positions.

References

1. Hodge, H. L.: *Principles and Practice of Obstetrics.* Philadelphia, Blanchard and Lea, 1864.
2. Igerslev, E.: *Die Geburtszamge; eine geburtshulfliche Studie.* Stuttgart, F. Enke, 1891.
3. Findley, Palmer: *Priests of Lucina.* Boston, Little, 1939.
4. Butter, Alexander: The description of a forceps for extracting children by the head. *Med. Essays and Obst. Soc., Edinburgh, 3*:320-322, 1735.
5. Chapman, Edmund: *A Treatise on the Improvement of Midwifery, Chiefly with Regard to the Operation,* 2nd Ed. London, J. Brindley, 1735.
6. Radcliffe, Walter: *The Secret Instrument* (the birth of the midwifery forceps). London, Heinemann, 1947.
7. Graham, Harvey: *Eternal Eve. London,* Heinemann, 1950, p. 671.
8. Lusk, W. T.: *The Science and Art of Midwifery.* New York, Appleton, 1892, p. 361.
9. Aveling, J. H.: *The Chamberlens and the Midwifery Forceps.* London, Churchill, 1882.
10. Chapman, Edmund: *A Treatise on the Improvement of Midwifery, Chiefly with Regard to the Operation,* 2nd Ed. London, J. Brindley, 1735.
11. Lusk, W. T.: *The Science and Art of Midwifery.* New York, Appleton, 1892, p. 362.
12. *Ibid.,* p. 363.
13. *Ibid.,* p. 364.
14. *Ibid.,* p. 364.
15. *Ibid.,* p. 364.
16. Simpson, Sir James Young: *Obstetrical Memoirs and Contributions,* edited by Priestly, W. O., and Storer, H. R., 2 vols. Edinburgh, Black, 1855-56. (Also an American publication of the above, viz: Priestley, W. O., and Storer, H. R.: *Obstetrical Memoirs and Contributions of Simpson, Sir James Young,* 1st and 2nd series. Philadelphia, Lippincott, 1855-56, p. 494.)
17. Findley, Palmer: *Priests of Lucina.* Boston, Little, 1939.
18. Ricci, J. V.: *Genealogy of Gynecology.* Philadelphia and Toronto, Blakiston, 1950, p. 350.

19. Dill, L. V.: *The Obstetrical Forceps.* Springfield, Thomas, 1953.
20. Findley, Palmer: *Priests of Lucina.* Boston, Little, 1939.
21. Hirst, B. C.: *Text Book of Obstetrics.* Philadelphia, Saunders, 1918, p. 744.
22. Hodge, H. L.: *Principles and Practice of Obstetrics.* Philadelphia, Blanchard and Lea, 1864.

Chapter XIII

AGE OF REASON AND SCIENTIFIC OBSTETRICS

(A.D. 1700-1800)

THE 18TH CENTURY was the Age of Reason, so-called because they looked for the causes of the ills of the universe and for the remedies by doubting and questioning all accepted ideas and beliefs; in other words, they wished to solve all world problems on a rational or reasonable basis. This principle was accompanied by a profound religious skepticism. Before this only the political structure of the church was attacked. Now, in the 18th Century, there prevailed a disbelief in and contempt for religion itself. It was John Locke (1632-1704) who started, in England, this principle of rational thinking to solve all problems. He represented the spirit of the modern age, of individualism, of independence, of criticism and of democratic government.

The rich and perplexing heritage from the 16th Century had to be assimilated, for although science had taken tremendous strides during the 17th Century, medicine still tagged behind; but with such men as Harvey, Leeuwenhoek, Sydenham and others in the vanguard of the rear echelon medicine, it appeared only a matter of time before medicine would catch up to science. Alas, when they did catch up, they became confronted with another problem, and that was the inability of the practitioner of medicine to make proper use of the newly found medical sciences, because many of these new found basic medical sciences did not have any direct bearing on the practice of medicine, and it would be many years later before this knowledge would be able to be applied and thus put medicine on a truly scientific basis.

In the meantime, we have for the first time in medical history a replacement of empiricism by rationalism. It was slow in producing results, for there was an unreasonable mania for classification and theorization, a mania to explain life, health, disease and death according to some rigid formula. The net result was confusion. So many apparently simple systems made their appearance that it became impossible for the befuddled practitioner to make a choice. Whenever data became inadequate, logical analysis was used to cover up the gap. The result of all this was not only confusion, but a failure to apply these newer concepts in their bewilderment of such an array of facts that were constantly being promulgated. Menstrual function and its associated phenomena were considered with the same unscientific attitude of the past. They looked upon it as something unclean, a purifying bath was still considered necessary.

The 18th Century was also called the "Age of Humanitarianism," an outlook that had its inception with Francis Hutcheson (1694-1747) who propounded the formula "the greatest happiness for

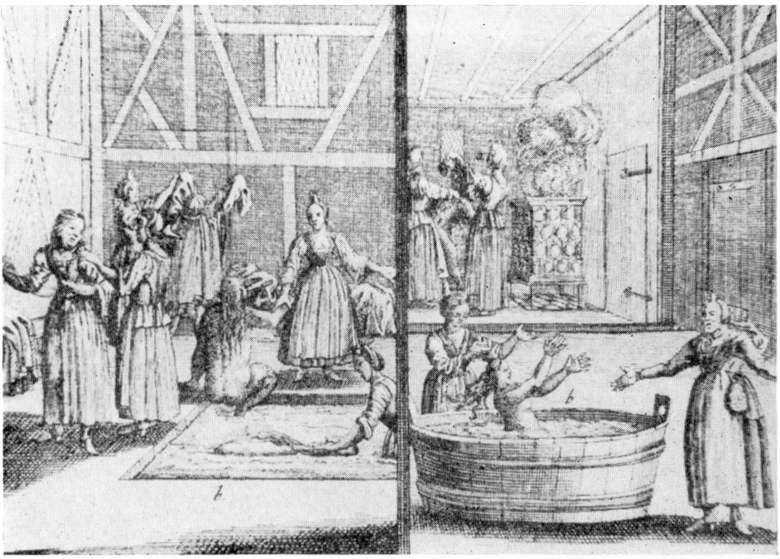

Fig. 119. Hebrew purification baths, circa 1726. (The Bettmann Archive.)

the greatest number." Until medicine reached the status of a science that it was certainly approaching, it remained temporarily bogged down; but it did serve to speed up social progress by its "humanitarianism," and its democratic movements. Even the humblest man had a right to happiness, society began to recognize its obligations toward the welfare of all its members. Such convictions broadened the field of medical care to include new groups: the poor, cripples, even political prisoners and criminals. Even the wealthier class joined the crusade, for practical as well as charitable reasons; sick and impoverished workers meant economic waste, waste reduced the ability to produce goods, and undermined a nation's wealth. The physicians of the 18th Century was the group most imbued with this spirit of humanitarianism and reason, in fact the physicians of this time have been referred to as the most charitable members the profession has ever had.[1]

As a result of this modern outlook, kingdoms toppled and governments crashed. All sorts of governing bodies, such as limited monarchies, republics and absolute rulers existed at the same time. The 18th Century began in the midst of the War of the Spanish Succession. The French were driven from the Holy Roman Empire, from all of Italy and the Netherlands. In the middle of the century we have the Austrian Succession and the Seven Years War. France and England fought on the continent, in North America and in India. Finally France sank into economic collapse and England rose to world dominion. This was still a period of monarchs, cardinals and nobles, until the latter part of the century when the bourgeoisie revolted. Thousands upon thousands of the aristocrats were led to the guillotine along with Louis XVI and Marie Antoinette. Thus ended the century with a Reign of Terror and with Napoleon, an achievement of the rational and reasoning mind.[2]

Some of the great minds who took up the cudgels under the banners of rationalism and reason for everything done were Voltaire (Francois-Marie Arouet, 1694-1778). He maintained a lifelong interest in the oppressed and the fight for toleration, and fought for political and religious reforms. His methods earned him the title of "Giant of Mockery." On a par with the philosophers came the scientists, the greatest of this century, the early part of it:

Isaac Newton (1624-1726) with his law of gravitation. Gabriel Daniel Fahrenheit (1686-1736), a German, developed the thermometer bearing his name. A Swede, Anders Celsius (1701-1744), originated the centigrade thermometer. Joseph Priestly (1733-1804) and Carl Wilhelm Scheele (1742-1786) isolated oxygen, and Sir Humphry Davy (1778-1829) discovered that nitrous oxide was respirable and intoxicating. Physicists Luigi Galvani (1737-1798) of Bologna and Count Alessandro Volta (1745-1827) initiated electro-physiology by studies of muscle-nerve preparations. Stephen Hales (1677-1761) gave the first notions of blood pressure.

Leadership in medicine was wrested from Italy in this century, by central Europe. Geographical limitations meant little; besides central Europe, where medicine was under the influence of Hermann Boerhaave in Leyden, we have the school at Edinburgh that the Monros helped to establish, and a medical center in London. More than this, it was in this century that medical advance spread itself to distant lands, and prominently among them was the establishment of the first hospital and the first medical school in America.

The University of Leyden

Hermann Boerhaave (1668-1738) was professor at Leyden for many years. His greatness rests not on his original works, which were wanting, but chiefly for the influence he cast among his students, who subsequently accomplished greatness. He was a voracious student, lectured four and five hours a day, and used sound teaching methods. His success was pre-eminent because of his simplicity, clarity and eclectic wisdom, personal warmth, and radiant personality and uncommonly good sense. He held a professorship in medicine, chemistry, pharmacology and botany. His most effective method of teaching was to bring students directly into the hospital. He was a superb orator, clear in diction and thoroughly systematic. As already mentioned his real accomplishment was to contribute great doctors to the medical world, who established or revitalized schools in Edinburgh, Vienna and Goettigen. His teachings reached as far as America. It was his pupil Gerhard van Swieten, who brought clinical medicine to Vienna; Albrecht von Haller, a Swiss, who established physiology at Goettigen; and Alexander Monro who began the reign of the "Monro Dynasty" in

Scotland. There is no doubt that Shippen and Morgan in America had come under the influence of Boerhaave, even if indirectly.[3]

The School of Edinburgh

THE MONRO FAMILY: It was the Monro family of physicians who helped to establish Edinburgh as a great training center. It began with Alexander Monro in 1719, after which his family occupied the chair of anatomy for 126 years. Alexander was only twenty-two when he became professor of Anatomy. There were four Monros, each son succeeding the father. They made no lasting medical contributions, but they were instrumental in starting "Old Surgeon's Hall" in Edinburgh.

Alexander Monro was assisted by four other Boerhaave students in the teaching at Edinburgh. One of the men of distinction at Edinburgh, next in greatness to Boerhaave himself, was William Cullen (1710-1790). For science he did little, but for medical practice he did a great deal. An interesting theory of Cullen's was that nervous irritability was the cause of disease. When we, today, say someone is ill because of frayed nerves, we are harking back to Cullen. He ignored the advances in pathology and diagnosis that had been founded or at least broadened by such men as Morgagni, Lancisi and Auenbrugger. None of his works contained any originality. But his teaching inspired many men, among them being Samuel Bard of New York, and later, William Shippen, John Morgan and Benjamin Rush of Philadelphia, men who were instrumental in starting medical education in the United States; we can thus appreciate how widely Boerhaave's influence penetrated.

Medicine of England (London)

In London there was an air of expansiveness about the doctors of this period. They were both prosperous and likable, full of good fellowship and humor and outstanding as men and practitioners. There was established a close link between the intellectual elite and the medical practitioner in this golden age of literature. England's great poets such as Swift, Pope and Johnson counted doctors among their coffee house brethren. The symbol of the physician's rise in social standing was the gold-headed cane. This badge of honor was bestowed on the city's outstanding doctor by the College of Physicians. To walk or ride horseback now meant a serious loss of prestige, the gold headed cane plus a carriage was a sure index of professional prestige. Dr. John Radcliffe was the first to receive the gold-headed cane[4] and Dr. Richard Mead second. Neither of them made any original contributions; Radcliffe endowed the Radcliffe Observatory, Hospital and Library. While the barber surgeons did most of the surgery in central Europe, here in London they were curtailed. The hospitals of London, like St. Bartholomew, St. Thomas, Guy's and Chelsea Hospital, appointed young surgeons to their staffs, and not barber-surgeons.

Hospitals and Medical Schools

During the Byzantine period and latter Roman era, the clerics created sanctuaries for the wayfarer. The Christian hospitals were modeled after the Roman valetudinaria. In these havens the monks and nuns took it upon themselves to nurse, feed and clothe the homeless. Leprosariae and permanent homes for the old, sick and poor were established. Most of these offered nursing care but no medical aid. They were hospitals without doctors. The Middle Ages saw the rise of the monastic infirmaries. Here the modern hospital had its true origin, and to its growth doctors contributed greatly. These went on until the 11th Century when the secular School of Salerno challenged clerical dominance. So it was during the latter part of the Arabian era (11th Century) that a medical school was started in Salerno in southern Italy, the first medical school in Christian Europe. A woman physician named Trotula was mainly responsible for the Salernitan School.

If central Europe, which had wrested leadership in medicine from Italy, was dominating the field by virtue of her eminent systematizers, numerous independent advances were made without any geographical limitations. Medicine was becoming international, even America participated; the first hospital, the first medical school, and the first woman's medical school were originated in the United States in Philadelphia.

The First Medical School in America

In 1750, fifteen years before the actual inception of the first medical school in America, students were informally taught at "Charity

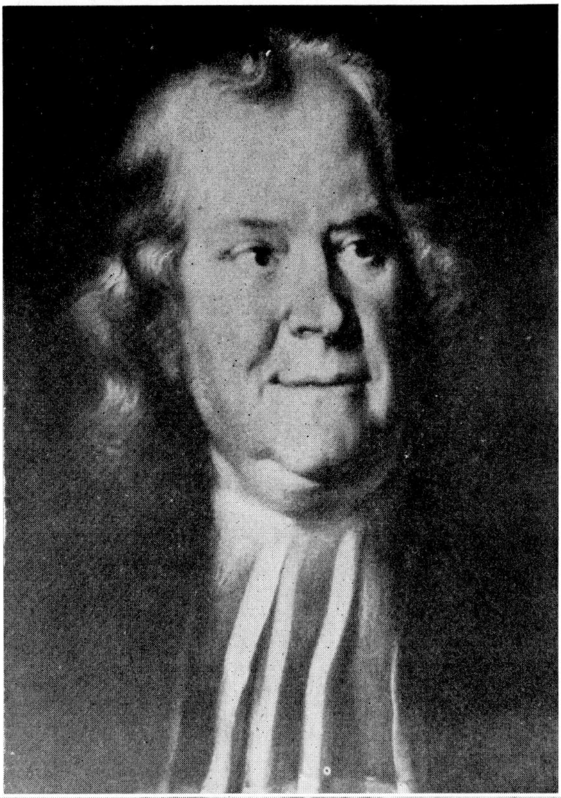

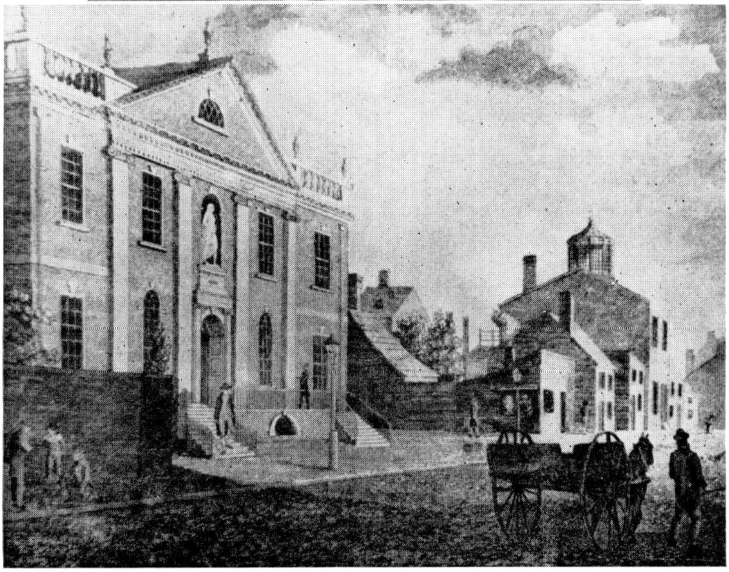

Fig. 120. H. Boerhaave. (The Bettmann Archive.)
Fig. 121. Library and Surgeon's Hall, Fifth Street, Philadelphia.

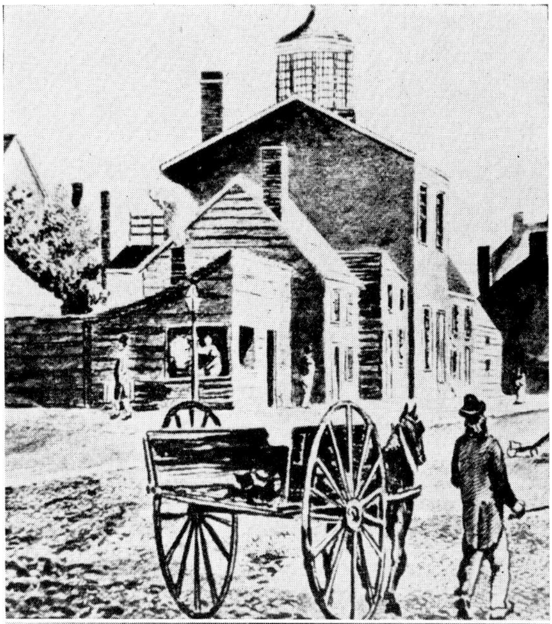

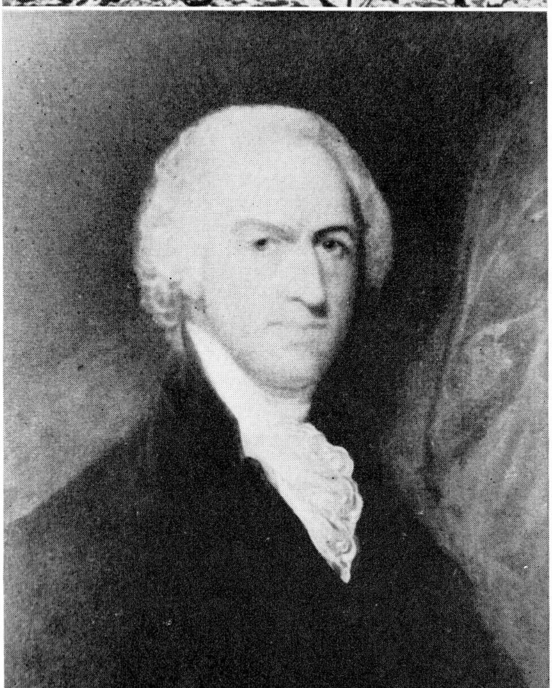

Fig. 122. Anatomical Hall.

Fig. 123. William Shippen, Jr. (Addison, Agnes: *University of Pennsylvania Medical School, Portraits.* Philadelphia, University Press, 1940.)

House," Fourth and Race Streets, Philadelphia. When WILLIAM SHIPPEN, JR. (1736-1808) returned to Philadelphia in November 1762 with an M.D. degree from Edinburgh, he began a course in anatomy and midwifery at the State House (later Independence Hall). Life-sized anatomical drawings, donated by Dr. Fothergill enlivened the discourses on anatomy, and gypsum case models helped to demonstrate the mechanics of childbirth. Some Philadelphians became suspicious when Shippen showed specimens from human dissections. One day a mob gathered, incited by the belief that the anatomist had obtained his specimens "via grave robbing." Dr. Shippen had to run for his life, but the uproar subsided eventually.

Meanwhile JOHN MORGAN (1735-1789), another medical student from the colonies who had obtained his degree in Europe and had met Voltaire and Morgagni in a post-graduate Grand Tour of the continent, put on paper his ideas for the establishment of an American medical school. Enthusiastically, the young doctor set to work immediately upon his return to Philadelphia to establish a medical college modeled after the Edinburgh school. His plan was received favorably, and, on May 13, 1765, the first School of Medicine in the new world was started. The Trustees of the College of Philadelphia appointed him Professor of Theory and Practice of Physick. On the day of founding of the new medical school, John Morgan gave a two-day inaugural address "Discourses upon the institution of Medical Schools in America," an address which served as the Magna Charta of medical education.

Shippen was made Professor of Anatomy soon afterwards. Morgan and Shippen became involved in a dispute as to who originated the idea of a medical school, in fact they actually came to blows. Shippen, who was the more influential, had Morgan removed as Director General of Hospitals, and took over the medical department himself. Morgan, who had had such an auspicious beginning, died a broken man.

First Woman's Medical College in America

Philadelphia bears the distinction of being the site of the first Woman's Medical College, opened in 1850, guided by Dr. Anne Preston. In 1857, the New York Infirmary for women and children

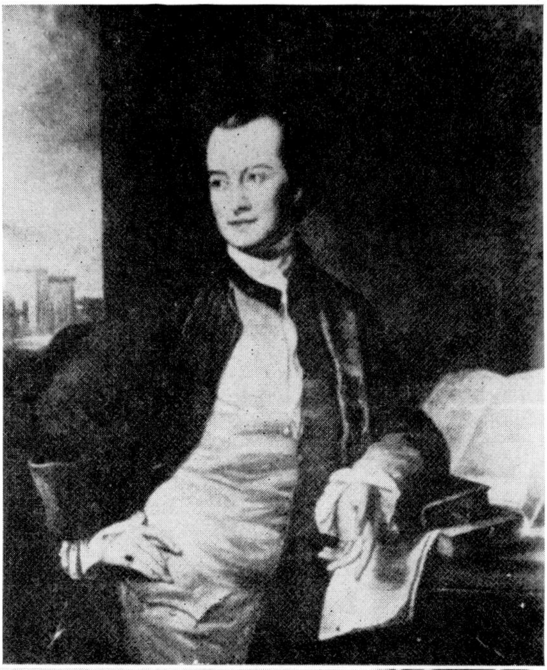

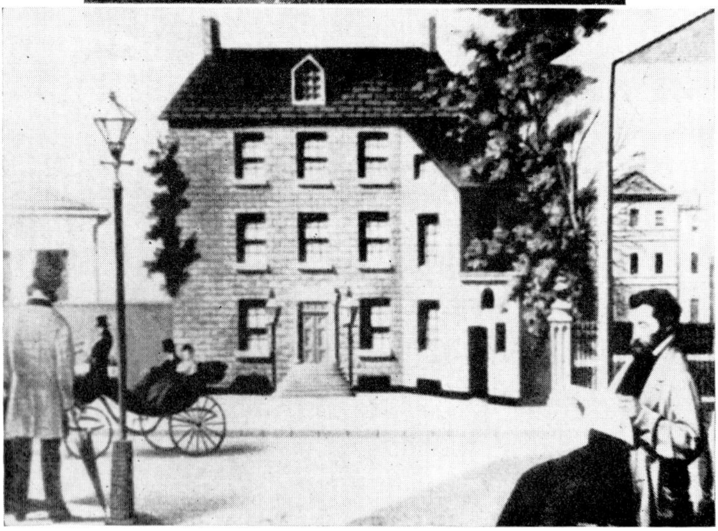

Fig. 124. Dr. John Morgan. (Addison, Agnes: *University of Pennsylvania Medical School, Portraits*. Philadelphia, University Press, 1940.)

Fig. 125. First Woman's Medical College, Philadelphia, 1850. (*MD Medical News* Magazine, Jan. 1958. New York, MD Publication, Inc. [MD Medical News Magazine Photo.])

was established by Dr. Elizabeth Blackwell, the first academically trained woman doctor, who graduated from the Geneva Medical College in 1849 after many rejections to matriculate in other schools.

Progress of women doctors began after the Civil War, in the face of much mockery. Dr. Mary Walker held a commission as Assistant Surgeon during the Civil War. She wore trousers (it was said by the sanction of Congress). She was the first woman to serve officially on the staff of any army in wartime. She was taken prisoner, exchanged for a soldier and awarded a gold medal.[5]

The First Hospital in America

In a pamphlet from the Department of Public Health, Ciudad Trujillo, Republica Dominicana, 1954, we have the following information:

> The hospital system of old Europe came to America when it was discovered, and it developed under the influence of Christian charity during the Spanish colonization. The Catholic King and Queen, through their laws of the Indies, as well as Christopher Columbus, saw to it that there were hospitals in the lands now belonging to them. Health was a noble goal in the crusade that had the greatest influence in the destiny of mankind and in the great historical transformations of the western hemisphere. Columbus, on his second trip had two surgeons with him, a Dr. Diego Alvarez Chanca and another (name unknown) who visited the Indian Chief Guacamari who feigned to be sick. These doctors remained behind to take care of the settlers.
>
> On March twentieth to twenty-ninth, 1503, Governor Ovando was ordered to build houses to be used as a hospital for the poor, both Christian and Indian. This gave birth to the first hospital in America, the San Nicolás de Bari Hospital, in the city of San Domingo. According to a document of the eighteenth century, the origin of this hospital was the charity of a pious negro woman who used the building (such as it was) which she owned, to take care of the sick from 1502 to 1503. Gov. Ovando took over, financed and erected the hospital. The original documents of the hospital disappeared during Drake's invasion in 1586. A written report, the same year the city was looted, gives the exact date of the founding of the hospital and other details such as accounts of authentic tax collections for it, and talk of the elders,

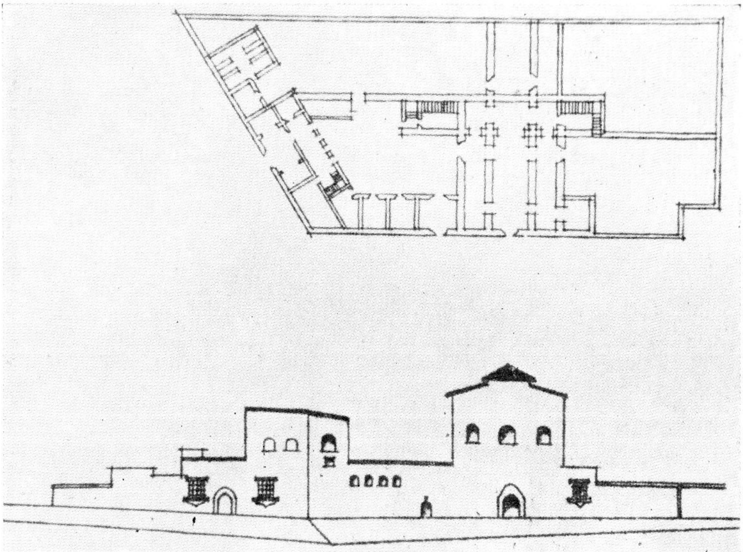

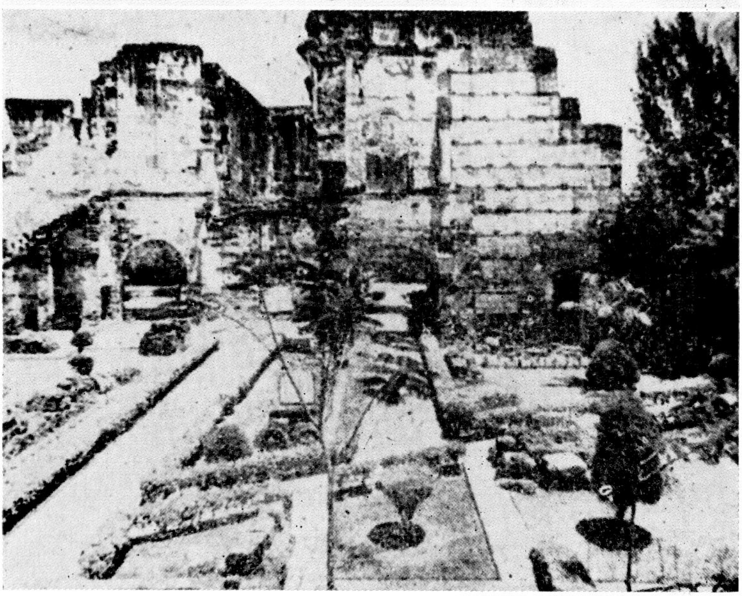

Fig. 126. Old plan of the "San Nicolás de Bari Hospital" (from *Plans of Architectonic Monuments of America and the Phillipines kept in the Files of the Indies*, by Diego Angulo Iniguez. (Comarazamy, Francisco: *The First Hospital in America*. Ciudad Trujillo [Dominican Republic], Department of Public Health, 1954.)

Fig. 127. Ruin of the "San Nicolás de Bari Hospital" (1503-1506). (Comarazamy, Francisco: *The First Hospital in America*. Ciudad Trujillo [Dominican Republic], Department of Public Health, 1954.)

> etc. that Nicolás de Ovando founded this hospital November 29, 1503. The hospital was limited to six beds, but a second structure was added to it in 1519 and completed in 1552 by a third addition. It now had a bed capacity of fifty to sixty, and cared for seven hundred patients annually. Many of these patients were sailors and passengers.
>
> The Bari Hospital became associated with the "Holy Ghost" Hospital in Rome, thus the first hospital in America became associated with one of the most venerable institutions in Europe. As a result of this affiliation, the order of the "double cross" was introduced in Hispaniola. Hospitals began to spread to the continent, e.g., to Columbia in 1551; to Mexico and Cuzco in 1560; Lima, Peru, in 1585. During the sixteenth century, the city of Santo Domingo had two more hospitals, the San Andres Hospital (nine years after the Bari Hospital); the other hospitals were for lepers. Interestingly it anticipated an ordinance of 1573 of the Laws for the Indies. The law read: "when a city or town is founded the hospitals for the poor and non-contagious diseases should be placed next to the church, but those for contagious diseases should be built on high places so that the wind going through them will not hurt the city or town.

Some historians believe that the first hospital in the new world was founded by Hernan Cortes in Mexico. This is disputed because the Aztec Empire was conquered between 1519 and 1521, whereas the San Nicolás de Bari Hospital was founded in 1503.[6]

Hospitals in the United States

The earliest institutions in the United States were poor houses and guest houses, resembling those of the medieval era in Europe. The first such hospital was at Henricopolis, Virginia in 1612; then came Blockley in Philadelphia in 1732; and later the Poorhouse in New York in 1736.

The first hospital of the nation that more closely approximated hospitals as we know them today was the Pennsylvania Hospital founded in 1751. Then came the New York Hospital in 1791, and later the Massachusetts General Hospital in 1821. They were better than most European hospitals of the same period.

Pennsylvania Hospital is therefore the oldest hospital in the United States. It was founded in 1751 by Benjamin Franklin and

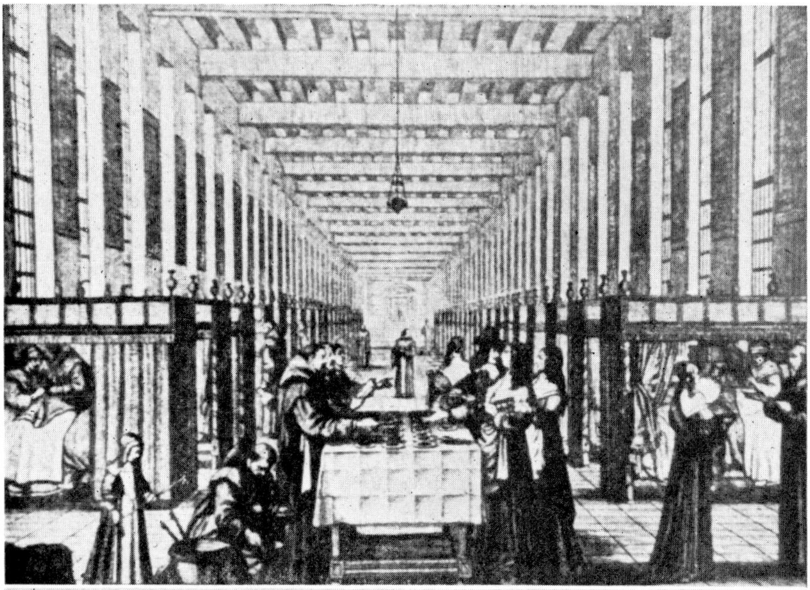

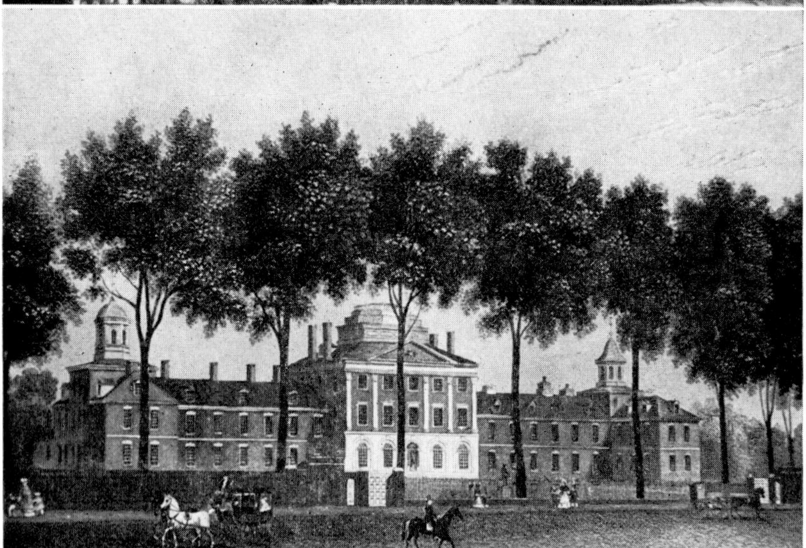

Fig. 128. Interior of the Hospital de la Charité at Paris (during the reign of Louis XIII). (Engraving in Carnavalet Museum.)

Fig. 129. Pennsylvania Hospital, Philadelphia. (Engraving by W. E. Tucker.)

Dr. Thomas Bond. No city in America possessed better facilities than Philadelphia to fulfill the postulates of Dr. Morgan that students be trained both in medical theory and at the bedside. The city's leading doctors and teachers volunteered as the hospital's consultants. To be admitted as candidates for a degree, students had to "walk the ward." From its very inception, the Pennsylvania Hospital has been an important educational center of medicine.

BENJAMIN RUSH (1745-1813) was one of the first Americans to gain world repute. He was born in Philadelphia, studied medicine in Edinburgh, and was apprentice to Dr. John Redman. He was an intellectual great. He was not a peaceable man, and in spite of his quarrelsome nature, he became an overpowering figure in American medicine. Shippen, Morgan and Rush comprised a formidable triumvirate. He seldom missed a day of rounds in forty-three years, at the Pennsylvania Hospital. He was a firm believer in bloodletting for which he was severely criticized. In 1793, when yellow fever was rampant, he was accused of killing more people by his bloodletting than all those who died of yellow fever. However, his popularity continued because people recognized that he was selfless in his devotion to the sick.[8]

Quite a number of ectopic pregnancies were reported in the 18th Century,[9] and most were discovered post mortem. Giovanni Battista Bianchi was the first of this century to attempt to classify ectopic pregnancy. In this entire century, no attempt was ever made to remove an ectopic mass.

JOHN BARD (1716-1799), father of Samuel Bard (1742-1821), who studied under Boerhaave in Edinburgh, was the first to report extra-uterine pregnancy in America. After its degeneration, it was incised at its most prominent part, a fistula resulted, and a large cavity was present (this was a full-time pregnancy). The cavity eventually (ten weeks) closed by the use of fomentations. According to 18th century records, this was an ovarian pregnancy. He was physician to George Washington and Benjamin Franklin. He moved from Philadelphia to New York City.

Pierre Duverney (1650-1728) in 1708 was the first to notice simultaneous extra- and intrauterine pregnancy. He also attempted original studies on the migration of the ovum.[10]

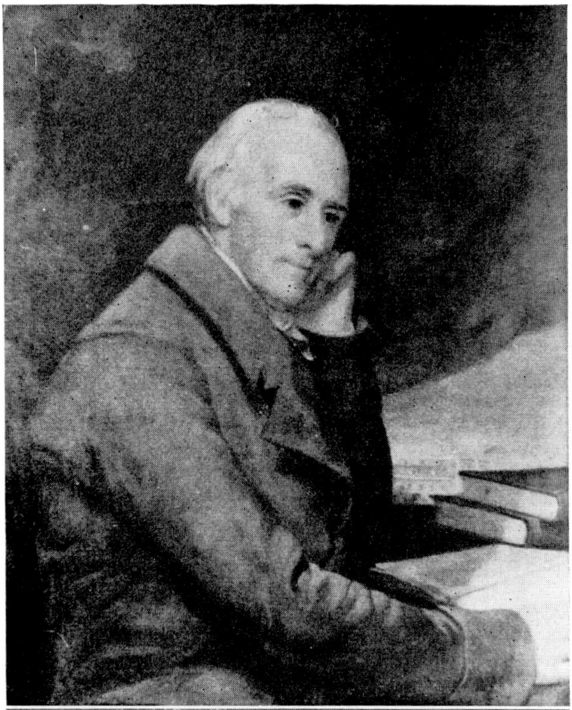

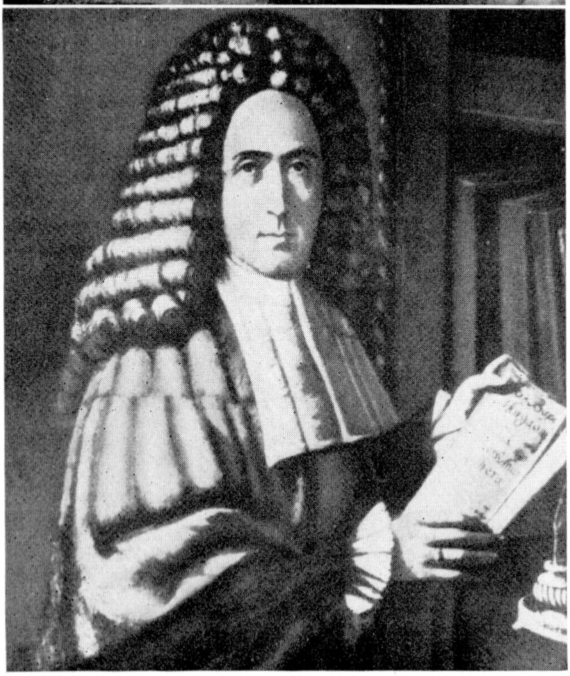

Fig. 130. Dr. Benjamin Rush. (Addison, Agnes: *University of Pennsylvania Medical School, Portraits*. Philadelphia, University Press, 1940.)

Fig. 131. G. B. Morgagni. (The Bettmann Archive.)

J. J. Courtial, Professor of Medicine at Toulouse, and Jouy, surgeon at the Hotel Dieu of Paris reported full-term abdominal pregnancies.[11]

Robert Houstoun in 1717 and Charles Kelly in 1763 made the diagnosis of full-term abdominal pregnancy. In neither case did the patient permit operation; they died years later, after the establishment of a fistula, at which time the diagnosis was confirmed.[12]

Smellie, in the 18th Century, abstracted the first case of ovarian pregnancy, a case that was operated by St. Maurice in 1682.[13]

Alexis Littre in 1701 found an early pregnancy of the left ovary.[14]

Varocquier in 1756 presented an ovarian pregnancy the size of a hen's egg, to the Academy of Science.[15]

G. Thom in 1781 described a case of ovarian pregnancy.[16]

Pierre Dionis gave the first clear description of interstitial pregnancy. He discussed the constriction of the tubal lumen, the size of the impregnated ovum and its arrest in the passage of the uterine cavity.[17]

Jean Astruc described a similar entity (constricted lumen at uterine end, etc.) but also gave as the cause of this accident, moral and mental influences.[18] This same sort of explanation is found in the early part of the next century by other authors; for example, Marc, in his book, says, "this patient heard the key of her door turn while in the arms of her lover."[19] Then there is Guillemot's reference "a stone was thrown through the window during intercourse."[20] Lallemand, "a stranger entered the woman's room immediately after intercourse."[21]

In this century, the concept of the physiology of reproduction was advanced but little. Nicholas Hartsoeker (1656-1725) was the first to describe peristalsis of the tube for propelling the ovum. Until Antonio Vallisnieri (1661-1730) settled the issue, all sorts of bizarre ideas prevailed as to the route of the sperm to meet the ovum; some believed the passage took place through the blood vessels, some did say that the tubes were the passageway of the sperm, and many traced its course through the wall of the uterus. They spoke of corpora lutea, and a good bit of original work was done by many investigators, however they did not get much further than von Graaf of the past century. In this century, they were quite concerned with the theories of generation, maturation of the follicle, ovulation, fertilization, nidation and fetal development. Most of the publications were a rehash of hackneyed ideas. The only original and epochal contribution in this field, at this time, was by Caspar Friedrich Wolff, after whom the Wolffian bodies were named, aroused no interest, not even by the great A. von Haller, to whom it was dedicated. It was the revival of the doctrine of epigenesis "the gradual building up of the parts," a theory hinted by Aristotle and advanced by Harvey. John Hunter in 1799 performed the first artificial insemination in a woman. Lazzaro Spallanzani, a few years earlier, 1780, successfully artificially inseminated a bitch.[22]

As far as menstruation was concerned, the only bit of knowledge contributed was that the bleeding came from a congested uterus; this was noted by Morgagni at autopsy, by Santorini, Smellie and, among the first to make this assertion, John Freund of England.

Anatomy and surgery offered very little over the past century. William Cowper (1666-1709) an English surgeon anatomist described para urethral glands now called Cowper's glands, in 1694. Such conditions as placental misplacements and its bleeding, abortal conditions and malpositions of the uterus were not appreciably elucidated during this period.

Malpositions of the uterus were noted as far back as ancient times, and were usually associated with pregnancy and given as the cause of difficult labor. In the 18th Century we find similar reference to malpositions complicating pregnancy, beginning with Deventer in 1701. The first observation, that an oblique uterus was usually to the right because of the sigmoid, was made by J. G. Günz. John Maubray in 1724 described the retroverted uterus. Hunter, Smellie and Hengeston are all associated with the early history of retroversion; Smellie advised the use of a pessary, which were in fairly common use at this time and were usually made of wood, leather, metal and cork; and to Hunter may be ascribed the first use of the term "retroversion," in 1770. Apparently retroversion and retroflexion were terms used interchangeably; it was Thomas Denman, the English obstetrician, who coined the phrase "retroflexion."

The origin of modern pathological anatomy occurred in this century; the two men most responsible were Bichat and GIOVANNI

BATTISTA MORGAGNI (1682-1771), who was really the founder of pathologic anatomy. Hydatid cysts of the ovary and broad ligament are named after him. In this century doctors tried hard to build valid systems in medicine; they made great strides in bedside teaching, but the scientific results remained poor, until the year 1761, when Morgagni published a book of two volumes that was to rejuvenate medicine with the spirit of observation. The title of this book was *de Sedibus et Causis Morborum*, and it dealt with the "seats" and causes of diseases. He was eighty years old when this work was published. He pronounced the organ as the seat of disease, then proceeded brilliantly to link up changes in function to pathological changes. Morgagni's erudite book established the high standards that made clinical pathology a leading discipline in the next century.[23]

MARIE FRANCOIS XAVIER BICHAT (1771-1802) in his short life, added invaluable information to our science by ascribing diseases to organic changes in the tissues, whereas Morgagni ascribed disease to the organs.

Leucorrhea was one of the commonest and most assiduously studied conditions during this time. They were absolutely in the dark concerning this gynecological disturbance. They considered it a symptom and also a disease. They believed it to be an elimination from the blood stream or the lymphatics. Their beliefs in this condition were awry because they had practically no knowledge of bacteriology and infection. Volumes were written on the subject; one of the largest texts on leucorrhea was written by Wenclsla Trnka de Krzowitz. In 1798, J. F. W. Seegert published a thesis on the subject. Humidity, climatic changes and soil dampness were the commonest causes. Also a "plentitude of humors and suppression of the menses" was a generally accepted cause by many of the 18th Century physicians who studied this condition, and most of them agreed it came from the pelvic organs. Some went so far as to minutely differentiate between discharge from the vagina as against that from the uterus.

Gonorrhea as against a pure "fluor albus" was likewise being tremendously discussed during this period. Some believed that a neglected leucorrhea usually led to a gonorrhea, while a chronic gonorrhea led to a luetic infection. A number of books were published on venereal diseases; they were by William Cockburn (1669-1739) who wrote *The Symptoms, Naute, Cause and Cure of a Gonorrhea*, London 1713. Cockburn was one of the few men of his time who believed that gonorrhea and syphilis were two separate entities. Jean Astruc, Benjamin Bell and John Hunter also wrote on the subject.

The use of the speculum received a mild forward impetus in the 18th Century; it was mentioned frequently, yet doctors never used it much or efficiently. Jean Astruc even wrote about the speculum in 1761, still it was not until the early 19th Century that Recamier reintroduced it to the medical profession. Its use goes back to ancient times, seemingly going through cycles of use and disuse, only to be revived at a later time. We might say of the speculum in the 18th Century that it was simply stirring.

JEAN ASTRUC (1684-1766) graduated from Montpellier, and then served on the staffs of Montpellier and Toulouse. He was an ardent student and critic of the Bible, especially the Old Testament. One of his first publications was on venereal diseases.[24] While the difference between gonorrhea and lues was not known by the majority of physicians of this period, Astruc clearly described the chancre, the secondaries and knew of its contagiousness. However, his greatest literary contribution was his six volume work on diseases of women *Traite des Maladies des Femmes*. It was a massive and exceedingly detailed work. Astruc was eighty-one years old when he completed this group of books. He was erudite and also a physician who had an extensive clinical experience. Like the others of his age, his writings were replete with theories and system. Instead of basing his studies on scientific observation, he had a logical cause for all phenomena. According to him, all genital pathology was the result of derangement of the uterine lymphatics. His volumes contained medical gynecology mainly, surgery was slighted to such an extent that his works could be captioned, and correctly so, as medical gynecology.

Most of the material found in his six volumes on *The Treatment of Diseases of Women* is the run of the mill information prevalent in that day. In other words, he contributed very little original material; in fact, much of his medicine goes back to the methods of the ancients, although not entirely. For example, he did not concur with rough methods for replacement of a prolapsed uterus as prescribed by the ancients, such as the application of a red hot iron near the organ, showing the patient a rat or any other means that might frighten her.

A relatively original paragraph is his reference to bimanual examination of the pelvis, and the value of the speculum. In all his writings one is impressed with the keen clinical observations. This is especially noticeable in his section on inflammatory diseases of the adnexa, which he describes accurately, but shows complete lack of understanding as to the method of extension and its etiology.

It seems as though he used the lymphatics to explain most everything, even cancer. He considered "schirrus" growths of lymphatic origin, and from it came the cancer ultimately. Again he refers to the lymph as the basis of menstruation, in which he avers that an accumulation and then a separation of lymph in the uterus is the cause of menstruation. He was the first to initiate the argument that menstrual blood was not an accumulation of bad humours, the current belief; instead, he said it was "laudable and good."

He applied the same principles, logic and thought in almost all known gynecological and obstetrical conditions of his time, such as sterility, miscarriage, abortions, fibroids and moles. As mentioned already, he rarely suggested or participated in surgical gynecological procedures.

Logic, reason and humanitarianism have, so far, been the basis from which medicine has evolved in this century. This designation is more properly applicable to obstetrics than to gynecology, for this is the period when obstetrics became, for the first time, a serious specialty. The only operative procedures tried during this century were the occasional attempt at repair of a third degree perineal tear, paracentesis of large ovarian cysts, and incision for imperforate hymen. While there appeared some interest in a cystocele and rectocele, very little surgery was done for these conditions except in very rare instances when suturing was performed. Instead of the word cystocele they spoke of hernia of the bladder, and for rectocele they used the term rectal hernia. It was in this century that enterocele was first noted and described. There was nothing done about malignant ulcerative processes; the subject, however, received much vocal attention, particularly toward the end of the century.

Uterine displacements were studied and the terms retroversion, retroflexion and anteversion were introduced in the literature. Prolapse and elongated, hypertrophied cervix was better understood; elongated cervix as such was never mentioned before this century. Surgery for prolapse was still a rarity. There was nothing new offered as far as fibroids are concerned; they did remove pedunculated and accessible fibroids from the vagina by using bizarre instruments. "Incontinentia urinae," meaning vesico-vaginal fistulae, a term not used in this century, received much attention. The surgical treatment of this condition was still very unsatisfactory; they cauterized or denuded the edges and approximated these raw surfaces with stay pins or sharp goose quills. Because bacteriology was still unknown, there was not much understanding of pelvic infections. In 1776, drainage through the abdomen of a huge pelvic abscess was recorded. Also in this century, an occasional incision through the vaginal cul de sac for abscess was performed.

Attempts at differentiation of discharges was made in this century without too much advance; they did begin to suspect the infectious nature of gonorrhea, and that it could involve the urethra and rectum and the eyes of the newborn.

Regner de Graaf's studies on the ovarian follicles and the corpus luteum stimulated the study of impregnation and sterility.

In obstetrics, Levret is considered by many the most important obstetrician of the 18th Century. Others have placed Smellie in this category. At any rate, both are responsible for placing the stamp of a science on obstetrics, and separating it from surgery. Their influence had spread throughout England and Europe, starting a chain reaction throughout the world in the science of obstetrics which had contributed to the advancement of this specialty. Because Smellie was a trifle earlier than Levret in his birth, it is fitting to begin a brief history of these two great men,[25] starting with Smellie.

William Smellie (1697-1763) was born in Lanarkshire, as was William Hunter, John Hunter and William Cullen. He studied medicine at Glasgow, did general practice for twenty years, and taught obstetrics in London. By some he was considered as uncouth and rough, and with big hands fit only to hold horses by the nose whilst they are shod. Some of his colleagues described him as the

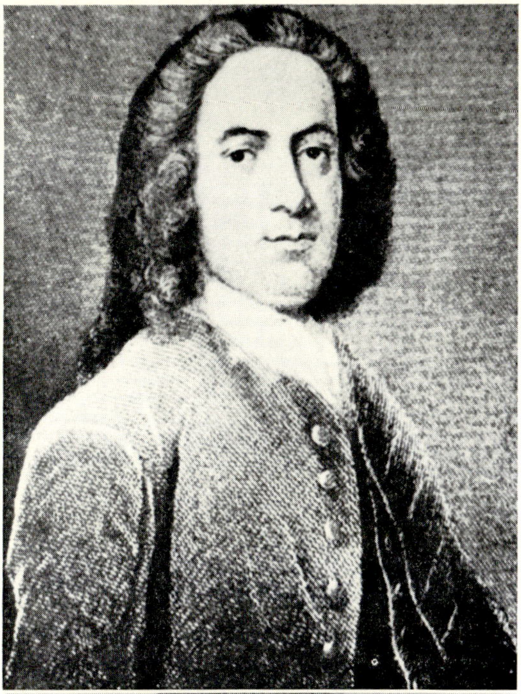

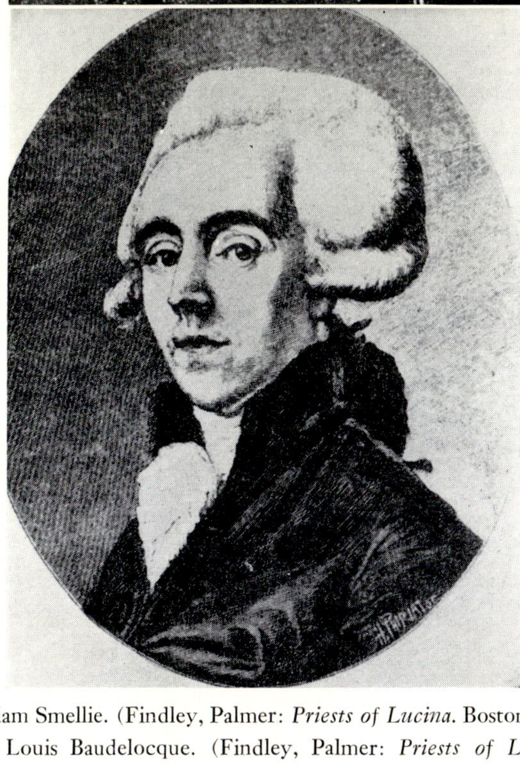

Fig. 132. William Smellie. (Findley, Palmer: *Priests of Lucina.* Boston, Little, 1939.)

Fig. 133. Jean Louis Baudelocque. (Findley, Palmer: *Priests of Lucina.* Boston, Little, 1939.)

"Master of British Midwifery" and one of the most important obstetricians of all times and countries. He had an apothecary shop in Pall Mall, where he privately taught obstetrics for a fixed fee.

In his practice he began the use of forceps with the Dusée type of instrument which was often confused with the Butter forceps. This he found mechanically inefficient, so he switched to Chapman's forceps, which also was unsatisfactory. So he had a very short pair of forceps made in boxwood with leather covering. The patient did not feel the cold metal and at the same time would not hear the click when the two blades were brought together. He felt that whenever possible the patient should not be aware of what was being done. So he taught his students to carry the blades in their side pockets, and to be drawn out secretly and applied under the covers. Manipulations under the bedclothes were still the mode, for there still was some prejudice against men midwives, and it was considered shameful for any man to glimpse the process of delivery.

It was not too many years before this when the obstetrician tied the corners of the top blanket round their necks. With no direct vision possible. Smellie in one of his deliveries divided the cord on the wrong side of the ligature so that a fair amount of bleeding occurred before he could again control the bleeding. Smellie, who had often been considered a very slow thinker, was quite quick witted in this instance; he explained to the midwives associated in the delivery that this was his method of preventing convulsions in the baby. He also invented a long curved forceps and covered the handles with leather (as noted before) for which he was roundly criticized because of infection.

In 1751, he introduced a steel lock forceps with the curved and double curved blades. He was the first to measure the diagonal conjugate manually, and was the first to add a pelvic curve to the forceps. The forceps which he developed with the lock and with the cephalic and pelvic curvature are basically the same forceps that are in use today with minor variations. Although he was accused of being overzealous in the use of the forceps, his figures show that he used it in only 1 per cent of his cases.

Another instrument that he devised was a crotchet. Smellie was a firm believer in knowing the mechanism of normal labor, and reduced interference to the necessary minimum. That is why he preferred a forceps with comparatively short blades, and one without too much mechanical advantage; that is, one that would only be of much assistance when the head was well down in the pelvis, thus minimizing damage to both mother and child. It is in this particular that he differed markedly from Levret, who felt the forceps should be one with the greatest mechanical advantage. He used his long forceps only for the aftercoming head and for breeches. He invented this long forceps in 1754, and never taught its use to his students because he was fearful of the damage it might cause.

He was the first to recognize the influence of rickets on the pelvis, and carefully described the deformity and how the sacrum was pushed toward the pubis. It was in such cases where his estimation of the internal conjugate by finger measurements stood him in good stead. He also spoke of the generally contracted pelvis.

Smellie and Levret also differed in the procedure of podalic version, Smellie used to introduce his hand outside the membranes so as to give the baby more room to move. Levret, on the other hand, introduced his hand inside the "water bag" so as not to dislodge the placenta. They applied forceps on the after coming head with the same maneuver used by Mauriceau.

Although his anatomical interest centered primarily on the bony structures, he did make important observations on the other structures. He concluded that neither the round nor the broad ligaments underwent any extraordinary extension during gestation; they were loose in the nongravid state so could readily expand or move up and out toward their points of attachment. Many, and Philipp Adolph Boehmer (1717-1789) in particular, thought otherwise.

There were numerous reports of ruptured uteri in the 18th Century, and these were taken from post mortem examination. Smellie was among these reporters. The first attempt to suture such a rupture was made by Lebas (1717-1797).

He was the first to refer to post-partum sulci tears of the vagina and laceration of the cervix.

He saw many cases of vesico-vaginal fistulae from childbirth and instrumentation. He rarely advised operation, instead he suggested the use of the inlaying catheter.

For uterine retrodisplacements and for prolapse he used a round pessary; he rarely suggested operation for prolapse except when gangrene was beginning and had not reached the area through which amputation was to be done. This was the accepted approach in this period.

His experience with ovarian pregnancy was limited, although he did abstract the first case on record, that of de Saint Maurice in 1682.

He was the first to suggest leucorrhea as a cause of sterility.

His views on menstruation are very interesting, for it seems he suspected what we know today, that the endocrines were the activators of the bleeding. Like his contemporaries he believed menstruation was initiated by a cyclic congestion of the uterus. He did not talk only of lymph, as did most of his confreres, but he actually stated that the uterine sinuses and small vessels were gradually stretched until rupture occurred. What concerned him particularly, and this was not mentioned by others, was that the same thing did not occur in the blood vessels of the nose, lungs, stomach and other organs. He did not know the answer but his thinking was in the right direction. He had noticed that delicate and well-fed women menstruated more frequently and in greater amounts than women who exercised much and perspired freely; he considered both normal, so in treating these patients he bled the profuse bleeders moderately just before the period and added cooling douches to his therapy. The scant bleeders he bled more, purged them, ordered warm baths and exercises.

With justification, Smellie may be considered the greatest pioneer in scientific obstetrics, one who so developed the forceps that it has not really been improved to this day, and one who may be called the founder of pelvimetry.

A Course of Lectures upon Midwifery in 1742 was his first publication. His most important books were *Treatise on the Theory and Practice of Midwifery* in 1752, and the *Set of Anatomical Tables* in 1754. The famous Rymsdyk drew most of the plates, but Smellie drew many of them himself.

ANDRE LEVRET (1703-1780) was born in Paris. He was to Paris what Smellie was to London. Like Smellie he invented a forceps with a pelvic curve, the difference as mentioned, in the paragraph on Smellie, being the mechanical advantage and compression obtained on the baby's head by Levret's forceps, something that Smellie did not approve. He also devised a crotchet. He did much work on the "normal tilt or inclination of the pelvic plane." Except for a few differences Levret and Smellie paralleled each other considerably in their work. In pelvic mensuration Levret deserves less credit than Smellie. Levret was one of the first to observe that retention of the placenta was not necessarily due to malformation of the uterus, as was thought, but could be due to irregularities of uterine contraction. Levret observed the three pelvic planes, the inlet, mid-pelvis and the outlet; their measurements and shapes were noted. Deventer, whom he tried to correct, Smellie and Levret —all three were pioneers in pelvimetry. The consensus of opinion favors Smellie as the most outstanding in this facet of obstetrics.

He wrote *Accouchemens Laborieux*, but his best known publication was in 1753. It was called *L'Art des Accouchemens demontre par les principes de physique et de mecanique.*

JEAN LOUIS BAUDELOCQUE (1748-1810) is ranged with Mauriceau, Levret and even Tarnier who was the greatest of French obstetricians. He was born at Heilly in the Somme. He became head of the Department of Midwifery in the Medical School of Paris, but he soon resigned because of the pressure from his private practice. He improved on Smellie and Levret's knowledge of the diameter of the pelvis in the living woman and interpreted more clearly the movements of the baby in its passage through the pelvis. Although he leaned greatly on the works of his predecessors, Smellie and Levret, he popularized and improved the best of their teachings.

His claim to distinction rests largely upon his development of the technique of measuring the diameters of normal and contracted pelves in living women and in correlating their relationships to the measurements of the fetal head. This was a noteworthy contribution and one that paved the way for a better understanding of the problems involved in obstructed labor. He first described the external conjugate diameter, now know as the "diameter of Baudelocque."

While Mauriceau would not perform cesarean operations except upon dead mothers, Baudelocque maintained that many such operations were performed successfully upon living mothers, and would do so if there was no other means of delivery. This attitude is interesting because he was sued, toward the end of his career, for the death of such a patient. It should be remembered that such an operative procedure involved extreme risks, and therefore daring on the surgeon's part, for the technique of this age included no anesthesia, only very little cleanliness (no knowledge of infection as yet), and only very little hemostasis was practiced.

His literary contributions were *L'Art des accouchemens*, Paris, 1775; *An in partu propter augustiam pelvis impossibili symphysis ossium pubis secunda*, Paris, 1776; and *Principles of Obstetrics*, Paris, 1775. His writings were translated into English and became very popular in the United States.[26]

When Smellie retired in 1759, he was succeeded by JOHN HARVIE (circa 1710-1770), who continued the Harvey and Smellie tradition in London. He emphasized the importance of protecting the perineum and the necessity of delivering the placenta without violence. As far back as the time of Soranus the importance of protecting the perineum was known, but the necessity of delivering the placenta without violence antedates Credé by ninety years.

In the meantime one of the most famous lying-in hospitals was being created in Dublin. It began with BARTHOLOMEW MOSSE (1712-1759) who graduated from the King's and Queen's College in 1742. He died at the early age of forty-seven years, and although the Rotunda in Dublin was not so called during Mosse's time, he certainly is responsible for its inception.

FIELDING OULD (1710-1789) was appointed Master of the Rotunda Lying-in Hospital in 1759, succeeding the founder and First Master Mosse. Ould was knighted and did an extensive obstetrical practice. He advanced the knowledge on the mechanism of labor. He delivered all his patients in the left lateral position, for he did not agree with Deventer and Mauriceau that the lateral oblique position of the uterus was the cause of many difficult labors. He further disagreed with Deventer's idea that the uterus becomes thinner as the pregnancy advances. Sir Fielding Ould, therefore, becomes the first important Irish teacher of midwifery.[27]

Other obstetricians of the early 18th Century who were associated with the forceps, as already mentioned in Chapter XIII, "History of the Forceps," are to be discussed at this point for their attributes other than those of the forceps, even though none of them made any great scientific contributions. A brief dissertation on these men at this time will at least maintain a chronological sequence in our story.

JEAN PALFYN of Ghent, who is best remembered for his forceps which was a reconstructed Chamberlen forceps, with which he had no success; in fact, no one paid any attention to it whatsoever.

He was a widely known obstetrician in his time; he wrote an anatomy text on midwifery, and was one of the early obstetricians to describe perineal lacerations and reported a hernia with its sac containing the bladder which had been displaced by a fibroid. He was almost completely forgotten soon after his death.

WILLIAM GIFFARD was an English obstetrician, also best known for his forceps. He was the first to suggest the Von Ritgen maneuver in 1731. He wrote *Cases in Midwifery*, a book that was revised and published by his friend Edward Hody, M.D., in 1734. In this book he discussed the difference between placenta previa and separation. He also described a case of mole. An unusual case of ectopic pregnancy with the fetal mass ulcerating through the rectum and being expelled through the anus, is also found in this book. It is so unusual and interesting that I shall quote this case and the autopsy report; the post-mortem examination was performed by Giffard and Mr. Nourse of St. Bartholomew Hospital.

> The Fallopian Tube on the right side, we traced from the Fundus Uteri almost to the Morsus Diaboli, where it open'd into, and was confusedly and closely united with a Sacculus, immediately to be described. The Ovary on this side, together with the Ligamentum latum, was dilated into a large Sacculus of an irregular form, extending itself behind the Uterus, (to the back part of which it adhered) and passing on towards the left side, was connected to that part of the Colon that terminates in the Rectum. In this Sacculus we found part of a Placenta, and the Remains of the lacerated Membranes; and besides the Aperture of the Fallopian Tube mention'd before, there was another about four inches in Diameter, into the middle of the Rectum.[29]

DUSÉE of Paris, and ALEXANDER BUTTER of Edinburgh, practiced obstetrics in the early 18th Century. Their historical importance depends strictly on their relationship with the forceps; this has already been discussed in Chapter XII.

EDMUND CHAPMAN also practiced obstetrics at this time. His fame rests entirely on his exposure of the Chamberlen secret when he published a detailed description of the forceps with illustrations.

JOHN BURTON (1710-1771) was an outstanding obstetrician of this century, even though he did not make any really important contributions. He is probably better known to the lay literary world than to medicine, thanks to Lawrence Sterne, an obscure country parson who wrote *Tristram Shandy* in which he cast Dr. Burton as "Dr. Slop." Burton was known as Dr. Slop even before Sterne wrote his book, so there is pretty good evidence that Burton and Dr. Slop are one and the same. Cruikshank,* the greatest satirist and caricaturist of this century, gave an assist in this presentation of Burton as Dr. Slop whom Sterne presented as a "little squat, uncourtly figure of about four feet and a half perpendicular height, with a breadth of back and a sesquipedality of belly which might have done honor to a sergeant of the horseguards."

Dr. John Burton was born in Colchester and received his medical degree from St. John's College, and later studied under Boerhaave in Leyden and Gregorie in Paris and receiving an M.D. in Rheims. He spent most of his life in New York where he founded a hospital. He was supposed to have invented a forceps, a modified old French type. He also invented a perforator extractor which he considered much superior to similar instruments used by men like Mauriceau and Deventer. His forceps was severely criticized by Simpson, who said "they are ingenious, but very unserviceable . . . working like a lobster's claw." Smellie must have partaken of such criticism, for Burton roundly berated Smellie for his "gross mistakes and dangerous methods of practice." This was put in a letter that was insolent and censorious but displayed the remarkable literary qualities of the author. One of the criticisms that he heaped upon Smellie was a repetition of other men's disapproval of Smellie's practice of wrapping leather round his forceps. One of the sentences of this critical letter stated:

* See page 253.

> Some part of the Blood and Water must be sucked up by the Leather, and lodge betwixt it and the steel work, where it will corrupt the stink, let the Maker be as careful as he will in covering it . . . and in some Cases, perhaps, may convey infection.

Of the many writings of Burton, his work of greatest interest to obstetricians and gynecologists was a book of four parts, anatomy and physiology of the reproductive organs, diseases of the pregnant woman, "preternatural labours" and lastly a part on abortions. At the end of his book he gives an illustrated description of his forceps. The name of this work was *Essay Towards a Complete New System of Midwifery, Theoretical and Practical, together with Several New Improvements whereby women may be delivered in the most dangerous cases with more ease, safety and expedition than by any other method heretofore practiced.* This was published in 1751. It never became popular, in fact it was severely criticized, and referred to in *Tristram Shandy* as "the five shilling book on midwifery."

Although Barton did not make any great original contributions to obstetrics, he was very influential in obstetrics in his day, even though it was thought that his practice of midwifery was simply a means to an end, and that was to be an antiquarian. His object was to make sufficient money in obstetrics to be able to afford to devote his energies to antiquarian research. However, he spent his entire life practicing obstetrics; a life full of controversies, and political and religious persecution.[30]

George Cruikshank (1792-1878) was an English artist, caricaturist and illustrator who found satiric material in all levels of life about him—in national, political and public events, in high life and low life, the follies of the great, everyday ills and misadventures. Many of his cartoons were colored by hand.[31]

William Hunter (1718-1783) was one of the greatest names in gynecology, as well as in obstetrics and anatomy. Together with William Smellie his predecessor and teacher, he is regarded as having established scientific gynecology and obstetrics in Great Britain. He was born in Lanarkshire, Glasgow. He studied for the ministry which he relinquished after five years, and went to Glasgow under the tutelage of Dr. William Cullen, who at the time was a

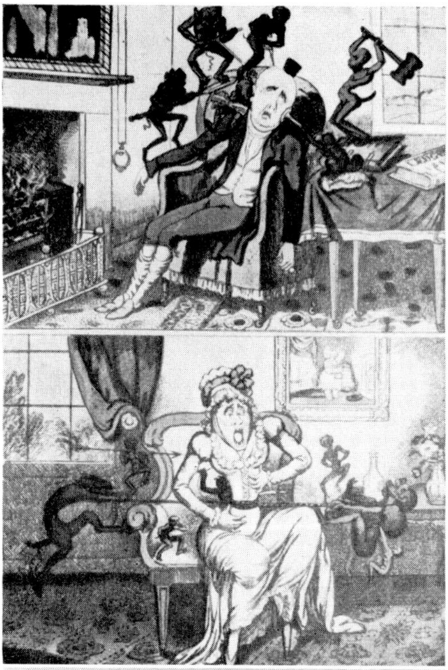

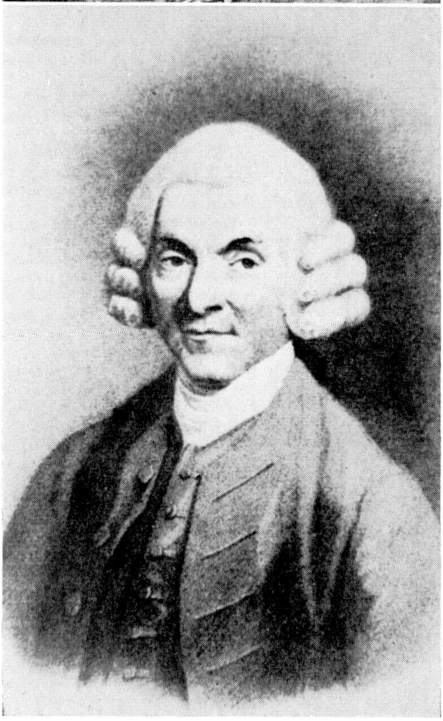

Fig. 134. Example of Cruikshank's art. (Dunham, J. S., ed.: *What's New*, No. 180, [The History of Medical Division, of the armed forces medical library]. Chicago, Abbott Laboratories, 1953, p. 12.)

Fig. 135. William Hunter. (Findley, Palmer: *Priests of Lucina*. Boston, Little, 1939.)

country doctor, but later became Professor of Medicine at Glasgow and afterwards at Edinburgh. They formed a partnership in which Hunter acted as Cullen's assistant. He also studied obstetrics with Smellie, and whereas Smellie was primarily interested in the clinical side of obstetrics, Hunter decided to study physiology and anatomy to use them as a basis for his clinical practice; he studied both in Edinburgh and in London, and it was here that he met Smellie, and, in fact, lived with him for a year.

While in London he studied and attended the lectures of Dr. Frank Nicholls. Then he went to live with a Dr. James Douglas, an anatomist of considerable repute, for whom he did innumerable dissections, and in the meantime he made trips to Paris and Holland to further his education. When he finally settled down for himself in London, in 1746, he advertised in a London paper that he would give lectures and instructions in anatomy. In 1749 he became surgeon man-midwife to the British Lying-in Hospital, having been appointed to a similar post the year before, to the Middlesex Hospital.

He gained lasting distinction when he taught anatomy because of his oratorical ability, thoroughness and because of his practical demonstrations. He lectured on medicine, surgery and physiology besides clinical obstetrics. While in Holland he learned to preserve bodies and specimens, from which many generations were taught. He had a passion for teaching anatomy. Said he:

> A man may do infinitely more good to the public by teaching his art than by practicing it. The good effects of the latter must center in the advantage of the few individuals that may be under his care as patients, but the influence of the teacher extends itself to the whole nation, and descends to posterity. Anatomy is the only solid foundation of medicine.

He was Professor of Anatomy in the Royal Academy of Arts, and three years later became its President. He endowed a professorship in anatomy, and founded the Hunterian Museum. He was obstetrician to Charlotte, Queen of George III. William Hunter was described as "a polite scholar, an accomplished gentleman, a complete anatomist, and probably the most perfect demonstrator, as well as lecturer, the world has ever seen." With his personal charm, his untiring energy and boundless ambition, he soon rose to high favor. He was esteemed as a friend by Samuel Johnson, James Boswell, Joshua Reynolds, David Garrick, William Hogarth, Thomas Gainsborough, and Oliver Goldsmith. His patients included many of the great women of England besides the queen, but many of the poor were also included in his list of patients. The women in particular were fond of him, the men thought he was conceited. He often said, "Now in my experience, etc., etc." which did not go over with the male element of the population. It was not long, however, before he replaced the prominent teachers of midwifery in London, for Douglas died, Manningham (who exposed the fraud of Maria Tofts, "the rabbit breeder") and Sandys were getting old, and Smellie was too crude to be favored with the patronage of the refined and fastidious.

He demonstrated the twofold nature of the circulation of the placenta, maternal and fetal. His brother John disputed his claim and tried to discredit him before the Royal Society. This feud separated the two brothers. Also, John claimed that the inner lining of the pregnant uterus was the product of inflammation, but William calling it decidua, held that it was nothing more than hypertrophied mucous membrane. William Hunter was the first to describe the round ligaments of the uterus and he named and defined the linea alba.

One of his greatest contributions was the proof that the lymphatics were not continuous with the blood vessels, as taught by his predecessors. He studied the embryo in its various stages of development. His anatomical researches, not his work as a clinician gave him his everlasting fame; the crowning work of his life, *The Anatomy of the Human Gravid Uterus*,[32] exhibited engraved figures; he started this work in 1750, and completed and published it in 1774. The pictures were engraved by the best masters; his brother John aided him in his dissections, from which the artists, Mr. Robert Strange, a Scotsman (who became Sir Robert later) and Van Rymsdyk made the engravings. The publisher was the Baskerville Press.

After Hunter's death, Matthew Baillie, his nephew, published (in 1794) an unfinished manuscript of Hunter's *An Anatomical Description of the Human Gravid Uterus and Its Contents*. Unfortunately Baillie used John's description of the decidua instead of

William's, thinking it was William's. Shortly after this publication by Baillie, a second edition of William Hunter's original work of 1774 was published by Lumley. Then a third publication by Cox was made in 1815. Some catalogues designate Lumley instead of Cox for this third edition*

One has only to see and examine these publications in order to appreciate their greatness and especially the remarkable engravings that illustrate them.** The neatness, the careful and methodical arrangement of its contents, and most of all the amazing engravings are extremely impressive. The more than thirty engravings are without a peer as works of art in this field. The illustrations are 19½ by 28 inches (covering both sides of the opened book). The pristine darkness of the ink gives a depth of tone that cannot be achieved by photography, and the selected details which the drawings contain are remarkable. Hunter, in the preface of one of these magnificent folios, indicates how much importance he attached to the engraver's art:

> The art of engraving supplies us, upon many occasions, with what has been the great desideratum of the lovers of science, an universal language. Nay, it conveys clearer ideas of most natural objects than words can express; makes stronger impressions upon the mind; and, to every person conversant with the subject, gives an immediate comprehension of what it represents.

The publisher deserves much credit for making up this beautiful edition, which we are discussing in some detail because one should be acquainted with the type of medical publications of this period, a sadly neglected art today. The cover of this book is a solid red, and in the center of the front cover is a black sticker four by five inches that contains a border of gold design, within which is a notation in gold lettering of varying sizes (see illustration).

The Title Page (see illustration) is divided in half by a horizontal line, the upper half is in Latin, the bottom half in English. Each half contains the title of the book and the author's name after which is the designation "Physician Extraordinary to the Queen, Pro-

* Mr. McDaniel, of the College of Physicians of Philadelphia, and the author checked catalogues and found that they differ as to the name of the publisher.

** The author owns one of the rare second edition Lumley publications and has therefore had ample opportunity to carefully study it.

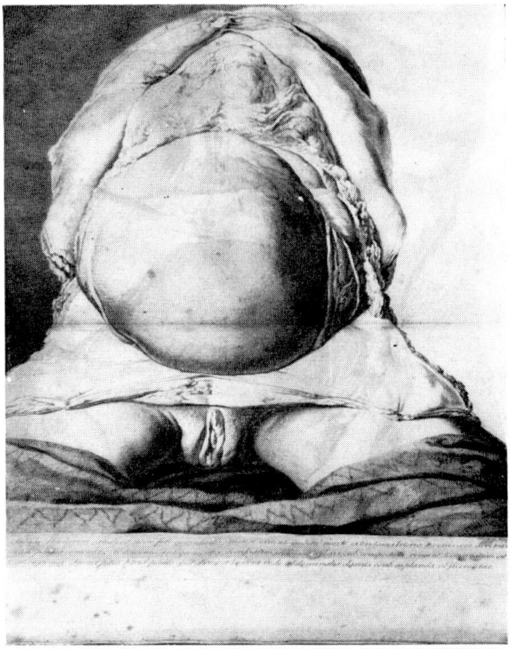

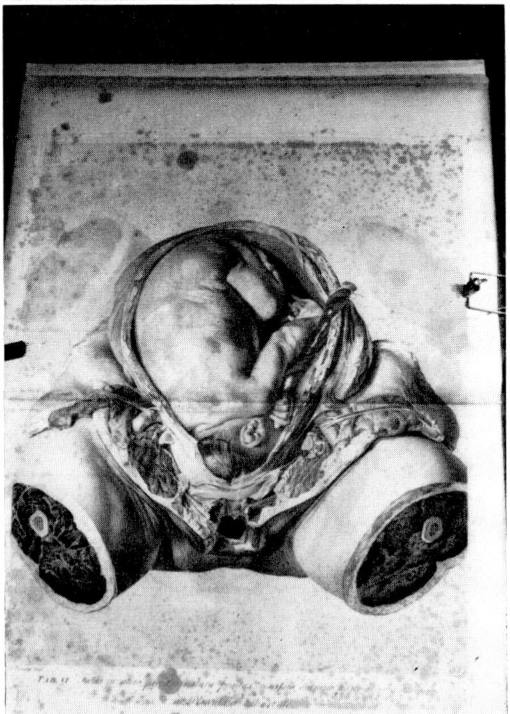

Fig. 136. Engraving from *Human Gravid Uterus* published by William Hunter. (Hunter, William: *The Human Gravid Uterus* [ed. of original 1774 text]. London, Lumley, 1798.)

Fig. 137. Engraving of fetus in utero from William Hunter's *Human Gravid Uterus*. (Hunter, William: *The Human Gravid Uterus* [ed. of original 1774 text]. London, Lumley, 1798.)

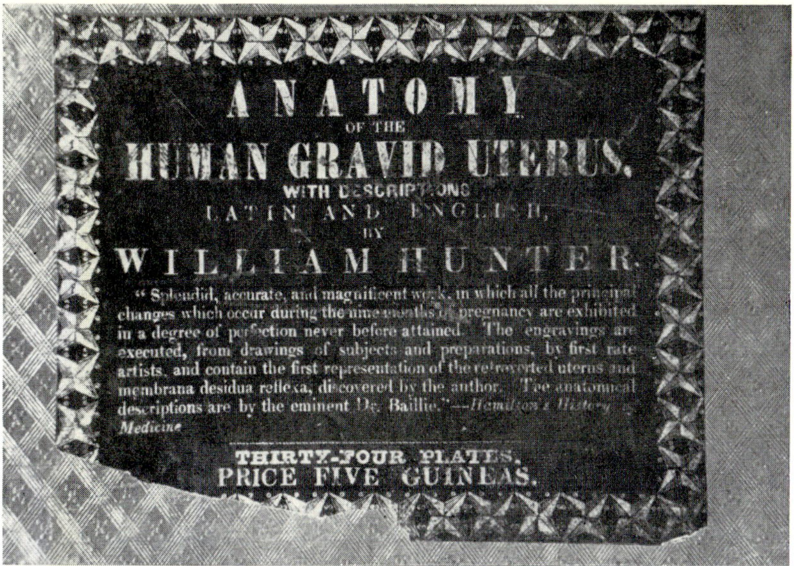

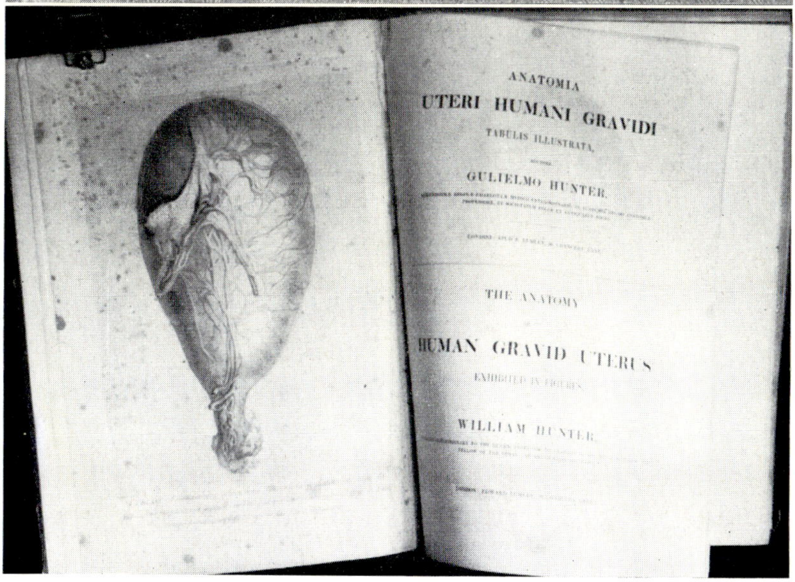

Fig. 138. Black and gold sticker on cover of Hunter's book *Human Gravid Uterus*. (Hunter, William: *The Human Gravid Uterus* [ed. of original 1774 text]. London, Lumley, 1798.)

Fig. 139. Title page from William Hunter's *Human Gravid Uterus*. (Hunter, William: *The Human Gravid Uterus* [ed. of original 1774 text]. London, Lumley, 1798.)

fessor of Anatomy in the Royal Academy, and Fellow of the Royal and Antiquarian Societies." The printed pages are divided in two by a vertical line; the left side is in Latin, the right in English. Each of the engravings, in almost every instance, occupies a spread of both pages, the right and left sides, making the drawings liberal in size.

William Hunter was conservative in his management of cases, and opposed many of the current procedures. In 1777 he published *Reflections on the Section of the Symphysis Pubis*, in which he cautioned against Camper and Sigault's proposal to sever the symphysis pubis in obstructed labor, for he said "the strongest joint in the body was weakened for an infinitesimal increase in space." Symphysiotomy never gained favor in England because Hunter disapproved. The use of the forceps which Smellie, his teacher, so strongly advocated, was considered of little use by Hunter, saying, "where they save one they murder twenty." He opposed cesarean section, and with reason, because the mortality was too high. His conservatism did get him into trouble. He counselled waiting, perhaps too long, before removing the placenta, and as a result of this principle the Countess of Suffolk died in delivery. As further evidence of his conservatism, his views on ovarian cysts are of interest, as far as his therapy was concerned. He was among the first, in 1775, to suggest tapping ovarian cysts, and later the same year recommended ovariotomy, yet he himself never did either of these procedures.

His views in obstetrics were so conservative that he influenced two generations of English obstetricians, who carried his policy of masterly inactivity to dangerous lengths. His life of self-denial is summed up by Stephen Paget:

> He never married; he had no country house; he looks in his portraits a fastidious, fine gentleman; but he worked till he dropped and he lectured when he was dying.

He was the first in Britain to apply enlightened methods of teaching and investigation to anatomy and, particularly, to the anatomy of obstetrics. He did as much for obstetrics as his brother John did for surgery.

Toward the end of the 18th Century, we began to see some light in a condition that was noted as far back as the time of Hippocrates, but did not become fully understood until the 19th Century. Hippocrates himself described the death of a patient from puerperal fever. William Harvey reported cases of high fever and offensive lochial discharges after an apparently normal delivery. Thomas Willis, in his 1660 edition of *De Febribus* used the phrase "puerperarum febris." Richard Morton, in 1691, wrote the phrase "febris puerpera." Others in the 17th Century dabbled with this condition which was not understood and its cause unknown.

In the 18th Century, Edward Strother, in 1716, wrote the *Criticon Febrium*—he called his cases "puerperal fever," so that it displaced the use of "child-bed fever" and "lying-in fever." Paul Jacques Maloruin in 1746, in the Hotel Dieu, described it clinically and post mortem. Thomas Kirkland, of London, in 1774, wrote a *Treatise on Child-bed Fevers*. Many other men had observed the train of events of puerperal infection. Among them were Clark, Denman, Burns, Young, Hamilton, Walker, Ramsbotham, Douglas and others. In the 18th Century the most important men who did outstanding work on "infection" are Alexander Gordon, Charles White and LUCAS JOHANN BOËR (1751-1835), who, after watching Denman and his contemporaries and particularly Charles White, introduced their methods, and with great success, in the Allegemeine Krankenhaus in Vienna. But it was not until the 19th Century that this issue became clarified and resolved through the efforts of Holmes in America and Semmelweis in Vienna. When Boër died, he was succeeded by a Johann Klein, whom Semmelweis assisted. By this time Boër had been forgotten and a high mortality in lying-in hospitals was accepted as normal. Semmelweis was also taught by Skoda and Rokitansky. It was Semmelweis who probably contributed the most. The complete 19th Century story of infection, which includes other illustrious names shall be taken up in the next chapter. For the present we shall discuss in more detail both White and Gordon of the 18th Century.

CHARLES WHITE (1728-1813) was born in Manchester on October fourth, the same year as John Hunter, the son of Thomas White, also a physician. He studied in London under William Hunter and also at Edinburgh. He had a collection of more than 300 specimens from which he lectured in anatomy. In 1772, he published a treatise for midwives based on a great number of patients he had seen; these cases were almost always in the most desperate of condition, for the midwives in Manchester, as elsewhere, were "ignorant women dominated by inveterate prejudices," and it was they who did most of the midwifery. The title of this work was *A Treatise on the Management of Pregnancy and Lying-in Women, and the Means of Curing, but more especially of Preventing the Principal Disorders to which they are Liable*, and it was dedicated to Dr. William Hunter. Of all his many treatises this one brought him the greatest fame. In this paper he made important recommendations on the conduct of delivery and the puerperium. He made a number of changes in what was then the accepted practice. He advised the use of baths during pregnancy and lactation, an innovation unheard of, being always considered dangerous under such circumstances especially. When the head appeared, he did not immediately grasp it and pull the baby out as was the usual practice, instead he allowed the shoulders to deliver themselves. Another of his suggestions, which we today think of as a modern innovation, was to allow the cord to stop pulsating before tying it. The most important practice that he instituted was to set the patient up in bed shortly after delivery, and often thereafter, this was one of his methods of attack on puerperal fever for it induced drainage; he said absorption caused this infection. To facilitate this maneuver he designed an adjustable bed and a chair; in this way he procured gravitational drainage. The same principle was evolved by Fowler a hundred years later, and was known as the "Fowler Position." He was most interested in prevention, and less in cure. He insisted upon absolute cleanliness of the lying-in chamber, adequate ventilation, and isolation of infected patients. Although this mode of approach to this devastating problem was not entirely new to White, he attacked the whole situation with more vigor and clarity than any of his predecessors. He seemed to recognize puerperal fever as a contagious disease. While this disease was rife and the death rate high, White had seen many cases but lost none.

He delivered his patients while they were in a horizontal position, on their left side, with the thighs drawn up, the accoucher placed at her back. It was the accepted custom to permit patients to do all sorts of gymnastics while in labor, such as standing, sitting, hanging by the arms between two persons, half sitting and half lying, either upon the bed or on the knee of an assistant. He thought such antics of service in expediting delivery, but he did not approve of the delivery of the child or the placenta in any position other than lying on her side, for they occasioned lacerations of the perineum and sphincter ani, prolapse of the vagina and anus, inversion of the uterus, retention of secundines, flooding, after pains, fainting and even death.

The same formula was used by most obstetricians, the following quotation from Alexander Hamilton, Professor of Midwifery in Edinburgh is offered as an example:

> The patient should be permitted to walk or rest in her usual postures till the os uteri is dilated, and the pains be frequent and pressing; she should then be placed on her side, with her knees drawn up; and in advanced labour they may be separated by a pillow and a resistance given to the feet by an assistant. Before she is placed in this position every indelicacy by frequent touching is highly improper.

It is not too many years ago that this position for delivery was used occasionally in some of the best obstetrical departments in the United States; however, this was not the rule.

In 1784, Charles White published *An Inquiry into the Nature and Cause of that Swelling in One or Both of the Lower Extremities, which sometimes happens to Lying-In Women.* This condition was known as "white leg." So to him goes the credit of being the first to describe "Phlegmasia alba dolens."

JOHN HULL (1761-1843) originated the name "Phlegmasia alba dolens" for "white leg" in 1800. He was born at Poulton, received his M.D. from Leyden University. In subsequent writings, Charles White called this condition "phlegmasia alba dolens puerperarum." John Hull had become physician to the Lying-in Charity. In 1801, he published *A Translation from the French of Two Memoirs on the Cesarean Operation by J. L. Baudelocque.* One of these copies fell into the hands of Dr. Jesse Bennett, in the United States. Baudelocque had reported thirty-one successes in over 1750 cases. John Hull shortly afterward reported on 73 cases, more than half of which were successful. Among his case reports was one by Jesse Bennett, who operated on his wife, at the same time sterilizing her; it was one of the first successful cesarean operations in the United States.

Toward the end of the 18th Century, cesarean section was such an explosive and controversial subject, that Manchester among other places was split into two extreme factions. Both White and Hull were severely criticized for approving the operation, because of its extremely high mortality. In the end, they, White and Hull, showed that a number of cases in which nothing was done because the crotchet or other means did not help; all died (mothers and babies). On the other hand, in some of the cesarean operations, either the mother or the baby was saved; so the results of cesarean were shown to be better than doing nothing and thus allowing both the patient and child to die. At any rate, to White and Hull goes the distinction of establishing cesarean section as a necessary and justifiable operation, especially in cases of gross deformity of the pelvis.

While Hull was famous for his stand on cesarean section, Charles White's fame rests on puerperal infection. White's influence spread throughout the world. Most important was his influence upon an Austrian named Boër, who against much opposition, introduced White's methods at the Vienna Lying-in Hospital.

Alexander Gordon (1752-1799). While Charles White was the very first to proclaim the doctrine of aseptic obstetrics, Alexander Gordon was the first writer to show clearly the infective nature of puerperal fever. He was born in Aberdeen, and studied at Marshall College, and later took up medicine at Aberdeen Infirmary and Edinburgh. In 1795 he wrote *Treatise on the Epidemic Puerperal Fever of Aberdeen* which showed how the disease was spread. Charles White in his treatise in 1773 showed how to treat this disease and made suggestions for its prevention. It must be conceded that Gordon's work probed deeper into the problem, and without this knowledge complete control was impossible. Gordon was influenced by Dr. John Clarke's observation made at the Store Street Lying-in Hospital, in which he related erysipelas to the epidemic disease of lying-in women. A break in the tissues permitted the entrance of the infecting agent (which they as yet did not know) and so erysipelas would result. They did not differentiate any wound that showed redness from true erysipelas. Gordon made an analogy with erysipelas and puerperal fever, because he realized that the fever did not occur in women until after delivery; in other words, wounds of entrance resulted from the childbirth. He realized that whatever the infective source was, one obtained it by being present in such a case, he even declared that he himself was the means of carrying the infection to a great number of women. He now realized that fresh air and cleanliness were not sufficient to eradicate the disease. Fire and smoke, in other words fumigation was his answer; so rooms, bedding, clothes of doctors and nurses should all be fumigated.

So by the end of the 18th Century all the knowledge needed had been accumulated, even if the actual offending organism was still unknown. Harvey had long ago recognized the large open areas after the placenta separated, Charles White stressed postural drainage and cleanliness, and Alexander Gordon contributed a new understanding of the mode of spread. Most physicians were slow to accept this knowledge, so many deaths continued in the early 18th Century. An abrupt change in results came in 1843, when Oliver Wendell Holmes presented a paper on the subject. Before this paper was presented, most doctors were harboring strong suspicions of the infectious nature of the disease, for they noted that one man would deliver scores of cases without incident, another would deliver just as many and most of them would develop the fever, especially if a physician had been called in consultation; in other words, the evidence pointed to a common carrier, but it was long before this was realized. The rest of the story of puerperal infection is part of nineteenth century history, so we shall continue with it in the next chapter.

Obstetrics had become so important and outstanding and scientific in the 18th century, that the dress of the newborn and even the wearing apparel of the pregnant woman was given serious consideration. It was during the 1740's that a group of pioneer pediatricians liberated babies from their life strangling bundles; a heavy, airtight wrapping of bandages, which was meant to keep the bad air out and the nourishing juices in, was applied to the newborn in the form of tight swaddling. This practice has gradually faded out, however, every now and then one comes across babies to whom this old-fashioned custom is still applied.

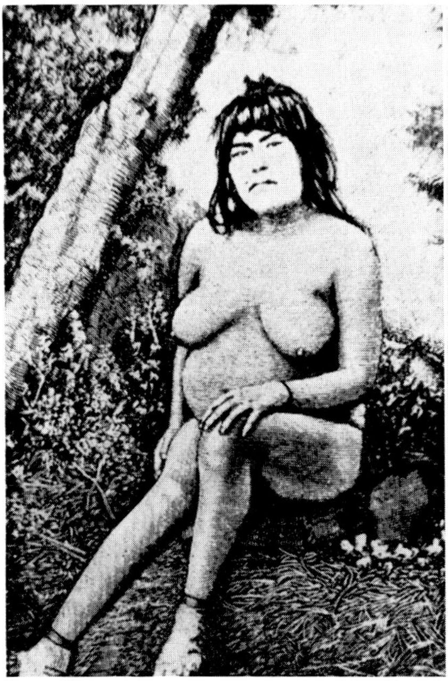

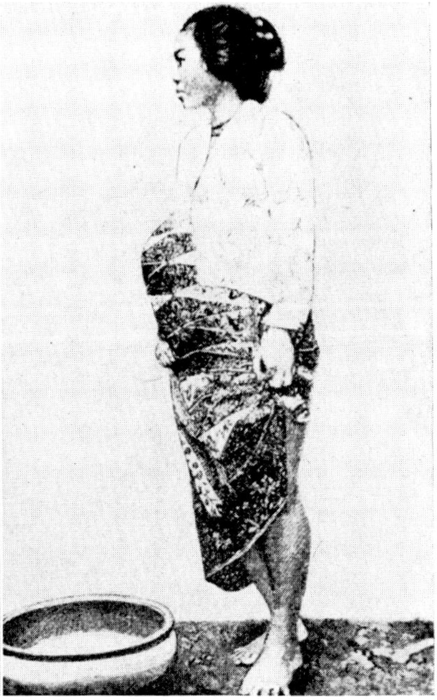

Fig. 140 A primitive woman. Living in a warm climate, no clothing was required. ([Ploss-Bartels] Hyades-Deniker.)

Fig. 141. A Javanese. Costume permits perfect freedom of body action. ([Ploss-Bartels] Neufeld & Henius.)

The type of dress, costumes or wearing apparel used by pregnant women has varied with the times. We can begin with the mode of dress in pregnancy in primitive times, or, more properly speaking, we should say undress since primitive woman living in a warm climate required no clothing. The Javanese wore costumes that permitted perfect freedom of body action, in contradistinction to the styles of the reign of Marie Antoinette, when women padded their skirts to keep pace with the Queen in her pregnancy. The styles of the middle-18th Century are stressed in obstetrical texts, and much was made in these medical books of the ill effects of improperly fitting garments and particularly corsets. In the middle of the 19th Century tight lacing was a custom that prevailed. In a book by

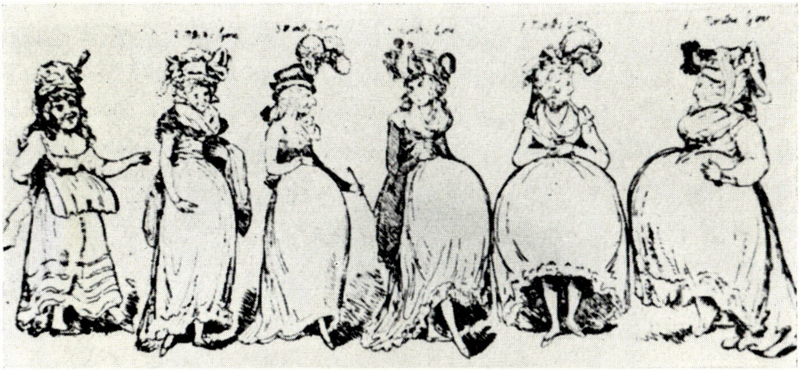

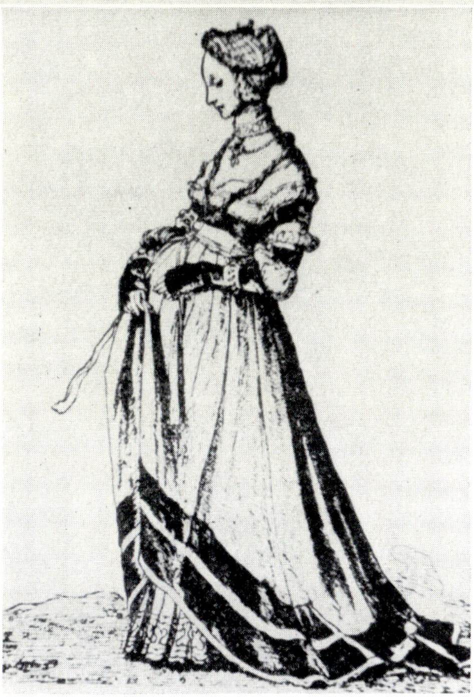

Fig. 142. "Whims of the day, or follies of fashion." In the reign of Marie Antoinette, women padded their skirts to keep pace with the Queen in her pregnancy. ([Witkowski] G. Steinheil, Paris.)

Fig. 143. Maternity costume of the Eighteenth Century. ([Witkowski] G. Steinheil, Paris.)

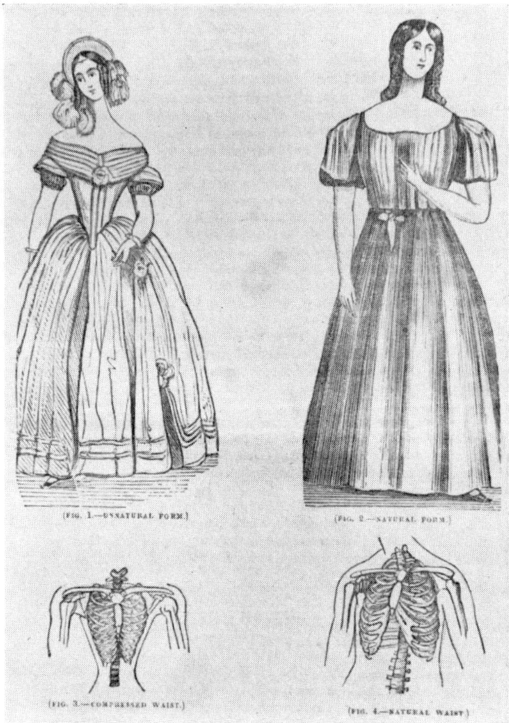

Fig. 144. Ill effects from tight corseting. (Beach, Wooster: *Improved System of Midwifery*. New York, Redfield and Savage, 1847.)

Beach[33] in 1846 he illustrates by drawing the ill effects of this lacing. Today we advise special maternity corsets, and sensible fitting clothes and shoes.

The 18th Century was definitely not a gynecological era; only a few advances were made, especially in anatomy and physiology. Obstetrics on the other hand, burst forth as a bona-fide specialty in this century for the first time; obstetric diagnosis was improved, the study of the contracted pelvis and introduction of pelvimetry took place. Despite the additions of surgical cleanliness, their management of incomplete abortion showed very little enlightenment. In retained secundines they used uterine irrigations of milk, wine water, vinegar water and alum. The vagina was packed with red clay, the white of egg and occasionally sow dung. The blunt hook or finger was used to grasp large fragments in the uterus. Podalic version and the use of forceps increased in this century.

First Occurrences and Outstanding Events

First time in history of medicine that rationalism replaced empiricism.
Physicians of this period referred to as the most charitable members the profession ever had.
Stephen Hales gave us the first notions of blood pressure.
John Radcliffe was the first to receive the gold headed cane from the College of Physicians as a sign of professional prestige.
First medical school in America, 1765, the College of Philadelphia, now the University of Pennsylvania.
First women's medical college in America, 1850, Philadelphia.
First academically trained woman doctor, 1849, Dr. Elizabeth Blackwell.
First woman to serve officially as doctor in army, Civil war, Dr. Mary Walker.
First hospital in America, the Bari Hospital in San Domingo, 1503.
First "poorhouse" in U. S., Henricopolis, Va., 1612.
First hospital in the U. S., Pennsylvania Hospital, 1751.
First American doctor to gain world repute, Rush.
First to classify ectopics, Giovanni Battista Bianchi.
First to report simultaneous extra- and intrauterine pregnancy, Pierre Duverney, 1709.
First description of interstitial pregnancy by Pierre Dionis.
First to describe peristalsis of Fallopian tube in 18th Century, Nicholas Hartsoeker.
First artificial insemination in 1799 by John Hunter.
First to use term retroversion, William Hunter
First to coin term retroflexion, Thomas Denman.
Morgagni was the founder of pathologic anatomy.
Obstetrics becomes a serious specialty for the first time, 18th Century.
First time enterocele was noted.
Greatest obstetricians of the 18th Century, Smellie and Levret.
Smellie, Master of British midwifery. In 1754 he invented the long curved forceps, therefore the first to add a pelvic curve; he was the first to measure the diagonal conjugate manually; and the first to recognize a ricketic pelvis.
Lebas made the first attempt to suture a ruptured uterus, 1769.
Smellie was the first to refer to postpartum sulci tears of the vagina and lacerations of the cervix.
Smellie was first to suggest leucorrhea as cause of sterility.
Smellie was the founder of pelvimetry.
Baudelocque was the first to describe the external conjugate diameter.

Wm. Giffard first suggested the Von Ritgen maneuver.

Wm. Hunter demonstrated the two-fold nature of the circulation of the placenta. He described the decidua as hypertrophied endometrium instead of inflammation, for the first time. He was the first to describe the round ligament and named the linea alba. He was the first to prove that the lymphatics were not continuous with the blood vessels.

Wm. Hunter was one of the first to suggest tapping and even removal of ovarian cysts. He never performed these procedures.

Charles White practiced the Fowler position 100 years before Fowler appended his name to it.

Charles White was the first to proclaim the doctrine of aseptic obstetrics. He was the first to describe "phlegmasia alba dolens, which was known as "white leg"—but

John Hull gave it the name of "phlegmasia alba dolens."

Alexander Gordon was the first to show the infective nature of puerperal fever.

References

1. Bettmann, O. L.: *A Pictorial History of Medicine.* Springfield, Thomas, 1956.
2. Ricci, J. V.: *Genealogy of Gynecology.* Philadelphia, Blakiston, 1950.
3. Bettmann, O. L.: *A Pictorial History of Medicine.* Springfield, Thomas, 1956.
4. Macmichael, William: *The Gold Headed Cane*, 3rd Ed. London, Longmans, 1884. Or
   Micmichael, William: *The Gold Headed Cane*, 7th Ed., with a foreword by Waring, J. J. and Kerr, W. J. Springfield, Thomas, 1953. Or
   Macmichael, William: *The Gold Headed Cane*, edited by Munk, William. London, Longmans, 1884.
5. Bettmann, O. L.: *A Pictorial History of Medicine.* Springfield, Thomas, 1956.
6. Comarazamy, Francisco: *The First Hospital in America.* Ciudad Trujillo, Republica Dominicana, Department of Public Health, 1954.
7. Wood, G. B.: *Founding of the Pennsylvania Hospital*, an address delivered June 10, 1851. Philadelphia, Collins, 1851.
8. Bettmann, O. L.: *A Pictorial History of Medicine.* Springfield, Thomas, 1956.

9. Campbell, W.: *Memoir on Extra Uterine Gestation.* Edinburgh, Black, 1840, pp. 29-60.
10. Leonardo, R. A.: *History of Gynecology*. New York, Froben, 1944, p. 216.
11. Ricci, J. V.: *Genealogy of Gynecology*. Philadelphia, Blakiston, 1950, p. 395.
12. *Ibid.*, p. 397.
13. *Ibid.*, p. 301.
14. *Ibid.*, p. 395.
15. *Ibid.*, p. 395.
16. *Ibid.*, p. 395.
17. *Ibid.*, p. 394.
18. Astruc, Jean: *Traité des Maladies des Femmes*, etc., 6 vols. Paris, Mequignon ainé, 1765, tome IV, p. 67.
19. Marc: Grossesse extra-utérine. *Dictionnaire des Sciences Médicales*, *19*:398-413, 1817 (Paris).
20. Guillemot: Prégnancy extra utérine. *Gaz. hôp., Paris*, *6*:17, 1832.
21. Ricci, J. V.: *Genealogy of Gynecology*. Philadelphia, Blakiston, 1950, p. 453.
22. *Ibid.*, p. 363.
23. Walsh, J. J.: *Makers of Modern Medicine; Morgagni the Father of Pathology*. New York, Fordham U. P., 1915, pp. 29-51.
24. Bettmann, O. L.: *A Pictorial History of Medicine.* Springfield, Thomas, 1956.
25. Findley, Palmer: *Priests of Lucina.* Boston, Little, 1939, p. 169.
26. *Ibid.*, p. 202.
27. Graham, Harvey: *Eternal Eve.* London, Heinemann, 1950, p. 302.
28. Findley, Palmer: *Priests of Lucina.* Boston, Little, 1939.
29. Ricci, J. V.: *Genealogy of Gynecology*. Philadelphia, Blakiston, 1950, p. 397.
30. Findley, Palmer: *Priests of Lucina.* Boston, Little, 1939.
31. Bethel, J. P.: *Webster's New Collegiate Dictionary*. Springfield, Mass., Merriam, 1949, p. 1019.
32. Hunter, William: *The Human Gravid Uterus* (ed. of original 1774 text). London, Lumley, 1798.
33. Beach, Wooster: *Improved System of Midwifery*. New York, Redfield and Savage, 1847.

Chapter XIV

OVARIOTOMY, EARLY 19TH CENTURY

IT WOULD SEEM that the accomplishments of the 18th Century, though minimal in themselves, were in the nature of ground work for what was to come in the 19th Century. Actually, there were no outstanding contributions in the 18th Century, but there was a constant, gradual probing of ideas and problems, a gentle seething, so to speak, of the medical men, as if they knew that great things were to happen in the next century, and for this they were quietly preparing. During the 18th Century, their attention was given to the problem of infection, puerperal infection especially; they learned from clinical observation and study; all that was lacking was the discovery of the offending organism. Obstetrics had already become a science, having made more contributions in the 18th Century than gynecology, which had made very little progress. However, in the first half of the 19th Century, gynecology began to move ahead, while obstetrics contributed very little. So by the middle of the 19th Century, when the "revolution" came, both obstetrics and gynecology were already moving along and fully prepared to utilize the tremendous discoveries of anesthesia, bacteriology and cellular pathology. These were the revolutionizing discoveries that skyrocketed obstetrics and gynecology to its present-day level.

The empirical advances of gynecology and obstetrics up to the mid-19th Century, furnished the clue to the stupendous discoveries that were to come. In a sense the work of Pasteur, Lister, Virchow and Morton (anesthesia to a lesser extent), only corrobrated the clinical (empirical) advances up to that time. However, we cannot deny that the mid-19th Century was a time of transition from a blind empiricism to an increasing scientific knowledge of pathological processes.

In the graph (in the front of the book) we notice a slight upward bend in the curve of progress commencing about the 16th Century. This could be explained by the discovery of the microscope by Leeuwenhoek, the founding of histology by Malpighi, the advances in physiology by Harvey, and pathology by Morgagni. The effect of these investigations had a universal effect on medicine. These factors did not influence the progress of obstetrics as much as the surge of gynecology. The progress of obstetrics was more dependent on the ability of man to analyze, deduce logically and profit by experience—that is, clinical experience. On the other hand, gynecology, which is a specialized form of surgery, was more dependent on scientific discoveries. As a result gynecology came into its own, and today it is basically the same gynecological surgery that prevailed in the latter half of the 19th Century, with improvements, modifications and refinements.

Until the early part of the 20th Century, "female troubles" in many of the schools were given only minor consideration. Because of this lack of importance attached to women's troubles, we find at the University of Pennsylvania, where the first chairs of medical instruction in this country were established in 1791, only one professor (William Shippen, Jr.) of anatomy, surgery and midwifery combined. In 1805, surgery was made a separate department, but Shippen continued to teach anatomy and midwifery until his death in 1808. His successor CASRAR WISTAR (1761-1818) was not interested in midwifery. Through his influence, midwifery was isolated and dropped from the list of subjects required for graduation. Thus, he taught only anatomy. There was, at that time, a lapse of two years without a head of obstetrics, until THOMAS C. JAMES (1766-1835), who was a graduate of the University of Pennsylvania, succeeded William Shippen, Jr., in 1810, as head of the Department of Obstetrics. This is the first such occurrence in the history of the United States, that is, a separate department of obstetrics with its own professor. Although James became head of obstetrics in 1810,

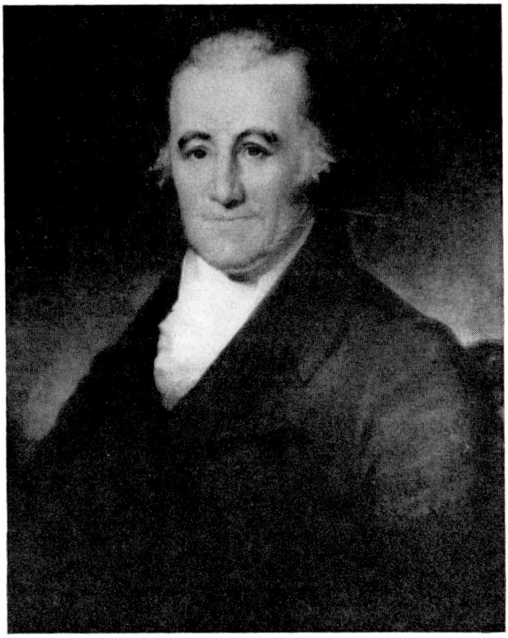

Fig. 145. Caspar Wistar. (Addison, Agnes: *University of Pennsylvania Medical School, Portraits*. Philadelphia, University Press, 1940.)

it was not until 1831 that the course in obstetrics was made a requirement for graduation. He designed his own forceps which was particularly good for compression rather than traction. It never became popular. He was succeeded, in 1834, as Professor of Obstetrics by WILLIAM POTTS DEWEES (1768-1841) who distinguished himself by the masterful use of the forceps. Although he favored the Baudelocque type of instrument, he laid no claim to obstetric forceps of his own design. However, there is a Dewees axis-traction forceps which Dr. Barton C. Hirst, also Professor of Obstetrics at the University of Pennsylvania in a later era, considered the best axis-traction forceps available.[1] Dewees resigned the professorship in 1835.

CHARLES D. MEIGS (1792-1869) was born in Bermuda, attended lectures at the University of Pennsylvania for three years, then

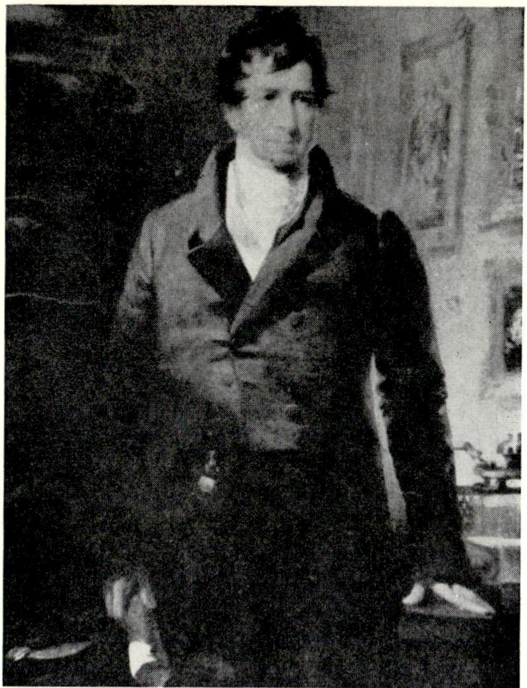

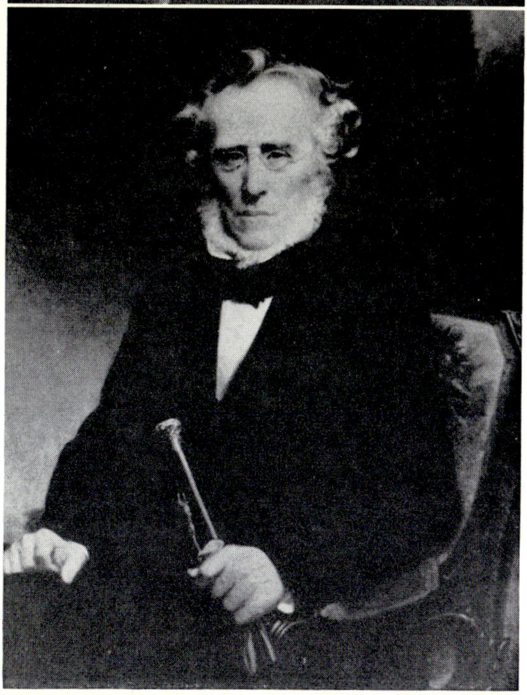

Fig. 146. William Potts Dewees. (Addison, Agnes: *University of Pennsylvania Medical School, Portraits*. Philadelphia, University Press, 1940.)

Fig. 147. Hugh Lenox Hodge. (Addison, Agnes: *University of Pennsylvania Medical School, Portraits*. Philadelphia, University Press, 1940.)

settled in Philadelphia. Among his many books and papers was a treatise on puerperal fever, which gained for him the "distinction" of reactionary. He was Professor of Obstetrics and Gynecology at Jefferson Medical College, Philadelphia. He believed that anesthesia did more harm than good. He rejected absolutely the theory of contagion; he did not see any relationship between puerperal fever and erysipelas as did others. He said that he should prefer to rely on Providence so long as we did not really know. He was an antagonist of the cesarean section. He detested the crotchet, and invented the embryotomy forceps to take its place. He is remembered as a controvertionalist and an exponent of conservative obstetrics. His favorite forceps was the Davis instrument. Nevertheless, he did much to further the science of obstetrics.

Hugh Lenox Hodge (1796-1873) was born in Philadelphia, and was graduated from the University of Pennsylvania. He occupied the chair of midwifery after Dewees resigned. He refused to subscribe to the prevalent belief that pregnancy should receive no help because it was a physiological process. His armamentarium in obstetrical cases went as far back as the fillet which he still used in breech presentations. He, of course, also used the blunt hook, vectis or lever and the forceps. In cesarean operations he held to a middle ground. Although he sided with Meigs in the controversy of contagiousness of puerperal fever against Holmes, he was never contentious in his attitude, as was Meigs. He devised a pessary which is still used today. Among a number of instruments he devised was a forceps that was extremely popular in his day.

He wrote much. Some of his contributions were *Observations Regarding Puerperal Fever*, 1833; *The Non-contagious Character of Puerperal Fever*, 1852; *Diseases Peculiar to Women*, 1860; and his masterpiece, *Principles and Practice of Obstetrics*, 1864. Just before he died he wrote *Essays upon Synclitism of the Fetal Head*, 1870-1871.

The influence that affected medicine was world-wide; the basic science discoveries such as bacteriology, and the invention of operations proceeded simultaneously in a number of countries. While Semmelweis and Pasteur performed epochal studies in bacteriology in Europe, Holmes was studying childbed fever in America. In

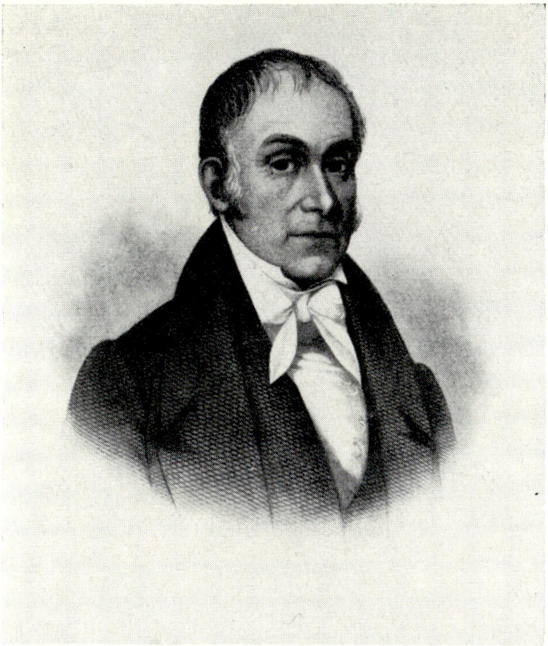

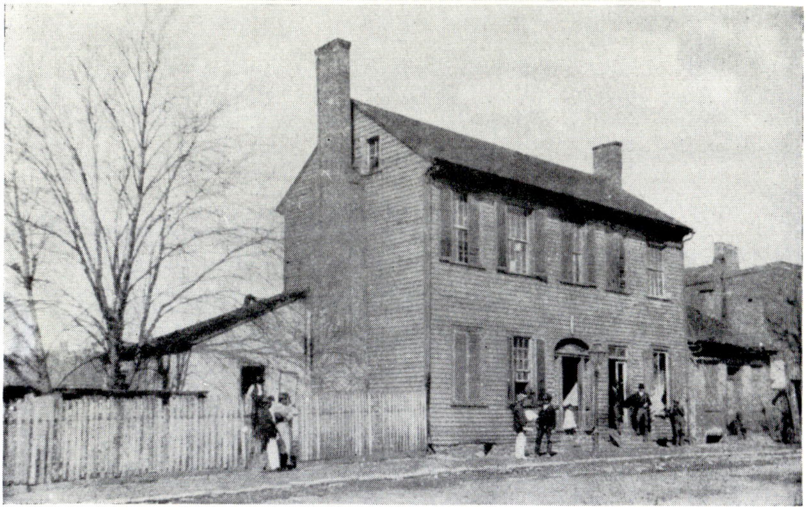

Fig. 148. Ephraim McDowell. (Ridenbaugh, M. Y.: *Biography of McDowell.* New York, Webster, 1890.)

Fig. 149. Old McDowell residence. (Ridenbaugh, M. Y.: *Biography of McDowell.* New York, Webster, 1890.)

1815 at Faenza, Doctor Emiliani was the first to perform ovariotomy in Europe, not knowing that this operation previously had been done in America by McDowell in 1809. While we in America credit Sims with the operation for vesico-vaginal fistula, which must have been about 1845, ten years after his graduation from Jefferson Medical College, John P. Mettauer (1787-1875) reported six successful operations for vesicovaginal fistula in 1838-47.

The 19th Century had an auspicious beginning when Dr. Ephraim McDowell did the first operation for a diseased ovary, one which paved the way for abdominal surgery, generally. This took place in a small Kentucky village in 1809. Mrs. Jane Todd Crawford, forty-seven years old, mounted and rode sixty miles into Danville to submit to this history-making operation, which was performed without anesthesia. She was suffering from a large and rapidly growing ovarian tumor.

EPHRAIM McDOWELL (1771-1830) was the ninth of eleven children born to Mary McDowell, née McClung, who was born in Ireland. His father, Samuel McDowell, was active in public life, had studied law, became a judge and later a governor. Dr. Ephraim McDowell was born November 11, 1771, in Rockbridge County, Virginia.

At the age of thirteen he moved to Danville, Kentucky. He was thoughtful and mature beyond his age. He was studious and preferred books to playing games. He developed into a tall, erect and commanding figure, was strikingly handsome, was a fine conversationalist, and had a ready wit that was most pleasing. He received his early education in a classical seminary of Messrs. Worley and James. He went to Virginia into the office of Dr. Humphrey of Staunton, as a medical student. Dr. Humphrey was a graduate of Edinburgh. Then he went to the University of Edinburgh in 1793 and 1794. While there he attended the private course of John Bell. That portion of his course in which he lectured on the diseases of the ovaries, dwelling on the inevitable death to which the victims were doomed, and merely suggesting the possibility of success attending any operation that might be attempted for removal of the organs, was certainly never forgotten by McDowell. He carefully stored in his mind the principles and suggestions at this time enunciated by the Master, together with other impressions, and sixteen years later attempted his first ovariotomy, an operation which has immortalized him and opened to the broad field of surgery the abdominal operations.

Upon his return to Danville in 1795, McDowell entered at once on the practice of his profession, assuming a top place in the field in his community despite the envy and jealousy of his confrères because of his superior medical advantages. In just two years he was considered the greatest surgeon north and south and west of Philadelphia. Together with J. Marion Sims, a native of South Carolina, no physician on this continent has contributed such far-reaching and potential influence toward advancing and enriching the resources of surgical science. These two great American surgeons founded the modern science of gynecology, which has brought to American medicine and American physicians so much of the renown and esteem with which they are regarded in all foreign countries.

McDowell had six children, owned a farm and raised livestock, and maintained slaves. He was a prayerful man, as an evidence of which we have the following invocation offered up by him to the Divine Master a few hours before the appointed time to make the first ovariotomy:

> Almighty God be with me, I humbly beseech Thee, in this attendance in Thy holy hour; give me becoming awe of Thy presence, grant me Thy direction and aid, I beseech Thee, that in confessing I may be humble and truly penitent in prayer, serious and devout in praises, grateful and sincere, and in hearing Thy word attentive and willing and desirous to be introduced. Direct me, oh! God, in performing this operation, for I am but an instrument in Thy hands, and am but Thy servant, and if it is Thy will, oh! spare this poor afflicted woman. Oh! give me true faith in the atonement of Thy Son, Jesus Christ, or a love sufficient to procure Thy favor and blessing; that worshiping Thee in spirit and in truth my services may be accepted through His all-sufficient merit. Amen.[2]

Remembering the prayer and writing it down with his own fingers, he placed it in his pocket, thinking some day that his faithful wife might accidentally find it—perhaps after his death, for threatening clouds were gathering about him as the time drew near for him to perform the operation upon Mrs. Crawford.

The operation: It was on the thirteenth day of December, 1809, after Dr. McDowell had been practicing his profession for fourteen years, that he was sent to see Mrs. Crawford, residing in Green

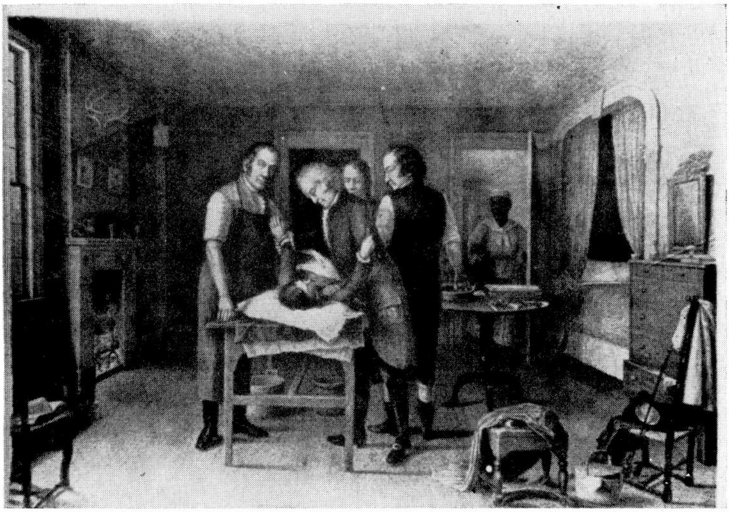

Fig. 150. First ovariotomy. (Ridenbaugh, M. Y.: *Biography of McDowell*. New York, Webster, 1890.)

County, Kentucky, some sixty miles from Danville. She was thought by her physicians to have gone long beyond her time in pregnancy, and to be the subject of extrauterine foetation. McDowell found her trouble to be an ovarian tumor, rapidly hastening to a fatal termination. McDowell informed his patient that the only chance for relief was the removal of the diseased mass. He explained to her with great clearness and fidelity the nature and hazard of the operation. He told her that he had never performed it, but that he was ready, if she were willing, to undertake it, and to risk his reputation on the issue. He added that it was an experiment, but one well worthy of trial.

He operated on this woman, who was possessed of unusual fortitude, without anesthesia; twenty-five days later she returned, on horseback, to her cabin in the hills. The cyst contained fifteen pounds of gelatinous material; the sac itself weighed seven pounds.

The patient made a complete recovery and lived to be seventy-eight. McDowell allowed eight years to elapse before publishing an account of this epoch-making operation and two subsequent cases of ovariotomy, likewise successful.

McDowell made a left rectus incision nine inches long, through the peritoneal cavity. The cyst was so large that he states in his description of the operation that it was not possible to remove the mass *in toto*, so he incised and drained it, and subsequently removed the sac. Before incising the cyst, he placed a strong ligature around the Fallopian tube near the uterus. He describes the large mass as the ovarium and fibrous part of the Fallopian tube very much enlarged. They removed fifteen pounds of dirty gelatinous substance, after which he cut through the "Fallopian tube" and extracted the sac, which weighed seven and one-half pounds. During the twenty-five minutes it required for the operation, the intestines were out of the abdomen. The patient was turned on her side to allow the accumulation of blood to escape. Then the wound was sutured, by interrupted stitches, leaving, at the lower end of the incision, the ligature which surrounded the "Fallopian tube." Adhesive strips were placed between the interrupted stitches.

Comment: It is not clear to the author what "Fallopian tube" means. Does McDowell confuse the pedicle, ovarian ligament, with tube? And the explanation of enlarged tube is confusing, could it have been a tubo-ovarian mass? In subsequent operations this ligated end was not sutured in the wound, but was allowed to drop into the abdomen.

Another point of interest: in all my research I have been unable to find a record of the exact medication used pre-operatively for analgesia. We know that no anesthesia was used as we do today, but it would be important to know whether spiritus frumenti, laudanum (which was given post-operatively according to records) was a much used drug at this time, or just what measures were taken to minimize the pain and permit operation.

McDowell was conscious at the time he was doing the operation, that an angry and excited crowd of men were collected in the street awaiting the result of his experiment of "butchering a woman," as they expressed it. Had she died under the operation, there was no law in those primitive days sufficiently strong to have protected him from the people who were clamoring for his life; determined men who would have shown no mercy, for they regarded it a duty to avenge the wrong inflicted on Mrs. Crawford.

McDowell did not possess an M.D. degree until 1825, when, entirely unsolicited on his part, the University of Maryland honored itself by conferring upon him its honorary diploma. It has often been wondered why he was so late in publishing his papers (his first ovariotomy performed in 1809 was published in 1817).[3] The condition of the country, the times in which he lived, and his great aversion to writing, palliate the seeming neglect of what appears to have been his duty; his failure to report the more minor operations that he originated has been the cause of failure to receive other honors. A prominent Brooklyn surgeon said that he knew from good authority that McDowell was the first to perform the cesarean operation in this country successfully (in New York City). No report of this case was made. He crossed the Atlantic three times to do the cesarean operation, and so great had become his reputation in surgery that he was called to operate upon President Polk for bladder stone and hernia later.

"Like all men of genius, the man destined to rise, must traverse the rank and foulsome sloughs of envious persecution, until victory carries him out of them," said Professor Tyndale. "A great theory has never been accepted without opposition. Such must always be the course of things so long as men are endowed with different degrees of insight; where the mind of genius discerns the distant truth which it pursues, the mind not so gifted often sees nothing but the extravagance which it avoids." He was persecuted, and his own profession denounced him as a cruel, wicked person, who had no sympathy for man or woman, that he gloried in cutting open the belly of a woman. (Remember, abdominal surgery was practically unheard of.) His most intimate professional friends avoided him, and the prejudice was carried so far that he was socially shunned by many. The Negroes of the village and the surrounding country being naturally ignorant and superstitious, whenever they spied Dr. McDowell walking in the distance, would rush into the nearest building, fearing that he might waylay and maltreat them. They feared him as they would some beast of prey. Indeed they could scarcely be induced to venture out after twilight, unless McDowell was absent from home. For this fear, their masters were, of course, responsible.

But he had his sport out of them. One afternoon as he was wending his way homeward, he met, in a solitary part of the road, a burly Negro face to face. The man looked an instant at the Doctor, and then attempted to run, but being ordered, halted. With wild, staring eyes, and terrified face, the Negro gave one unearthly groan and falling upon his knees offered up an appeal to God that would have touched a heart of stone. When he stopped praying, the doctor talked with him, trying to make the man understand his foolishness. The Negro stated that he had heard his old master say, "that Dr. McDowell was next to the devil, that he went about cutting people open and killing them." To the time of his death, the ignorant residents, both white and black, held such ideas of him, and no argument could disabuse their minds of the uncanny impressions.

A few quotations will show the attitude of some of the profession. It was Professor William Tod Helmuth who said that the national pride of every American physician is to find gratification "in pronouncing Ephraim McDowell 'the father of ovariotomy,' not of American ovariotomy, but of ovariotomy the world over. The endeavor has constantly been made in England to deprive the American people of the honor which belongs to them in this regard." In 1817, McDowell sent a report of his cases to his former preceptor, Mr. Bell, who was away on the continent at the time. Mr. Lizars, in charge of Bell's correspondence, put the reports away and so they were not noticed by Bell until seven years later, when Lizars recorded a case of his own, and McDowell's paper to Bell appeared as an appendix. Lizars' case proved to be not an ovariotomy, but simply the removal of an accumulation of fat. In England, priority in the performance of ovariotomy was given to a certain Robert Houstoun, of Glasgow. In Mr. Lawson Tait's latest work, 1883, the endeavor of the author to procure for Great Britain precedence in the performance of this operation is so apparent and indeed so overdrawn that the animus is plainly perceptible. The case of Mr. Houstoun which Mr. Tait refers to in the *Philosophical Transactions*, published in 1834, is Case XXVIII; the report therein is that of Margaret Millar, operated in 1701.[4] From a careful reading of this article, we may deduce that Mr. Houstoun did not perform a complete ovariotomy, as was thought by Dr. Tait. A Dr. R. S. Sutton of Pittsburgh suggested that Dr. Houstoun did not perform ovariotomy. Peaslee, in 1882, definitely says that Dr. Houstoun did not perform ovariotomy.

It was not too many years after McDowell's performance that a rash of ovariotomies spread throughout the world. Many of these operations were done almost simultaneously; whether McDowell was actually the spark that ignited this particular advance or whether all acted from a common stimulus, indirectly provided by the discoveries of Leeuwenhoek, Malpighi and Harvey, is not known.

Emiliani of Faenza in 1815 performed ovariotomy in Italy without the knowledge of McDowell's performance in 1809; McDowell's operation was published in 1817.

Chrysmar in Germany in 1819 did the first ovariotomy there.

Nathan Smith (1762-1829), Professor of Surgery at Yale, performed the second ovariotomy in the United States in July 5, 1822,[6] at Norwich, Vermont, without knowing that it had ever been done before.[6] His technique was an improvement over McDowell's in that he dropped the pedicle into the abdominal cavity instead of suturing it into the abdominal wall.

Alban G. Smith of Danville, who assisted McDowell in his operations, performed the third ovariotomy in this country on May 23 or 24, 1823.[7]

David L. Rogers of New York performed the fourth on September 14, 1829.[8]

J. Bellinger of Charleston, South Carolina, successfully performed the operation on December 23, 1835. His first attempt in 1828 was unsuccessful.[9]

While the above operations were being done successfully, quite a few attempts were made in the United States that did not succeed. Some of them were:

Joseph A. Gallup of Vermont, in 1824.[10]

Dr. Trowbridge of New York, in April 1827.[11]

Dr. R. D. Mussey, Professor at Dartmouth, in July 1828, at Vermont.[12]

Dr. J. C. Warren of Boston, in November 1830.[13]

After these performances, the first successful attempt was made in 1843 by John Light Atlee (1799-1885), who did a revised form of McDowell's operation, giving a new impetus to its performance. Then WASHINGTON L. ATLEE in 1844, associated with his brother John, in Lancaster, Pennsylvania, did his first ovariotomy, unsuccessfully. Nevertheless, he persisted through a storm of abuse, and in thirty-four years performed 387 ovariotomies.

RANDOLPH PEASLEE of New York did four successful ovariotomies in 1851,[14] the first one in February.[15]

In the United States, up to October 10, 1871, there were 739 ovariotomies with 68.63 per cent of successes.

LIZARS in Scotland, Bell's associate, attempted ovariotomy on October 23, 1823, but failed.[16]

In England, the first successful operation was performed by WILLIAM JEAFFRESON of Framlingham on May 8, 1836. D. H. WALNE, on November 6, 1842, did the first successful operation in London.

CHARLES CLAY of Manchester, a graduate of Edinburgh, and pupil of Lizars, did ovariotomy after twenty years of surgical experience. In his first year, 1842, he did four cases, saving three. He became the most distinguished ovariotomist living. He is credited more than anyone else for placing this operation on a sure foundation. By 1866 he had done 137 cases with 95 recoveries.

T. SPENCER WELLS, born in 1818, one of the greatest gynecologists in Great Britain during Simpson's days, did his first ovariotomy in 1858. By 1871, he did the operation 440 times with a recovery rate of 74.5 per cent.

THOMAS KEITH of Edinburgh did his first case in 1863, and by 1872 had done 136 cases with 81.6 per cent recovery.

In Great Britain a total of 377 cases with a 60 per cent recovery rate, and by 1870 the number of cases ran up to over a thousand cases.

In France the Academy of Medicine virulently opposed the operation in 1856. Only four cases were reported up to that time:

DR. WOYEIKOWSKY of Quingez (Doubs) who performed the first operation in France on April 29, 1844.[17]

M. VAULLEGEARD of Conde-sur Noireau (Calvados) on September 15, 1847, did the second.[18]

Other Frenchmen credited with ovariotomy are EUGENE KOEBERLE (1828-1915) in 1862, supposed to be the first French surgeon to do the operation; he was followed by JULES PEAN (1830-1898) who performed the first ovariotomy in Paris in 1864.

The procedure in France was definitely established by AUGUSTE NELATON (1807-1873), who was among the leading French surgeons and gynecologists in the pre-Listerian epoch of the 19th Century.

Among the German performers was ALFRED HEGAR (1830-1914). Curiously, ovariotomy was not extensively practiced in Germany until 1872, when Hegar introduced it chiefly to check the bleeding of fibromas. This practice was discarded in favor of x-ray at a later date when perfected.

CHRYSMAR did the first case in 1819. Others who attempted it with but fair success were Heyfelder, Nussbaum, Siebold, Kiwisch, Dieffenbach and Langenbeck.

By 1852, according to Kiwisch's statistics of fifty-four cases, fifty-one died.

Up to 1857, ovariotomy had been completed but four times in France, with 50 per cent success. In the meantime, in the United States, it had been done 97 times, with 54 successes. In England it was done 123 times, with 71 recoveries, and in Germany 47 times with 13 cures and 34 deaths.

First Occurrences and Outstanding Events

First time in the U. S. that a professor (Thomas C. James) became head of the department of Obstetrics (at the University of Pennsylvania).

H. L. Hodge devised a pessary that is still in use today.

McDowell did the first operation (ovariotomy) for a diseased ovary, in 1809. He was known as the father of ovariotomy the world over.

Emiliani, first ovariotomy in Italy.

Chrysmar, first ovariotomy in Germany.

William Jeaffreson, first ovariotomy in England.

D. H. Walne, first ovariotomy in London.

Woyeikowsky, first ovariotomy in France.

References

1. Hirst, B. C.: *Text Book of Obstetrics.* Philadelphia, Saunders, 1918, p. 744.
2. Ridenbaugh, M. Y.: *Biography of Ephraim McDowell,* New York, Webster, 1890.

3. McDowell, Ephraim: Three Cases of Extirpation of Diseased Ovarii. *Eclectic Repertory and Analytic Review*, 7:242, April 1817 (Philadelphia).
4. Houstoun, Robert: A Dropsy of the Left Ovary Cured. *Philosophical Transactions* (from the year 1719 to 1733), Abridged and Disposed under General Heads, 7:541-546, Case XXVIII, 1834.
5. Smith, Nathan: Case of Ovarian Dropsy Successfully Removed by a Surgical Operation. *Am. M. Recorder*, *5*:124, 1822 (Connecticut).
6. Smith, Nathan: *Med. and Surg. Memoirs*, ed.: Smith, N. R. Baltimore, Francis, 1831.
7. Smith, Alban G.: An account of a case in which an ovarium was successfully extirpated. *North American M. and S. J.*, *1*:30, 1826.
8. Rogers, D. L.: Case of Ovarian Tumor Successfully Extirpated. *New York M. and Physical J.*, 2:284, 1830.
9. Bellinger, John: Extirpation of an Ovarian Tumor, complicated with Hydrops uteri—recovery. *South. J. Med. and Pharm.*, 2:241, May 1847.
10. Gallup, J. A.: Case of extirpation of ovarian sac, designed for the care of Hydrops Ovarii. *New England J. M. Surg.*, *14*:358-364, 1825.
11. Trowbridge, Amasa: Diseased ovarium cured by an operation. *Boston M. Intelligencer*, *5*:337-339, 1827.
12. Mussey, R. D.: Successful Operation for Ovarian Disease. *Am. J. M. Sc.*, *21*:380, 1837.
13. Warren, J. C.: *Surgical Observations on Tumors, with Cases and Operation.* Boston, Crocker and Brewster, 1839, p. 589.
14. Peaslee, E. R.: *Ovarian Tumors, Their Pathology, Diagnosis, and Treatment.* New York, Appleton, 1872.
15. Peaslee, E. R.: Report of a case of ovariotomy, one of double ovarian dropsy. *Am. J. M. Sc.*, *21*:321, 1851.
16. Lizars: Observations on extirpation of the ovaria, with cases. *Edinburgh M. and S. J.*, *22*:247, Oct. 1824.
17. Woyeikowsky: Extirpation avec succès d'une tumeur ovarique. *J. Med. et. chir. prat.*, *18*:145-148, Paris, 1847. (Cited by Ridenbaugh, M. Y.,[2] p. 128.)
18. Vaullegeard, M. L.: Ovariotomie; succès; le premier cas, peut-être, d'ovariotomie pratiquée en France. *J. d. conn. méd.-chir. Par.*, *15* (2): 224-230, 1847-48. (Cited by Ridenbaugh, M. Y.,[2] p. 128.)

Chapter XV

ANESTHESIA

A. DISCOVERY OF ANESTHESIA

IT REMAINED for the 19th Century to see the virtual banishment of pain, an accomplishment that the human race had been seeking from the beginning of time, practically. The discovery of anesthesia was one of the greatest and most far reaching events in the history of medicine. Without it surgery could never have attained it's goal. As far back as ancient times, all kinds of measures were used to lessen pain; this practice was rarely tried on the pains of labor because of the erroneous idea of the natural basis for such pains, with which man had no right to interfere. In ancient times, physiotherapy measures, such as the use of hot and cold water, amulets in the form of tattooing, ear rings and nose rings in aboriginal tribes, incantations and magic to remove the demon pain from the body, were used. Then the religious healers invoked prayers. As far back as 2250 B.C. there is evidence in the clay tablets of the Babylonians, of the use of herbs such as powdered henbane. The Greeks and Romans used drugs; Galen, in his time, experimented with "mandragora." In 1562, in the Englishman William Bullein's *Bulwarke of Defence Against all Sickness*, there is this account of mandrake:

> The juice of this herbe pressed forth, and kepte in a close yearthen vessel, accordying to arte; this bringeth slepe, it casteth men into a trauns or depe tirrible dream. . . .

In Bullein's time, it was the common drug used for "cutting for stone." This drug, together with "hemp" which was used almost as much as "mandragora," began to lose popularity about the 16th

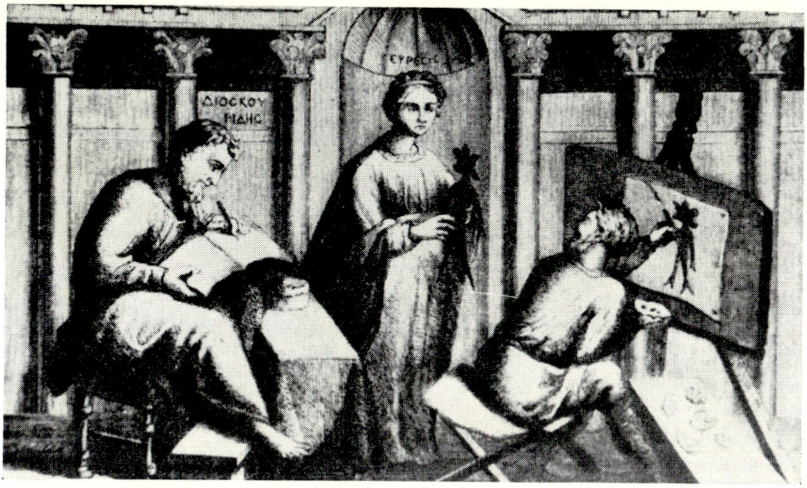

Fig. 151. Mandrake, used up to the Sixteenth Century. (The Bettmann Archive.)

Century. Then for the next two centuries alcohol and opium plus some strong-arm tactics became the popular "anesthetic."

In the 13th Century a Raymond Lullius, an alchemist of Spain, discovered a white fluid he called "sweet vitriol." In the 16th Century, Valerius Cordus made a similar discovery. In 1730, a German rechristened it "ether." Then Franz Anton Mesmer of Vienna, brought out mesmerism in 1765. He eventually was labelled a quack, and by the end of the 18th Century it finally petered out as a serious method of "anesthesia."

During the early part of the 18th Century, Joseph Priestly performed many experiments with gases. These were carried out with mice and even himself. He evolved nitrous oxide or laughing gas. When Priestly died, shortly after coming to America, Humphry Davy continued the experiments on himself with this gas. He suggested its use in surgery in 1800. However, most people were taken up by its "laughing" propensities. In 1844, Horace Wells had a tooth pulled with nitrous oxide (Dr. Riggs did the pulling). He passed all this information to his friend, Dr. William T. G. Morton of Charlton, Massachusetts, who, in turn, explained it to Dr. John C. Warren of Harvard Medical School.

Morton worked with a doctor who was also a chemist, named Jackson; Dr. Jackson had showed Morton that ether dropped on

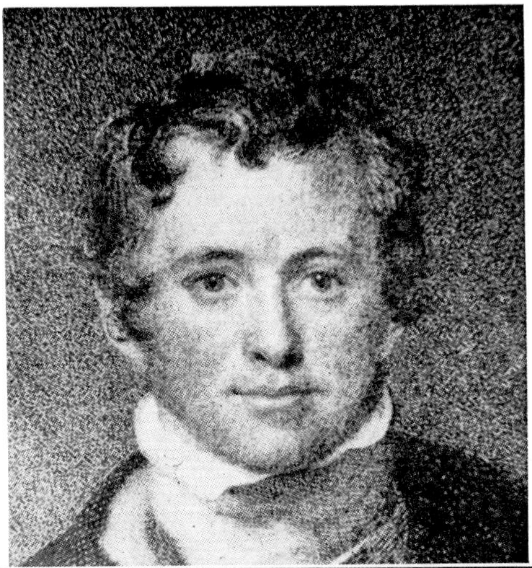

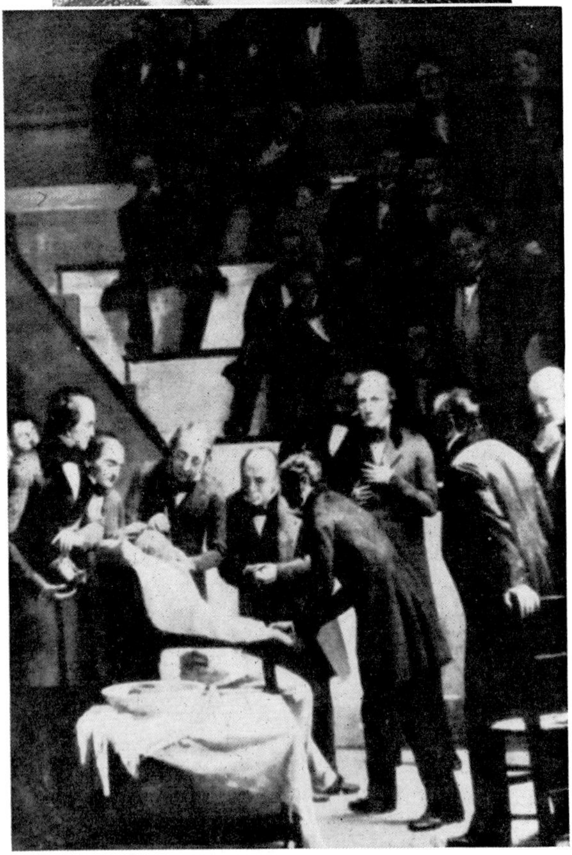

Fig. 152. Sir Humphry Davy, who recommended the use of nitrous oxide in surgery. (Culver Service.)

Fig. 153. Wm. G. T. Morton gave ether anesthesia while Dr. Warren operated; Boston, October 16, 1846; the first reported use of ether. (The Bettmann Archive.)

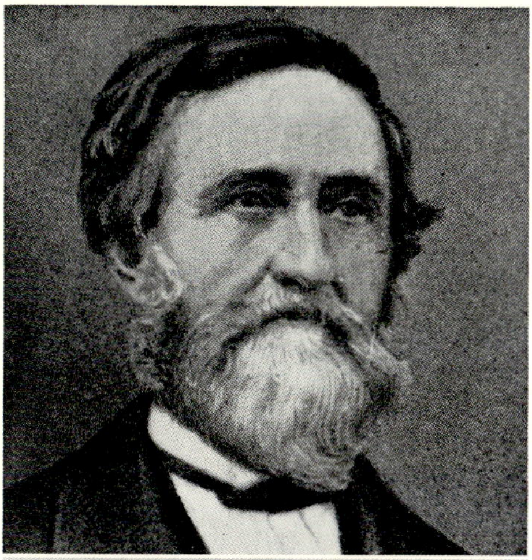

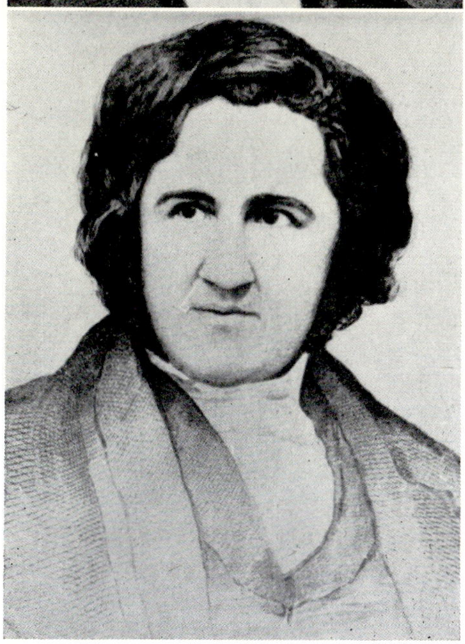

Fig. 154. Dr. Crawford Long used ether in 1842, but failed to report his results until years later. (Culver Service.)

Fig. 155. Sir James Young Simpson. (Findley, Palmer: *Priests of Lucina*. Boston, Little, 1939.)

the skin would anesthetize it. As early as 1805, Dr. Warren gave it to consumptives; it had been used for asthma and migraine. As a matter of fact, ether was quite well known at this time, but not its uses. Morton, fresh from Wells' exhibitions with nitrous oxide, used it to numb the face in placing fillings in teeth. Michael Faraday, a student of Humphry Davy's had already used ether experimentally in 1818, and knew that it would keep a person anesthetized for many hours. Of this, Morton knew nothing. Nevertheless, he used ether to extract a tooth from one of his patients. On October 16, 1846, he gave ether for Dr. Warren to remove a cyst from the jaw of a patient. It was immediately used, beginning the next day, on many surgical cases, especially for dental extractions. A few months later it was used in France, and a few days after this, it was tried in England.[1]

Dr. Crawford Williamson Long, of Georgia, a graduate of the University of Pennsylvania, used ether for his surgery four years before Morton, in 1842, but he did not publish his work until 1849, in the *Southern Medical and Surgical Journal*.[2] Morton's work had already appeared in the *Journal* in 1846.[3]

A Dr. William E. Clarke removed a tooth under ether anesthesia in Rochester, New York, in 1842. In fact, attempts in the use of ether go even farther back than this. Dr. Henry Hill Hickman of Ludlow, England, had written a paper on his experiments with ether with the view of using it in surgery. But his work failed to convince anyone. Bolstered by the opinions of S. Weir Mitchell, William H. Welch, and Oliver Wendell Holmes, Morton received credit for the discovery of anesthesia.

B. ANESTHESIA IN LABOR

It was not long after the discovery of ether that the problem of anesthesia in labor began to be discussed. In *An Essay on the Means of Lessening Pain in Facilitating Certain Cases of Difficult Parturition*,[4] William P. Dewees, forty years before chloroform was discovered, advanced the unique hypothesis that pain in parturition must be regarded as a disease having its origin in the changes produced by civilization and refinement. Most of the obstetricians, according to a paper by Dewees in 1819, used opium in the form of laudanum to relieve the pains of labor. He disapproved because it lessened the efficiency of the pains. Another procedure used was to bleed. This was Dewees' favorite. It was Simpson, in England, who began and popularized chloroform in obstetrics.

James Young Simpson was born on June 7, 1811, and died in 1870. He was born in Bathgate, close to Edinburgh. He graduated from the University of Edinburgh; at the age of twenty-eight he succeeded James Hamilton to the chair of Midwifery. The chair of Midwifery was now on a par with Surgery and Medicine, having achieved this distinction when Hamilton, his predecessor, was given the chair. Up to that time no instruction in midwifery was required by medical students, a situation comparable to that which existed at the University of Pennsylvania about the same time. Simpson obtained the chair by the slightest of margins, his jealous adversaries believing him an ignorant and uncultured male midwife. As it turned out, he became the most honored professor of the entire faculty.

Although he was the first to use chloroform in obstetrics, he did not discover this chemical; it was found by Soubeiran of France and Liebig of Germany in 1831 in independent experiments. When Simpson began to fight for anesthesia, he had almost unsurmountable odds against him, for he encountered not only the enmity of the profession who claimed that operating a patient under the effects of the anesthetic did the patient more harm than good. Besides, the objections on moral and religious grounds were even greater.

Simpson's *Text Book*, Vol. II, (1855) contains copies of the correspondence with the public about anesthesia, most of it with ministers who considered the use of anesthesia in labor a sin and therefore unacceptable.

> Pain during operations is, in the majority of cases, even desirable! its prevention or annihilation is, for the most part, hazardous to the patient. In the lying-in chamber, nothing is more true than this: pain is the mother's safety, its absence her destruction. Yet, there are those bold enough to administer the vapor of ether, even at this critical juncture, forgetting it has been ordered, that "in sorrow shall she bring forth."[5]

One of the principal dissenters was Dr. Meigs of Philadelphia. Here are the objections he wrote to Dr. Simpson:

1. In deliveries requiring "chirurgical intervention," and especially in forceps operations, on the ground that the sensations of the patient afford us our best aid for the introduction of the instrument.

Simpson's answer, in brief, was that Meigs implies the lack of anatomical knowledge which is not true of Meigs, and therefore is simply a prejudiced afterthought only.

2. Anesthesia in natural labors is objectionable, because pain of natural labor should not be annulled because pain is calculated to promote the safety of the mother.

Simpson reminds Meigs that in many of his publications he describes the labor of a woman as indescribable and not comparable to any other form of pain, and that it is the contractions of the uterus and not the pain that is essential for the progress of the labor. So long as chloroform does not obviate the contractions, the objection then is not valid; for Meigs himself among his many writings describes methods to avoid pain in other conditions.

Simpson further states: "Like other physicians, you deem it, I doubt not, your duty to wield the powers of your art, in order to free those that submit themselves to your medical care, from these and from other similar sufferings. But if it is right for you to relieve and remove these pains, why is it not right for you also to relieve and remove the pains accompanying the act of parturition? I cannot see on what principle of philosophy, or morality, or humanity, a physician should consider it his duty to alleviate and abolish, when possible, the many minor pains to which his patients are subject, and yet should consider it improper to alleviate and abolish, when possible, pains of so aggravated a character, that, in your own language, they are 'absolutely indescribable and comparable to no other pains,' 'Pains for which there is no other name but Agony.' "

3. Anesthesia in natural labor is objectionable because natural labor is "a physiological pain."

Simpson answered this by reminding Meigs that the contractions and not the pain is needed to aid the baby along in its journey. But everything new was considered, philosophically, as subversive of the Christian faith, even optical glasses, the telescope and the microscope were thought to be atheistical inventions because they perverted our organs of sight (D'Israeli). Simpson reminds Meigs that he would not relish a foot journey from Philadelphia to Baltimore for instance, instead of the use of the train (invention, too) since he believes walking "a desirable, salutary, and conservative manifestation of life-force." Further how can anyone assume it to be physiological when the labor is obstructed and therefore requiring the use of forceps, which of course is attended with pain. He quotes many other such similes.

4. The objection in labor, because the mother, in escaping by it from the "pangs and agonies of labor," may, in a few rare cases, be thus made to encounter danger to her own life.

Logically, according to Simpson, man should then give up traveling by rail, steamboats, etc., for these are questionable attempts, according to Meigs, to abrogate what he calls "one of the general conditions of man, viz., his original pedestrianism." The entire practice of medicine, thinking in the same vein, should be abandoned for man (doctors) are interfering with the processes of nature and in so doing human lives are often lost from the mistakes, or the passiveness, or the want of knowledge and skill, on the part of the physician. And there are such arguments, many quoted in the celebrated work of Raynald. In his preface:

"There is no anything so absolute and perfecte, but by the occasion of the abuse thereof at one tyme or other, may and doth ensue great daunger and damage to mankynde. Fire and water, two right necessary elements to the use of man, without the whiche he could not lyve, yet sometimes, by fyre hath ben consumed and devoured whole cities and countreys. Meate and drynke, to the moderate users thereof, doth minister and maynteyn life; and contrary, to the unmeasurable and unsatiate gourmanuntes and gluttons, it hath full many thousand types brought surfetes, and sickenesse, and at the last, death. . . . But should man, for the avoydyng al these forsade inconveniences, and for the reasons above sayde, condempe and bannysh fyre and water, forsake theyr meate and drynke? No, 'it were but madness once to thinke it.' "

5. Anesthesia was objected to by Meigs because he did not consider that the mother encounters danger to her health or life from the endurance of the pains.

Simpson says that he sincerely believes that the human constitution is so that it cannot endure pain, particularly when that pain is long in duration, or severe in degrees, without being more or less affected and injured by it. As far back as Paré it was considered that pain was deleterious and could cause depression of the heart, syncope and sudden death.

(Author's note: We know today that deep anesthesia is preferable to light anesthesia, let alone no anesthesia whatever, because complete nerve block of impulses is essential to prevent shock.)

Simpson further states that he proved, in the use of anesthetics in surgery, that recovery occurred in a larger proportion when anesthetized than those who had similar operations without ether. He believes the same applies to obstetrics.

It was Bacon who said, "I esteem it the office of a physician, not only to restore health, but to mitigate pain and dolors."[6]

Ether's acceptance by such a man as Dr. Warren and also Dr. Henry J. Bigelow, who published the first paper on ether anesthesia, made its acceptance by the surgical world inevitable. In December of 1846, the same year that Morton published his paper on the use of ether in a case at the Massachusetts General Hospital operated by Warren, the "Yankee dodge to make men insensible" was used on a patient of Robert Liston's in London, and pronounced by that excited surgeon to "beat mesmerism hollow." Simpson discussed the new anesthetic (ether) with Liston and, less than a month later, used it successfully in delivering a woman of her second child. He continued to use ether, and in March (1847) published a paper recording his results. Yet, Simpson was not satisfied; he kept experimenting with many different drugs, noting their effects on himself, and occasionally making himself very ill. On the night of November 4, 1847, Simpson and his two assistants, George Keith and Matthews Duncan, after trying several other substances without effect, unearthed a bottle of a heavy oily liquid, recently sent him by a Liverpool chemist. Sitting around the dining room table, each inhaled the fumes from a tumbler. At first stimulated, they one by one toppled over insensible. The new liquid was chloroform. Promptly trying it on his maternity patients, Simpson felt it to be more satisfactory than ether. His first patient was so grateful that she named her baby girl "Anesthesia." The skeptical public did not fully accept this new blessing until six years later when chloroform was used by Queen Victoria at the birth of Prince Leopold.

Besides the memorable accomplishment of anesthesia, Simpson, made other important contributions to his specialty. He invented a uterine sound and an obstetrical forceps that retained its popularity to the present time.[7] A description of the Simpson forceps and explanation of its use can be obtained in the section under "Forceps."

Simpson's last work, which was left unfinished at his death, was a protest against "hospitalism." Though unaware of the causes, Simpson realized that "a man laid on the operating table in one of our surgical hospitals is exposed to more chances of death than the English soldier on the field at Waterloo." The introduction of anesthesia, by increasing the number and variety of operations, augmented this evil. Septic poisoning was an ever-present horror, often supervening in the slightest operation; the stench of pus filled every ward, and phagedena was rarely absent. Pestilence followed in the footsteps of the most careful surgeon, and often the number of patients carried out of a hospital corresponded to the number of patients who had entered. Simpson, appalled, urged the hospitals to be abolished altogether, or else that they be constructed of iron in order that they might frequently be taken apart and moved, or rebuilt and renovated. Still he had so little idea of how to combat this menace that, when a young colleague in Edinburgh University tried to point the way out, Simpson was one of the conservatives who opposed the carbolic spray antisepsis of Joseph Lister. His attitude toward Semmelweis was the same; he lent him no encouragement whatever.

He wrote numerous papers on anesthesia mostly, but also on other subjects such as certain aspects of puerperal fever, duration of human pregnancy, determining the cause of labor, and many others.

He died on May 6, 1870, of angina pectoris.

A name closely associated with that of Simpson's is WALTER CHANNING (1786-1876). The first professor of midwifery at Harvard, he was also on the staffs of the Boston Lying-in and the Massachusetts General hospitals. He was a graduate of the University of Pennsylvania. He was a descendent of a famous and illustrious family, being the grandson on his mother's side, of William Ellery, a signer of the Declaration of Independence. His father, an attorney, had been Secretary of State. A brother, Edward T. Channing, was Professor of Rhetoric at Harvard.

He was one of the men who, with Simpson, championed anesthesia. He was likewise one of the first to use ether anesthesia in maternity cases. He wrote a paper, "A Treatise on Etherization in Childbirth," in 1848, one year after Simpson's use of ether in labor. His work in this respect is of vast importance because it contained a careful study and analysis of 581 cases. The result of this study was extremely helpful in the cause of anesthesia, which was receiving such rebuke from religious quarters and from the perennial dissenter in anything new, Dr. Meigs.

He wrote on puerperal sepsis. This, with his investigations in this field, had a profound effect and stimulation on Oliver Wendell Holmes' decision to write his famous paper on puerperal fever.[8]

First Occurrences and Outstanding Events

A. Discovery of Anesthesia

"Sweet vitriol" was discovered in the 13th Century by Lullius of Spain. In 1730, Frobenius rechristened it "ether."

Long used ether in 1842, but did not publish his experience until 1849. Morton is credited with the discovery of anesthesia (Ether), in 1846.

B. Anesthesia in Labor

Simpson discovered chloroform anesthesia (for obstetrical cases) in 1847.

He invented the Simpson forceps and the uterine sound of his design.

References

A. Discovery of Anesthesia

1. Graham, Harvey: *Eternal Eve*. London, Heinemann, 1950.
2. Long, C. W.: An account of the first use of sulphuric ether by inhalation as an anaesthetic in surgical operations. *South. Med. and Surg. J.*, 5:705-713, 1849.
3. Morton, W. T. G.: Circular. *Morton's Letheon*. Boston, Dutton and Wentworth, 1846.

B. Anesthesia in Labor

4. Dewees, W. P.: *An Essay on the Means of Lessening Pain in Facilitating Certain Cases of Difficult Parturition.* Philadelphia, Oswald, 1806.

5. Simpson, Sir J. Y.: *Obstetric Memoirs and Contributions*, 2 vols., ed. by Priestly, W. O. and Storer, H. R. Philadelphia, Lippincott, 1855-56, vol. 2, p. 547. (Also an ed. Edinburgh, Black, 1855-56, in 2 vols.)

6. Simpson, Sir J. Y.: *Obstetric Memoirs and Contributions*, 2 vols., ed. by Priestly, W. O. and Storer, H. R. Philadelphia, Lippincott, 1855-56, vol. 2.

7. Lusk, W. T.: *The Science and Art of Midwifery*. New York, Appleton, 1892.

8. Findley, Palmer: *Priests of Lucina.* Boston, Little, 1939.

Chapter XVI

INFECTION

It was in this, the 19th Century, that many, in fact nearly all the operations of today, were devised; at least the basic principles were discovered. In this list are included vaginal hysterectomy, abdominal hysterectomy (for fibroids especially), and cesarean section, which was brought up to date. But before discussing these procedures, it seems pertinent to present at this point, a matter upon which the development was largely contingent. As a matter of fact, we have already discussed two of these factors, namely the beginning of abdominal surgery that was started by McDowell's ovariotomy, and the discovery of anesthesia. Many of the operations were in the process of "bursting" forth as a result of these discoveries. Most of them, however, came to fruition when the question of infection became solved. Since infection and contagion played such a big part in the advance in gynecological surgery, we shall forthwith proceed with the history and discovery of organisms, the streptococci in particular, before going into the history of the various surgical procedures.

As stated in the previous chapter, infection, contagion and more exactly puerperal fever, was beginning to be well understood (except for its specific cause) in the latter part of the 18th Century through the work of such men as Gordon of Aberdeen and Charles White and others. Even as far back as ancient times when filth and ignorance of the cause of infection persisted, a few attempts were made that might be considered the beginning of asepsis. The ancient Greeks, by their insistence on cleanliness and sunshine, were able to heal some wounds by first intention. However, the teachings of the Middle Ages were the cause of retrogression in this matter. It was not until the 18th Century that intelligent investigation of this problem began to produce results. There was Charles White (discussed in the previous chapter, 18th Century) of Manchester, who noted that in one town where two men were the only midwives, "one of them loses several patients every year from puerperal fever, while the other never so much meets with the disorder." Gordon of Aberdeen, in 1795 said, "Every person who had been with a patient with the puerperal fever became charged with an atmosphere of infection, which was communicated to every pregnant woman who happened to come within its sphere." This pronouncement was not taken very seriously, however it did recall to some of the readers' minds the work of Charles White, some short time previously. The same kind of writing and talk occupied many others. Among them was Robert Collins (1801-1896), master of Dublin Lying-in Hospital from 1826 to 1833, who began a system of chlorine disinfection so thorough that during his entire term not one patient was lost by puerperal fever.

Oliver Wendell Holmes (1809-1894) the greatest exponent in America, of the contagiousness of puerperal fever, crystallized this entire problem that was being discussed in the United States and abroad for some time, when he read to the Boston Society for Medical Improvement his paper on "The Contagiousness of Puerperal Fever."[2] His presentation was not the result of research or any original work; it brought the matter to a head only because it was so ably presented. He was a great writer, and the essay on puerperal fever was his greatest.

Oliver Wendell Holmes was not an obstetrician, he was a teacher of anatomy and physiology at Dartmouth, and for thirty-five years at Harvard. He was Dean of the Harvard faculty; his greatest renown probably comes as a poet, essayist and lecturer. Everybody remembers "The Autocrat of the Breakfast Table." Holmes had a genius for satire; this, plus a severe logic which may be noted in his contention: "The practical point to be illustrated is the following: The disease known as puerperal fever is so far contagious as to be frequently carried from patient to patient by physicians and nurses." Most physicians took umbrage at this statement, particu-

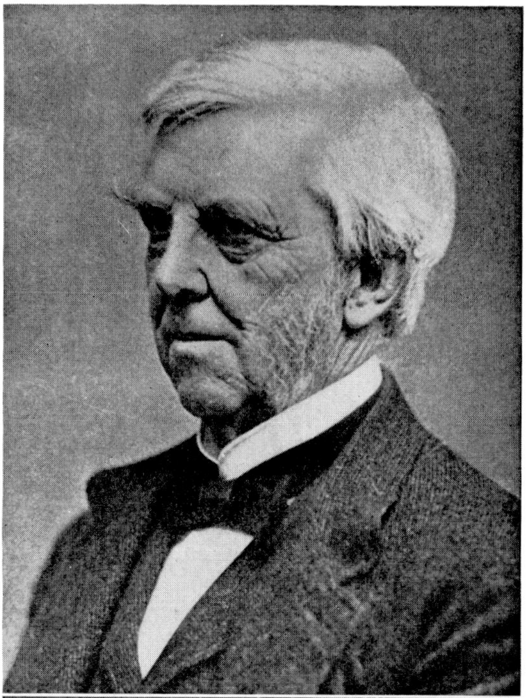

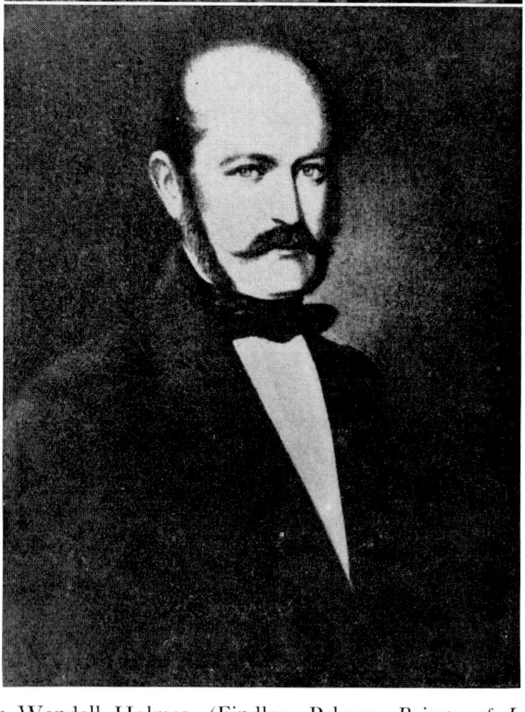

Fig. 156. Oliver Wendell Holmes. (Findley, Palmer: *Priests of Lucina*. Boston, Little, 1939.)

Fig. 157. Ignaz Philipp Semmelweis. (Findley, Palmer: *Priests of Lucina*. Boston, Little, 1939.)

larly Hodge and, more so, Meigs. But Holmes continued his satiric lectures, and however much they tried to disbelieve him, they were, in a way, much impressed against their will. His lectures were always well attended, what with such remarks as the following (during a lecture on the female pelvis): "The pubic arch is that underneath which every youthful candidate for immortality must pass." Another famous remark was that Philippe Ricord, an authority on venereal diseases, was such a skeptic of the morality of the human race that he would have ordered a course of Blue Pills for the Vestal Virgins.

His famous essay which was published in April 1843, warned against spreading the contagion, and advised doctors not to treat other patients if they had been taking care of a case of puerperal fever, and more so if they had attended or especially if they had assisted at a post-mortem examination of such a case. He cited the instance of Simpson, who had never seen a case of fever until he performed or assisted in a post-mortem examination on one of them, after which five of his patients were taken down with this contagion. Holmes was only thirty-four years old when he wrote this essay from which he became known as the "Contagionist." Twelve years later, in 1855, he published his essay which he called *Puerperal Fever as a Private Pestilence*.

In the Allegemeine Krankenhaus in Vienna, great strides were being made in this scourge, mainly by Semmelweis. In Holmes republication of 1855, he cites Semmelweis and the wonderful work he was doing. So we see that now this condition was being attacked vigorously both in America and Europe. Physicians of the late 18th Century had started, those of the early 19th Century were beginning to wind it up, so to speak.

It is perhaps to Semmelweis to whom we are most indebted, his clinical observations were epoch making; the greatness of his work was ultimately corroborated by the discovery of Pasteur, and the further practical application by Lister.

Ignaz Philipp Semmelweis (1818-1865). In the entire history of medicine, the work of Semmelweis rates as one of the greatest and most important in its effect and immediate blessings to the human race, by saving of life and the prevention of suffering. Twenty-five years after Semmelweis wrote his *Die Aetiologie, der Begriff*, *und die Prophylaxis des Kindbettfiebers* (1860), Fritsch of Breslau proclaimed in 1884 the Semmelweis Doctrine in the following words:

> In the history of Midwifery there is a dark page, and it is headed "Semmelweis." What man could close his eyes to the powerful impression of his book? Even now at the present time there are whole pages of his deductions which might stand in the most modern work. And the annihilating logic of his statistics. We younger men for whom antipathies were unthinkable, to whom the reading of coarse tirades about "genius misunderstood," was only tedious, we often find it incomprehensible that the logical conclusions of the doctrine of infection were nowhere drawn: I mean the local treatment; it was the keystone of the arch, the crown of the whole structure. . . . The efficient application of disinfection midwifery owes without doubt to surgery: most certainly it ought to have been the reverse. If the conclusions of Semmelweis had been followed, then the truth of his doctrine would have been demonstrated in the compelling language of statistics, and so perhaps Obstetrics would have stood in the forefront of the greatest advance of Medicine which has been made since physicians and physic came into existence.[3]

He was born July 1818 at Ofen or Buda (now part of the city of Budapest, son of a shopkeeper. He was Hungarian, was educated in public elementary schools and grammar schools, and attended the University of Pesth two years. He almost became a law student, but switched to medicine before the school year began. He studied medicine at the University of Pesth and Vienna, graduating in 1844. Six months later he obtained the degree of Master of Midwifery.

Semmelweis worked in the Lying-in Division of the General Hospital in Vienna. The General Hospital in Vienna (Das Allegemeine Krankenhaus) was sponsored by Emperor Joseph II who enlarged the Lying-in department so that the two services were active, the First Obstetric Clinic and the Second Obstetric Clinic. Joseph II sent Lucas Johann Boër to Paris and London where he became associated with Denman and his contemporaries in order to learn all about English midwifery. On his return in 1788 he was appointed professor and director of the new lying-in hospital. In his last year at the Vienna Hospital, 1822, the deaths among 3066 patients amounted to 26, a mortality of 0.84 per cent.

Boër was succeeded by Klein, a former assistant who proved unworthy of the post. The mortality rate during his regime jumped up again to 7.8 per cent. It was under Klein that Semmelweis took service as full assistant in 1846.

Semmelweis was one of the best prepared assistants ever appointed; he had studied pathology under Rokitansky, a world-famed pathologist. He helped Klein in his operations in the first clinic, did autopsies in the second clinic, and during the same period he had the privilege of working anywhere in the hospital. Emphasis on two clinics is made because they formed the basis and were an important factor in solving the enigma of the cause and nature of puerperal fever. One of the clinics was for medical students, the other for midwives; superficially the two clinics appeared identical.

In his first year at the hospital, Semmelweis noticed that the First Clinic (for medical students) had a mortality of 460, in the Second Clinic 105 deaths. This was casually accepted by the older associates of the hospital. Semmelweis, however, was unable to accept this mortality with indifference. Questions which constantly recurred to his mind were concerned with the cause, prevention and treatment of puerperal fever. He spent many hours in the library, death house, and at the bedside.

Before Semmelweis, many peculiar theories as to causation were being bandied around, none of them satisfactory to him. Except for Boër, who had studied in England, all continental physicians believed in the many theories that were as much as 200 years old in some instances. They all, more or less, agreed that there were two etiological factors, an external and an internal, depending upon the condition of the organism during pregnancy.

As far back as 1662, Willis, for the first time, wrote about *Febris puerperarum.*

As late as the middle of the 18th Century, anomalies of the lochia was blamed; Smellie was the chief proponent of this idea and he probably got it from Mauriceau.

That it was milk fever (many diseases were blamed in the same way) was the theory held by many prominent teachers. Among these was Boër, who picked up this idea from the English and taught it at the Vienna School with some modifications. Other theories were the "lucus a non lucendo" which was a mixture of the lochia and milk theories, the gastric-bilious fever theory which had a considerable vogue in England, and the peritonitis theory with Hunter and Baudelocque as its chief exponents. Then erysipelas was associated with puerperal fever. This explained the idea of contagion more readily, a factor that many were beginning to appreciate now (mid-18th Century). In 100 years, the middle of the 19th Century, they were considered identical. The pioneers of our modern pathology of the disease harked back upon a "specific something," an "unknown something," and the "divinum aliquid," perhaps a specific primary change in the blood producing the local lesions known to the pathological anatomist. The external factors were still more vague and even incomprehensible; such as atmospheric, cosmic and mere weather change, and the resulting injurious entity blamed was called miasma. They believed that a contagion represented a specific virus which could take its origin only in the diseased organism, and that it could be conveyed by propinquity or actual contact. In some minds the contagion assumed the form of a mysterious halo or aureole which clung to the unfortunate practitioner who came under its malign influence.

A theory which prevailed close to the time of Semmelweis was the "doctrine of crasis," in which special changes in the blood occurred with an increase in fibrin (which occurred in the pregnant woman), all of which might increase so as to finally deposit in the form of exudation on the inner and outer surfaces of the uterus spontaneously. This might go on to pyaemia, bloodcrasis, or a spontaneous blood dissolution. Among the supporters of spontaneous origin were Virchow in 1861, and Barnes in 1875. This condition might also be produced by the external factor, the miasma. Pyaemia was similarly explained by the older surgeons. The latest and most acceptable idea was that, generally speaking, there existed a specific virus, and this virus was identified with that of erysipelas. In Europe, the miasma theory was the most acceptable, while in England the theory of contagion was more readily considered.

In the works of Semmelweis we find that all infection comes from without; his problem was to prove this. He showed that all of the above causes could not explain the difference in the two clinics;

three times as many deaths occurred in the First Clinic as in the Second Clinic. Rough examinations and too many examinations by the students were blamed, and as a result all foreign students were expelled so as to cut down the number. Still the mortality rate did not change. Religion, emotional disturbances of all sorts, and fright from the ordinary routine of hospital practice were blamed. Even the wounded modesty of the patients was blamed. Early rising in the puerperium was blamed, yet Charles White wrote a paper in which he credited his low mortality in part to early ambulation. Street births (Gassengeburt) and premature cases seldom got the infection; the Gassengeburt were placed in special places in the hospital and were not examined as were the regularly admitted cases.

Semmelweis gathered all this information and could not come to an intelligent conclusion until he realized that the students came to Clinic I from the dissecting room. The thought occurred to him that bits of cadaveric tissue might cling to their fingers even though they washed their hands with soap and water. So he ordered every student to wash his hands with "Chlorina liquida" before making an examination. This was in 1847. A rapid and pronounced drop in the mortality occurred. Diligently following the practice of washing with chlorinated lime (substituted because it was less expensive), the mortality rate of the First Clinic dropped to 1.27 per cent and in the Second Clinic 1.33 per cent by 1848. This was the first time in the history of the Vienna Lying-in Hospital that the mortality in the First Division fell below that of the Second Division. This also explained the difference in the mortality in the two divisions up to this time. The system of instruction for midwives was such that neither teachers nor pupils had much occasion to manipulate the cadaver, and thus render their hands unclean. Hence, the comparative immunity of the Second Division from puerperal fever.

The discovery of the causation of puerperal fever was now complete: the three sources of infection mentioned throughout his "Aetiologie" and "Briefe" were established facts in the mind of Semmelweis. It was the division of the Vienna Lying-in to two groups that served as an experimental ground for this discovery. His doctrine firmly established, and one that he never changed, amounted to this: "That puerperal fever was caused by a decomposed animal organic matter conveyed by contact to the pregnant, parturient or puerperal woman without regard to its origin, whether from the cadaver or from a living person affected with a disease which produced a decomposed animal organic matter." To his original theory he added as a further explanation that "the conveyance of a foul exudation from a living organism may be one cause which produces the puerperal process, e.g. filthy discharge from a leg ulcer, infected medullary sarcoma of the uterus."

The early supporters of his theory were his three friends Hebra, Skoda and Rokitansky; also, Haller, Michaelis of Keil, Lange of Heidelberg who applied his theory and publicly announced their debt of gratitude to Semmelweis. Klein, his former chief, became hostile, and went so far as to encourage students to obstruct the exact and thorough application of the method of prophylaxis introduced by Semmelweis. Léon Le Forte, Tarnier, Meigs, Denham of Ireland and Scanzoni all disagreed with Semmelweis.

Among the earliest and most important criticism was the article by Breisky, an assistant at the Lying-in Hospital of Prague. Like many others, it is typical of his adverse critics. Breisky takes exception to the self-consciousness of Semmelweis; after years of silence, says Breisky, Semmelweis proclaims his discovery as the Koran of a puerperal creed which he preaches with fanatical zeal and enters into battle with threatenings of fire and sword for the unbelievers. He is very sarcastic about the discoverer of the "eternally true" etiology of puerperal fever. He has not produced anything like an exact and complete demonstration of the truth. He has not proved the identity of pyaemia and puerperal fever. He destructively criticizes the three lying-in hospitals to which he so often refers. Even infection by want of cleanliness of bedding, etc., at the St. Roche Hospital at Buda-Pesth is questioned (Semmelweis was a chief there for five years, where he also decreased the mortality rate). Hardly any obstetrician except Semmelweis has observed any advantage from the method of prophylaxis recommended in the book, and the conclusion is therefore reached that cadaveric infection cannot be the cause of puerperal fever even in such cases as those described.[4, 5]

A friend of Semmelweis, Markusovszky, took it upon himself to reply to Breisky, whose outburst hurt Semmelweis immensely. He wrote:

> The investigation into the etiology of the fever is not yet complete, even if everyone agreed that puerperal fever is due to decomposed animal matter. Much of his definition is provisional and still subject to further research. The exact chemical composition of the infecting material, how it gains access to the organism and many other points must be cleared up. But all this does not make his doctrine false . . . we certainly cannot demand from the relatively new knowledge, and from a single individual, the solution of all the questions to which answers can only be obtained with the aid of all the branches of natural science. . . . Breisky has made no reference to the lifesaving discovery and the favorable results already obtained: he has only though it right to raise a series of objections of doubtful value, and to demand from the obstetrician such a full and complete development of his Doctrine in all directions as can be reached only by the cooperation of physiology, chemistry, physics and histology, when in the course of time these branches of science have made further advances.[6]

Of course a prolonged and acrimonious controversy followed his publication of *Die Aetiologie*, and while his friends spread the doctrine by correspondence, Semmelweis remained curiously quiet. In a reply by Simpson to a letter he received, Semmelweis says:

> This letter was filled with abuse; Simpson said that without the letter he knew in what a lamentable condition midwifery in Germany, and especially in Vienna, still remained; he knew for certain that the cause of the high mortality lay only in the unbounded carelessness with which patients were treated; as, for example, when they put a healthy lying-in woman into the same bed in which another patient had just died, without changing the bedclothes and linen.

What Simpson said about conditions of uncleanliness was admitted to be true by Semmelweis. Simpson was abrupt in his reply because he honestly believed that the Englishmen had practically propounded the theory that Semmelweis was now proclaiming, which of course was not true and which Simpson eventually admitted. Nearly all the English medical men were in sympathy with

Semmelweis and afforded him the honor he deserved.

In William Sinclair's Book on Semmelweis appears the following quotation:

> v. Balassa, professor and distinguished Hungarian general surgeon, was mistakenly accused of saying that he did not think it worth the trouble to adopt the antiseptic method of Semmelweis. Tiberius v. Gyory states that the incident of v. Balassa assisting Semmelweis at the first ovariotomy performed in Hungary, in 1863, was not merely an isolated act of collegial courtesy, but that v. Balassa himself rigidly applied the Semmelweis antiseptic method in his surgical work "Sondren ein jedes Mal auch die dort gelehrten antiseptischen Maasregeln genau befolgte." v. Gyory possesses contemporary evidence in writing that at least from 1858 onwards in Hungary the chlorine disinfection was rigidly practiced not only in the Obstetric Clinics but also in the Surgical.[7]

This fact is of remarkable interest historically inasmuch as it proves that before the work of Pasteur was known, and before Lister introduced his methods of preventing wound fever, and long before anyone elsewhere thought of routine antiseptic midwifery, the systematic use of antiseptics in midwifery, gynecology and surgery had been regularly practiced in Buda-Pesth.

The antiseptic employed was chloride of lime, but there can be no doubt that with further experience some of the newer chemical substances would have been brought into use. So we may, without violence, claim for Semmelweis that it was he who introduced antisepsis as a prophylactic measure both in obstetrics and gynecology.

By 1863, when he was only forty-five years old he began to have periods of depression with periods of excitement. By 1865, he was regarded as insane. He had been operating until the time of his admission to an insane asylum on August 1, 1865. One of the attendants noticed an injury of his right hand, a minor cut, probably sustained in one of the last gynecological operations he had performed. Just as cadaveric poison killed Professor Kolletschka, whom Semmelweis used as a case in point for his theory, so died Semmelweis. While practically the whole world mourned his death in reverence, Germany and Austria in their brief reference to his death showed only animosity to this great man.[8]

He died young (forty-seven), and he never saw the complete vindication of this theory. But it was shortly after this, that the doctrine became firmly and irrevocably entrenched as truly the cause of puerperal fever; this came as a result of the work of still another great scientist, Pasteur.

The supplementary knowledge which Markusovszky prophetically declared to be essential to complete the understanding of puerperal fever was soon to be revealed; the medium was bacteriology, the mediator was Pasteur.

LOUIS PASTEUR (1822-1895) was a French chemist. He was born in Dole, son of a tanner. He graduated from the École Normale in Paris in 1847. Words like miasma, humors, and spontaneous generation did not exist in his vocabulary. He sincerely believed that specific microbes were at the root of specific diseases, and that such diseases could be combatted by their own causative microbes in weakened form; all the microbes had parents, they did not burst upon the scene spontaneously. He deduced all these facts from his association with industrial chemistry, e.g. the wine, the vinegar industry, and silk. He developed vaccines against anthrax and rabies.

Pasteur's greatest contribution to puerperal fever was his discovery, in 1860, of the streptococcus; in 1879 he demonstrated the "hemolytic" streptococcus as the cause of puerperal infection. When he recovered the organism from a case of puerperal fever in 1860, Ogston of Aberdeen identified, for the first time, the organisms in surgical pyemia.[9, 10]

Scientists soon began to make innumerable contributions in bacteriology. It was started by Mayerhofer in 1863, who had isolated organisms from the air in the wards and from the lochiae of puerperal women who were sick. Dr. Hausman, in 1868, showed the same organisms in the vaginal secretions of well women, and argued therefore of their innocence as causative of infection.

It was left for Joseph Lister to apply these discoveries to the prevention of infection in hospitals, so together with Pasteur the study of infection was placed on a scientific basis.

JOSEPH LISTER (1827-1912) was born in the London borough of West Ham. He graduated from the University of London in 1852, and went to Edinburgh to study surgery under Syme, whose daughter he later married. He became professor of surgery at the

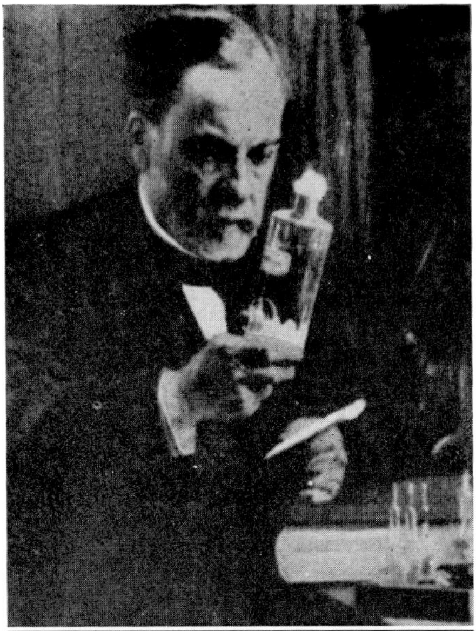

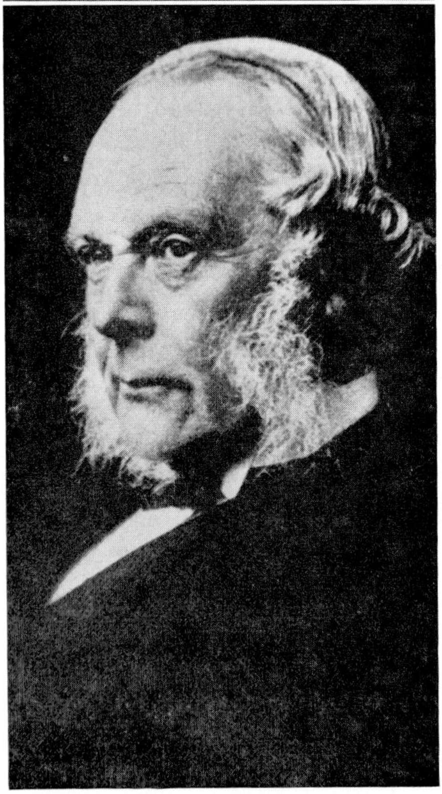

Fig. 158. Louis Pasteur. (The Bettmann Archive.)

Fig. 159. Joseph Lister. (The Bettmann Archive.)

University of Glasgow. In the record of amputations, from 1864-1866, Lister found 45 per cent of fatalities from infection, although he had used scrupulous care as to cleanliness, and Syme's technique of silver wire sutures, drainage and frequent change of dressings. He did not know much about Semmelweis and believed that suppuration was caused by putrefaction from exposure to the air, and this in turn caused blood poisoning. These conclusions were the result of his observations that compound fractures were nearly always fatal, whereas simple fractures healed. He undertook to perfect a dressing soaked in a solution of crude carbolic acid on the wound of a compound fracture. Sloughing of the skin resulted but the patient recovered.

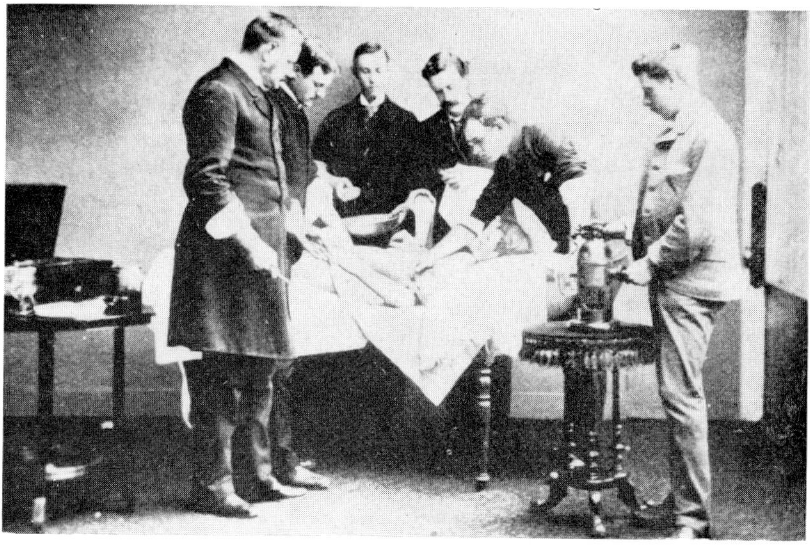

Fig. 160. Carbolic spray used in operation. (The Bettmann Archive.)

It was in the same year, 1865, that he learned of Pasteur's discovery of bacteria in the air causing putrefaction. With this information, he experimented with a great variety of dressings to disinfect wounds, and performed his operations in a room where carbolic acid had been sprayed. This unpleasant and not too safe procedure was a real progressive measure and paved the way for asepsis, and from this time forward surgery became relatively safe. In 1867, he published a paper "*On the Antiseptic Principle in Surgery*." This epoch-making address was frankly based on the work of Pasteur.

As usual, the Listerian doctrine and methods met opposition, chiefly in the person of Simpson. Except for this, the objection did not last for thirty years as was the case with Harvey, Jenner and Semmelweis. As a whole, it can be said that the adoption and success of Lister's methods were immediate and universal. It stimulated much original work in bacteriology. Waldeyer, of Breslau, in 1871 contributed the bacteriology of puerperal fever. Among the greatest was Doléris, who, in 1880, published a thesis that popularized antiseptic midwifery in France, and then largely in Europe.[11]

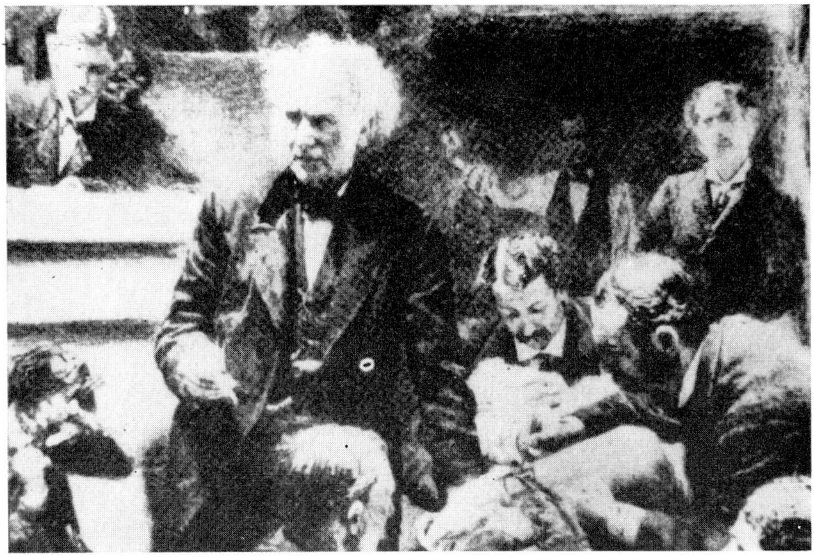

Fig. 161. Samuel D. Gross Clinic; operating in frock coats. (The Bettmann Archive.)

Gynecologists were slow to adopt and apply the principles of antisepsis. While the operators, especially the Americans, showed native ingenuity and pluck, operating in the McDowell tradition, there was no marked progress in the prevention of infection. Frock coats still prevailed in the operating rooms. Apparently the Americans were not overly impressed with Listerism. In fact, when Lister came to America for the 1876 Centennial, he was merely received politely. In contrast, Samuel D. Gross was lionized in Paris, and Dr. Marion Sims, great gynecological surgeon, was said to be so famous that he could settle in any capital of Europe and immediately be swamped with patients. It was not until the 1880's that Listerian principles were established, at Mt. Sinai Hospital, New York, through the pioneer work of Dr. Arpad Gerster.

So antiseptic methods began to improve, based on all the recent

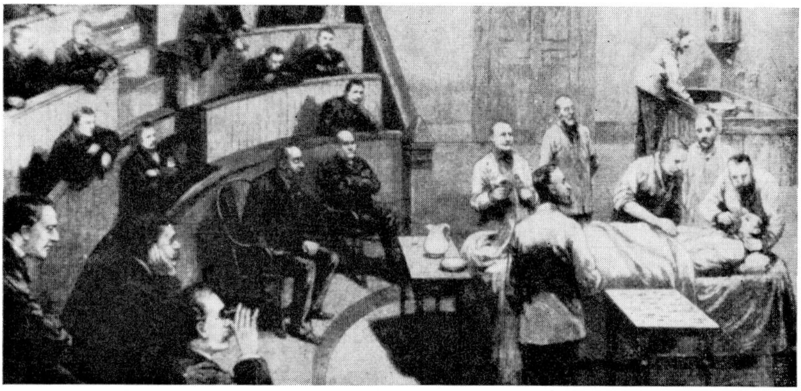

Fig. 162. Operation in Massachusetts General Hospital shows trend toward asepsis. (The Bettman Archive.)

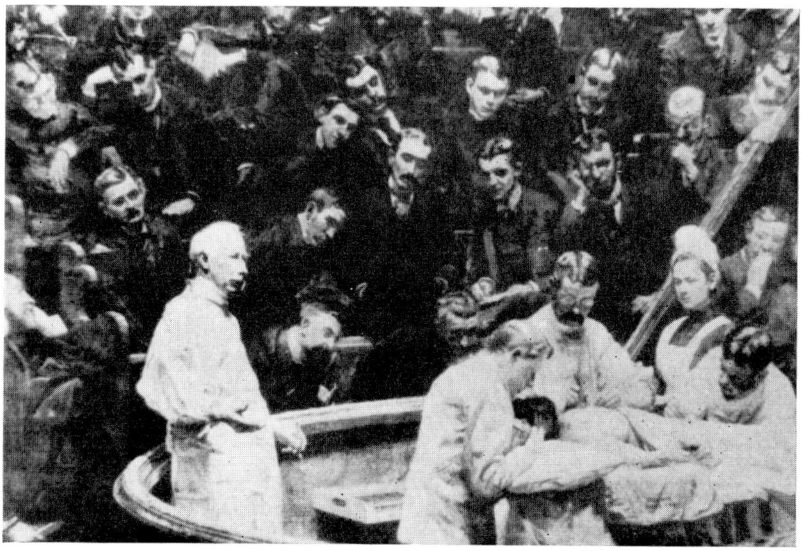

Fig. 163. David Hayes Agnew Clinic; no frock coats but also no gloves. (Addison, Agnes: *University of Pennsylvania Medical School, Portraits*. Philadelphia, University Press, 1940.)

discoveries pertaining to infection. Instead of spraying the operating room, generally, they began to concentrate the spray in the region of the diseased tissue. A few years later asepsis began to assume greater importance; linens were cleaned (no rubber gloves yet, see illustration) and operating room techniques showed improvement in many details pertaining to asepsis. The early 20th Century showed still more progress. In the Mayo clinic (illustration) they wore gloves but no mask. This progress continued until we come to the scrupulous asepsis of today.[12]

Our modern understanding and differentiation of the various types of pelvic infections is due primarily to T. GAILLARD THOMAS (1831-1903), attending surgeon at the New York Women's Hospital, in 1872. For fifteen years he was the foremost gynecological surgeon of America. Between 1841 and 1872, he published numerous works on infection of the pelvis; their true nature was never understood, except perhaps by EMIL NOEGGERATH (1827-1895), who was born at Bonn. He studied at the University of Bonn until 1852. He came to New York in 1857, and became Professor of Obstetrics and Diseases of Women at the New York Medical College. He founded the *American Journal of Obstetrics* in 1868, and, together with Abraham Jacobi, he edited this journal for five years. He was the founder of the American Gynecological Society. He had already published his famous observations on gonorrhea in the female (in 1872), but it was not accepted too generously. At the first meeting of the American Gynecological Society, 1876, he read a paper on "Latent Gonorrhea, Especially with Regard to its Influence on Fertility in Women." Again he was criticised, but he replied that he expected this reception, and asked the dissenters to withhold their opinions for at least five years, after which time he said that they would appreciate his work and agree with his views. His paper maintained that this disease was practically impossible to eradicate, and that it might remain latent for long periods before causing serious complications and that it was one of the chief causes of sterility. His paper continues:

> The complexity and latency (chronicity) of the disease, with the pelvic involvement which was never properly understood, explains

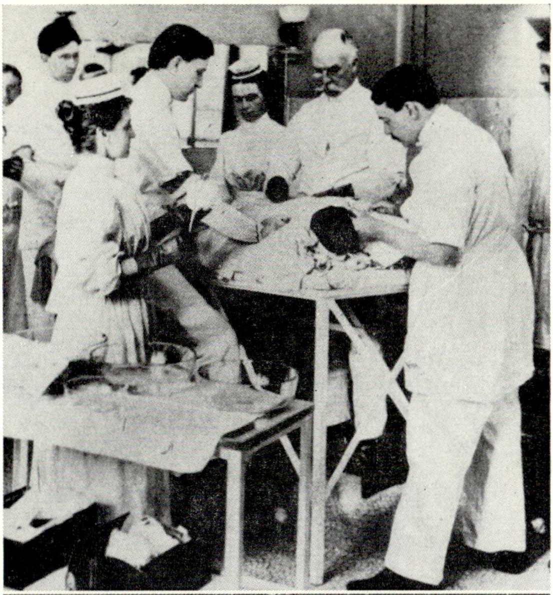

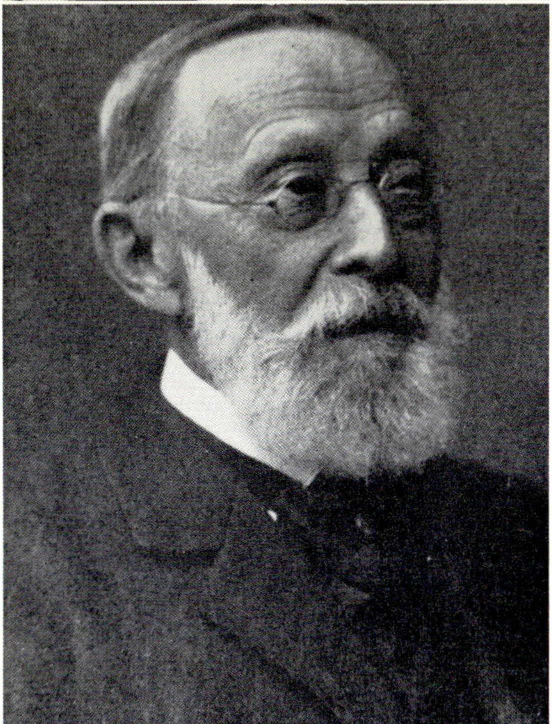

Fig. 164. The Mayo Clinic; gloves but no masks. (The Bettmann Archive.)
Fig.165. Rudolph Virchow. (Culver Service.)

> a. Why so many healthy, blooming, young girls, begin to suffer and fail as soon as they enter the bonds of marriage.
>
> b. Why so many apparently healthy young women remain sterile.
>
> c. Why the patient labor of our best physicians is so often thwarted in the attempt to cure certain affections of the female genital organs. It explains to some extent the prevalence of uterine diseases in large cities.
>
> As to the treatment applicable to these affections, the result of latent gonorrhea, I will make only one remark: I have found that an obstinate catarrh of the womb, which would not be influenced by remedies, yields pretty rapidly when the husband of the patient is also taken care of, especially where the signs of stricture and mucopurulent discharge have been very evident.[13]

In spite of the faithful description of the signs and symptoms of gonorrhea, he admitted the lack of direct proof. It was 1879, when this proof came, it was Neisser's discovery of the responsible organism, the gonococcus. And yet as late as 1888, there were some prominent physicians who refused to accept these findings. Such a person was Charles Carroll Lee, chief of the venereal wards of the New York Charity Hospital (now City Hospital).

Complete understanding of gonorrhea arrived only after centuries of fruitless groping, confusion, and tragedy. Some knowledge of it goes back to the time of Galen, about A.D. 150, who considered it a seminal discharge. In fact a smattering of information even further back may be noticed in the early civilizations thirty-five centuries ago. In all these centuries ignorance of etiology, clinical significance, prevention and cure reigned supreme. It was RICORD in 1838 who showed that gonorrhea and syphilis are distinct; NOEGGERATH in 1872 who pointed out the clinical character of this disease; NEISSER in 1879 who discovered the gonococcus, and TAIT who by his modern methods of abdominal surgery provided the opportunity for pathological study of this disease.

While the problem of infection was being solved, another discovery was made. This was Virchow's doctrine that the "cell" was the essential element of the living body, and completed the triad of revolutionary discoveries of the 19th Century which were to be the foundations of the present-day status of medicine (gynecology and obstetrics). This triad was anesthesia, infection and cellular pathology. William H. Welch called the cellular theory the greatest advance ever made in pathology. According to Howard A. Kelly, Dean of American gynecology, the cellular pathology doctrine of Virchow is the very groundwork of all that is scientific in our work.

RUDOLF VIRCHOW (1821-1902) was a tireless proponent of laboratory medicine. He was a kindly, busy man who lunched on a bottle of beer and two sandwiches, amidst skeletons and skulls (see illustration). He was the founder of the great scientific magazine *Archiv für Pathologische Anatomie*. It was in 1858 that he published his revolutionary work on "*cellular pathology*." He pronounced the cell the essential element of the living body and defined disease as the cell's reaction to altered conditions.

His views of the cell in pathology are an advancement on the ideas of Morgagni, who made the first contribution to pathology in 1761, when he defined the lesion responsible for death as being in a particular organ; he considered the organs as separate and complete entities. Bichat, soon thereafter, went a step further and described the site of disease (and, therefore, the entity) as the tissues. Then came the addition of Virchow's theory, that the cell was the entity. There had been some preliminary work done on the cell by Mathias Jakob Schleiden, who, in 1839, considered the cell formation elementary; that the ovum and the sperm were single cells from which all others developed. Cellular pathology continued to advance for fifty years, after which the cells were shown to have components such as the nucleus and nucleolus, so Virchow's tenets have had to be modified somewhat by the exploration of intercellular structures.

He trained hundreds of pathologists, and among other things collected and mounted 23,000 specimens, and was very interested in anthropology.[14, 15]

First Occurrences and Outstanding Events

Holmes published his essay on Puerperal Fever in 1843.

Semmelweis published his *Aetiologie* in October 1860, proving that foul organic material caused infection.

Pasteur discovered the streptococcus in 1860, as the cause of puerperal fever.

Lister, in 1865, applied knowledge of other men, by direct experimentation.

T. Gaillard Thomas was the first to explain pelvic infections.

Noeggerath was the first to understand gonorrhea and its complications clinically.

Neisser discovered the gonococcus in 1879.

Ricord showed gonorrhea and syphilis to be different, in 1838.

Virchow showed the cell as the essential element of the living body, 1858.

References

1. Graham, Harvey: *Eternal Eve.* London, Heinemann, 1950.
2. Holmes, O. W.: The Contagiousness of Puerperal Fever. *Boston Quart. J. Med. and Surg., 1*:503-530, 1842-43.
3. Sinclair, Sir W. J.: *Semmelweis, his Life and his Doctrine.* Manchester, Manchester Univ. Press, 1909, p. 1.
4. Sinclair, Sir W. J.: *Semmelweis, his Life and his Doctrine.* Manchester, Manchester Univ. Press, 1909.
5. Graham, Harvey: *Eternal Eve.* London, Heinemann, 1950.
6. Sinclair, Sir W. J.: *Semmelweis, his Life and his Doctrine.* Manchester, Manchester Univ. Press, 1909, p. 234.
7. *Ibid., p.* 358.
8. Findley, Palmer: Semmelweis and others on infection. *Am. J. Obst. and Gynec.*, pp. 700-710, April 1948.
9. Bettmann, O. L.: *A Pictorial History of Medicine*, Springfield, Thomas, 1956.
10. Walsh, J. J.: *Makers of Modern Medicine.* New York, Fordham Univ. Press, 1915.
11. Graham, Harvey: *Eternal Eve.* London, Heinemann, 1950.
12. Bettmann, O. L.: *A Pictorial History of Medicine.* Springfield, Thomas, 1956.
13. Leonardo, R. A.: *History of Gynecology.* New York, Froben, 1944, pp. 244-249.
14. Bettmann, O. L.: *A Pictorial History of Medicine.* Springfield, Thomas, 1956.
15. Walsh, J. J.: *Makers of Modern Medicine.* New York, Fordham U. P., 1915.

Chapter XVII

FISTULA AND SPECULUM

A. VESICO-VAGINAL FISTULA

JAMES MARION SIMS[1] (1813-1883) graduated from Jefferson Medical College in 1835. He was born in Lancaster County, South Carolina. His achievement of curing vesico-vaginal fistula came not too long after McDowell's accomplishment of ovariotomy, which opened the way to abdominal surgery, and may be considered a contribution to gynecology and to humanity second only to ovariotomy. The tragic history of these cases was long known, but the medical profession had been unable to cope with it. D. Hays Agnew, of Philadelphia, and Johann Friedrich Dieffenbach, of Königsberg, had written grim phrases to describe this condition, one that usually doomed the victim to isolation and seclusion. Physicions hardly ever attempted to cure a fistula; the usual comment was: "Why try, since they never heal?" Alfred Velpeau, Paris, remarked that all the procedures so far suggested or attempted could have no other result than to cause unnecessary suffering to the patient. Nevertheless, some attempts had been made to help these women before Sims found the answer.[2] These were:

Indwelling catheters, pessaries and truss fittings were tried by Desault.

Nitrate of silver and of mercury and tincture of cantharies were applied to the fistula by Lallemand of France in 1825, and by Roux in 1829.

Different types of sutures, pins and wires were tried by Naegle of Heidelberg.

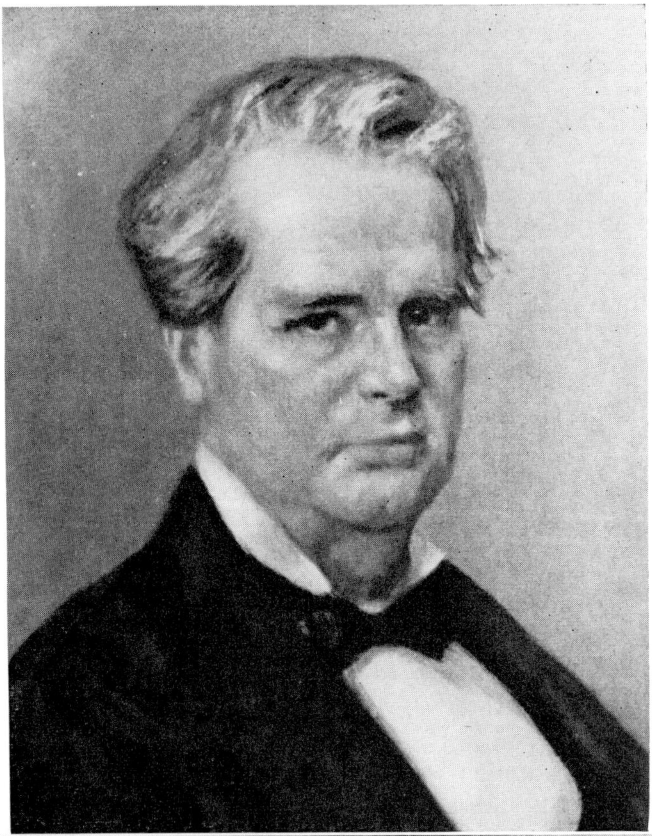

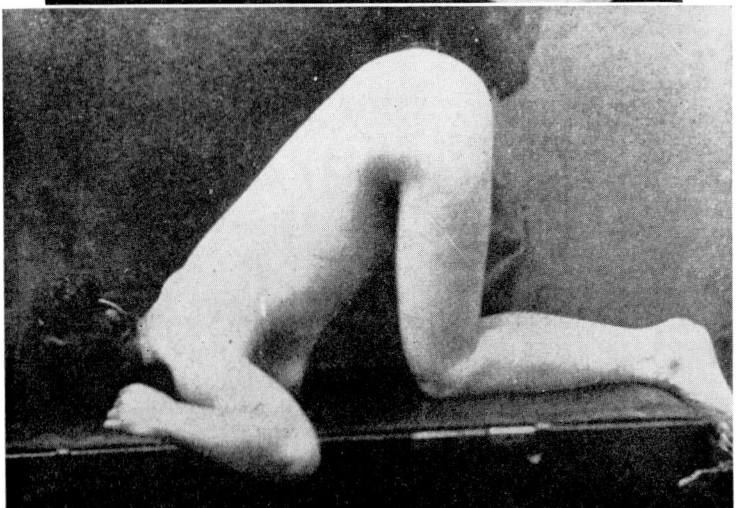

Fig. 166. James Marion Sims. (*Lederle Bulletin, 17*:No. 3, Aug. 1952. New York, Lederle Laboratories Division [American Cyanamid Co.].)

Fig. 167. Knee-chest posture. (Hirst, B. C.: *Text Book of Obstetrics*. Philadelphia, Saunders, 1918.)

In 1832, DeCassis tried the drastic expedient of obliterating the vagina, without success.

In August 1828, Malagodi of Bologna had success by excising the edges and using three special twisted sutures.

Jobert de Lamballe, of Paris, operated on four cases, with one success by doing a plastic repair with flaps of fresh skin from the labia majora or the buttocks.[3]

C. W. Wutzer of Bonn operated on twenty-eight cases from 1838 to 1852, with only two successes. He used suprapubic drainage. Thus far all the men used the lithotomy position.

Samuel Hobart of Cork had a single cure in 1825. The patient was placed in the knee-elbow position and a special speculum was used.

M. Gossett of London, using the same position, had a cure in 1834. He used gilt silver wire to which he attributed his success. A number of other men reported individual successes with silver wire and, in one instance, by the use of silk sutures.

John Peter Mettauer[4] of Virginia, in 1838, reported a success; he used leaden wire sutures.

George Hayward, Massachusetts General Hospital, did a case in 1839, and nine more in 1855 with good results.

The enumeration of the above cases is to show the status of vesico-vaginal fistula in the early 19th Century, just before the contribution of Sims. In going back still further in the history of this condition which existed in all eras, we cite the story of Queen Henhenit, wife of King Mentuhotep, 2050 B.C. A large vesico-vaginal fistula was discovered by post mortem examination of her mummy.[5] Hippocrates[6] referred to vesico-vaginal fistula, and Avicenna in A.D. 1037 was first to recognize incontinence of urine in women as the result of fistulae produced in labor. Felix Plater, in 1597, and Pinaeus in 1650, described this condition, and both deduced it as resulting from forceful labor.

Hendrik van Roonhuyse of Amsterdam, in 1663, was the first to give any practical suggestion for its cure. In his *Heelkonstige Aanmerkkingen*[7] he was the first to propose a scientific operation for the cure of vesico-vaginal fistula in which he advocated exposure of the fistula with a retracting speculum and the patient in the lithotomy position, vaginal denudation of the tract, exclusion of the bladder wall and approximation of the denuded edges of the fistula by means of quills fastened with silk threads. In 1676, thirteen years later, and again in 1684, Johannes Fatio[8] performed this operation. The patient healed in fourteen days. For 150 years this information was forgotten. Then, as already mentioned, followed the early 18th Century attempts at cure by cauterization, dressings, and catheters.

Sims performed the operation with history making results in 1849, by the use of the knee-chest position, the spoon speculum and silver wire. It was in 1852, when the operation was published in the *American Journal of the Medical Sciences*. He had been practicing general surgery, and had been called in consultation many times in cases of vesico-vaginal fistula, always refusing to operate before; like everybody else, he did not feel the results justified the attempt. In spite of his refusals patients persisted in getting his help; one patient who was sent to him by her owner had to travel a long distance. After Sims refused to operate he permitted her to remain for the evening before starting on her journey home. The following morning he was called to attend a woman who was thrown from horseback. What took place is best told by John Allen Wyeth, in *With Sabre and Scalpel*, who says:

> I have often wondered over what womankind would have suffered through all these years, had not that immortal Alabama hog laid itself down to sleep in that particular fence corner by the roadside on that eventful day in June 1845. The animal, awakened and frightened by the nearness of a lady on horseback, started up with considerable noise; the horse sprang from under its rider, who struck heavily upon her pelvis. She was carried to her home and, when Dr. Sims reached her, she complained of great pain in her back and pelvic organs. A careful examination revealed a backward displacement of the uterus.* Placing her in the genu pectoral position (knee chest posture) and in the further manipulation to replace the uterus, the accidental advent of atmospheric air dilated the cavity (vagina) and at the same time suddenly restored the uterus to its normal position. The quick eye of the genius at once took in the entire significance of this

* It is worthy of our attention that today we do not believe that displacement produces any such disturbance as quoted herein.

> accident. Almost overcome with the discovery, he said to himself, "If I can accomplish this by the use of atmospheric pressure, why can I not employ the same agency in attempting to relieve these incurable cases of vesico-vaginal fistula?" Enthused with this idea, he hurried back to his office, stopping only at a hardware store on the way to buy a large pewter spoon, and from this was evolved at once the speculum which bears the name of its inventor.[9]

The patient who was to have left the next day was placed in the position described with an assistant on either side to retract. From the rush of air into the vagina, the vaginal walls distended and the rugae disappeared, visibility became unbelievably clear, "the whole surface was seen at one view, for the first time by any mortal man." The fistula and its relation to its surroundings was noticed as never before possible, and from the words of Sims, "the principles of the operation were presented to my mind as clearly as at this time (of examination)."

He sought other cases of vesico-vaginal fistulae, whereas like everyone else before, he had been avoiding them. He attempted the operation many times after this initial success but failed in each instance. His friends began to despair, but for four years he persisted, trying all sorts of modifications in technique. He used lead shot instead of knots, silver quills, lead sutures and silk. Success came again when he used a fine thread of silver, cure after cure resulted, and his fame spread quickly and far.

In his paper published on the subject, he claimed originality for the operation because he discovered a method (spoon and knee-chest position) of exposing the lesion through the vagina; he introduced the suture material (silver) with a special apparatus for introduction, and a self-retaining catheter that he devised.

The special clamp suture which he devised is a modification of the quilled suture. For details, reference is suggested to any of the works on Sims, or to Graham's book *Eternal Eve.*[10]

In 1845, Sims introduced his double-ended duckbill speculum; this was four years before the successful performance of his operation. It is ordinarily called a bivalve speculum although only one end is inserted into the vagina (either end), the other being used as a handle. He also developed two other types of this speculum,

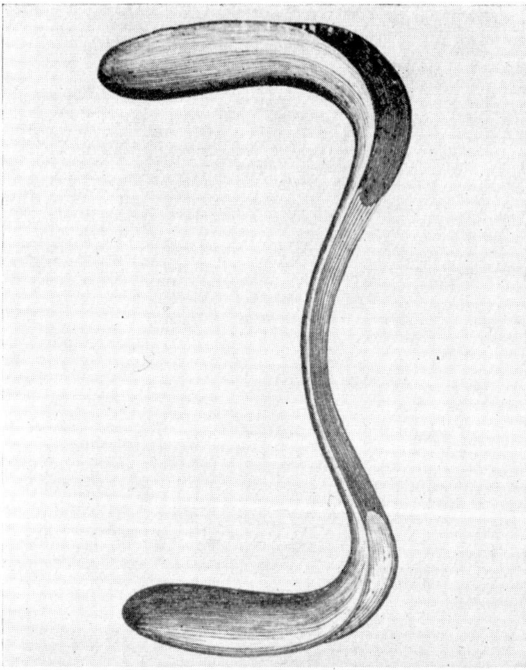

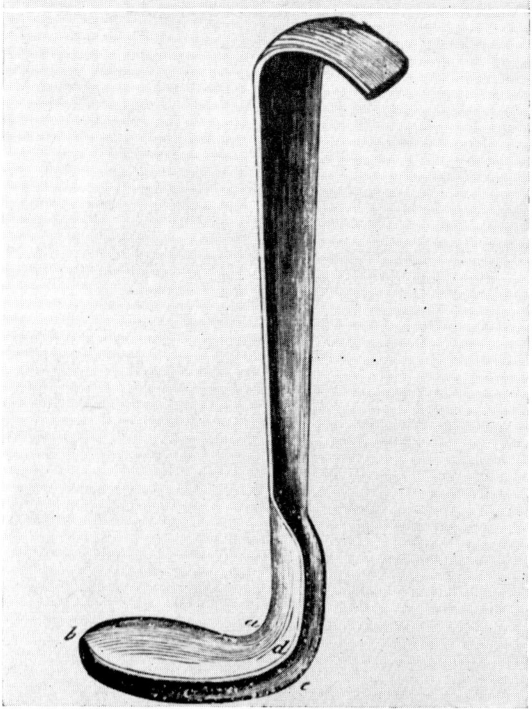

Fig. 168. Duckbill speculum of Sims. (Leonardo, R. A.: *History of Gynecology*. New York, Froben, 1944.)

Fig. 169. Lever speculum of Sims. (Leonardo, R. A.: *History of Gynecology*. New York, Froben, 1944.)

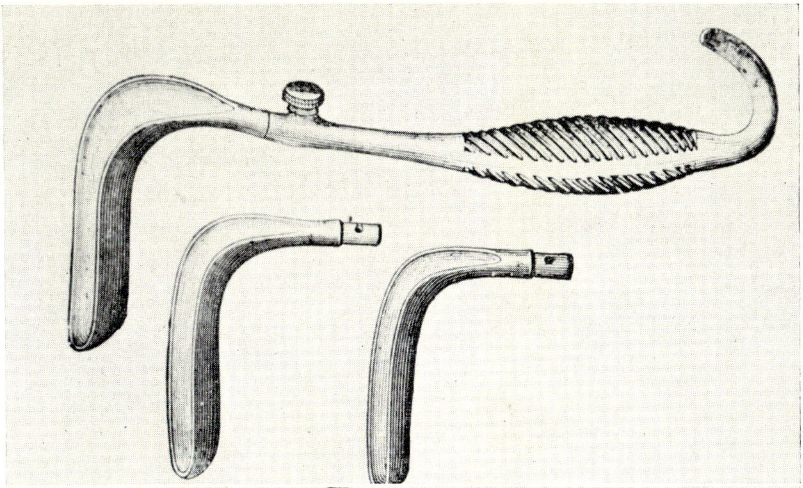

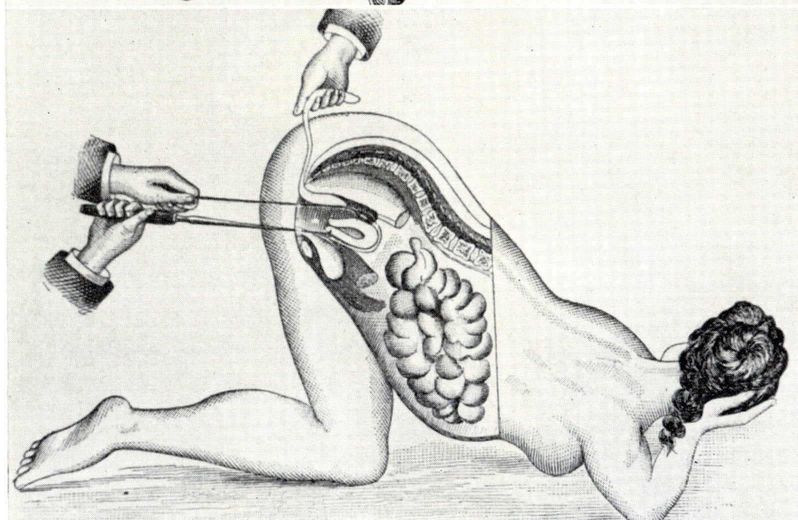

Fig. 170. Sims' specula. Detachable blades of varying sizes and handle. (Hirst, B. C.: *Text Book of Obstetrics*. Philadelphia, Saunders, 1918.)

Fig. 171. Replacement of retrodisplaced uterus by means of the uterine repositor, Sims' speculum and the knee-chest position. (Penrose, C. B.: *Diseases of Women*. Philadelphia, Saunders, 1897.)

the "lever speculum" and "the single detachable blade used with depressor" (Nott's).

The ordinary specula in use before the discovery of Sims, simply separated the vaginal walls mechanically, and thus exposed the uterus. Sims' instrument, on the other hand, elevates the posterior vaginal wall, which allows the entrance of air to distend the whole passage; the woman lies on her side in such a manner that the cavity can be probed with the most perfect ease. This is the Sims position. In this position the hips are on a higher level than the upper abdomen (diaphragm), toward which the abdominal contents drift causing a vacuum around the vaginal vault and thus bringing about the ballooning of the vagina, effacing most of the rugae seen in a collapsed vaginal canal. Sims' speculum simply separates the orifice allowing air to enter. The experience needed, however, to use this

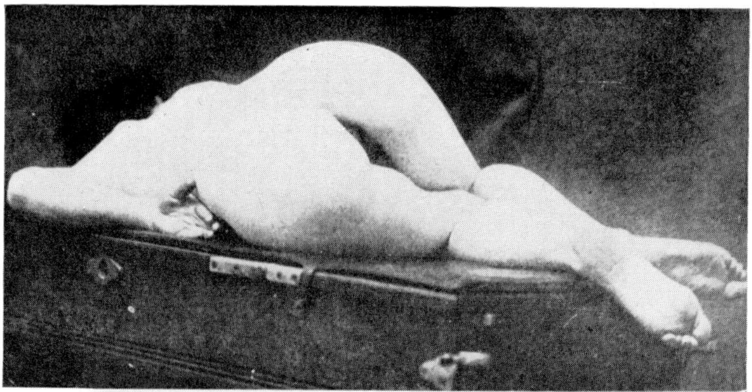

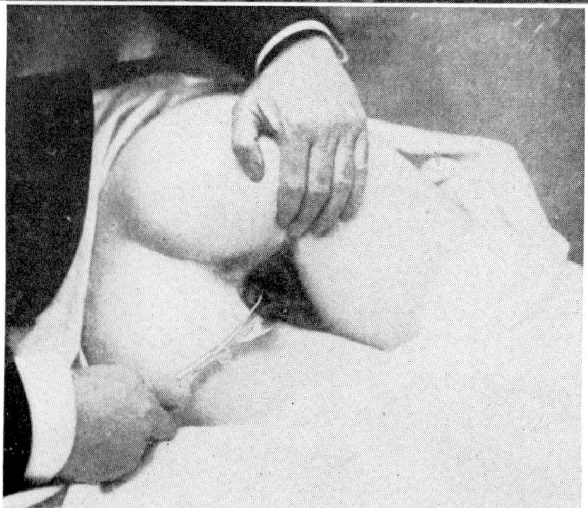

Fig. 172. Sims' position. (Hirst, B. C.: *Text Book of Obstetrics.* Philadelphia, Saunders, 1918.)

Fig. 173. Introduction of Sims' speculum. (Hirst, B. C.: *Text Book of Obstetrics.* Philadelphia, Saunders, 1918.)

speculum with advantage, and the disadvantage of its requiring aid of a nurse, will prevent its universal or even very general adoption.

Many thought that Sims was the inventor of the vaginal speculum because of his statement made in describing his findings when he first used his famous pewter spoon. The statement was, "I saw everything as no man had ever seen before." This belief was increased by what Emmet had to say regarding the value of the Sims speculum:

> From the beginning of time to the present, I believe that the human race has not been benefited to the same extent and in a like period, by the introduction of any other surgical instrument. Those who did not fully appreciate the value of the speculum itself, have been benefitted indirectly to an extent they little realize, for the instrument in the hands of others has probably advanced the knowledge of the diseases of women to an extent which could have have been done for one hundred years or more without it.[11]

Another of Sims' achievements was the establishment of a hospital exclusively for women at 83 Madison Avenue, New York, in 1855. A bigger hospital became necessary so The Women's Hospital in the State of New York, as it was named, replaced the old and original building, in recent years there was again a change of site, and the Waldorf Astoria Hotel now stands on the old ground. Not only was this the first hospital for women, but it marked the origin and recognition of gynecology as a modern specialty.

This hospital was preceded by a clinic, the first of its kind, for diseases of women, established by Dr. Guming S. Bedford, in 1841, who held the chair of Obstetrics and Gynecology in the New York University Medical College.[12] Before this a gynecological unit for the special care of women only was established by Evory Kennedy, Master of the Rotunda Hospital, in 1835. Then in 1851, the Philadelphia Woman's Hospital was started; in 1852, a similar hospital, the New England Hospital; and in 1871, the Women's Hospital of the State of Illinois.

While Sims was teaching and operating at the Women's Hospital, the Board of Managers limited the number of spectators of any one operation to fifteen. According to the Board, due regard for the modesty of the patient demanded such restriction. When Sims pro-

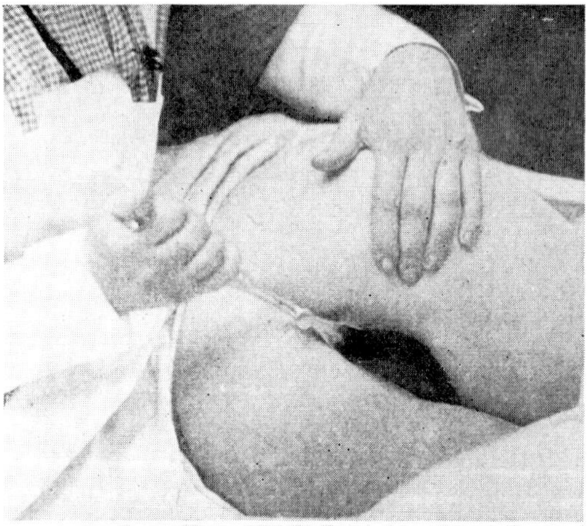

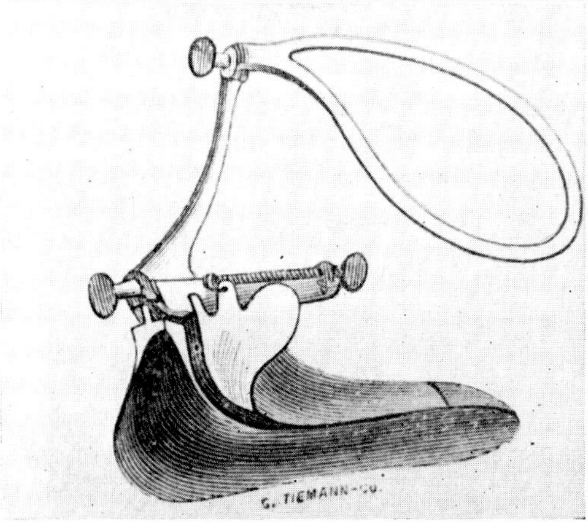

Fig. 174. Sims' speculum introduced and held by a nurse. (Hirst, B. C.: *Text Book of Obstetrics*. Philadelphia, Saunders, 1918.)

Fig. 175. Emmet's speculum. (Ashurst, John, Jr.: *Principles and Practice of Surgery*, 5th Ed. Philadelphia, Lea, 1889.)

tested and the Board adhered to its resolution, Dr. Sims tendered his resignation.

Thomas Addis Emmet (1828-1919) was Sims' able assistant until 1862, when he succeeded him as chief at the Women's Hospital. His skill and judgment eventually equaled that of Sims. When Emmet was Sims' assistant he often took complete charge because of the frequent absence of Sims who was forever taking European trips, operating for some of the great men, among them Simpson. Emmet made notable contributions to the field of plastic gynecology.[13] He showed the necessity of repairing also the deeper tissues in cases of cystocele and rectocele; in fact the modern operation for these conditions are based on Emmet's principles and teachings. He also devised a speculum that could be fixed to the patient so that an extra assistant would not be necessary, as was the case with Sims' speculum.

B. HISTORY OF THE SPECULUM

We have discussed the speculum of Sims at such length that it might be well to review the history of the speculum from the beginning. At the time of the Egyptians, the period of earliest recorded history, there is no evidence that the speculum existed. The first evidence that the speculum was used in antiquity is found in the Talmud about 1300 B.C., 800 years before Hippocrates. This speculum was a cylinder made from bamboo or the stem of a gourd, and later of metal. It was used more to determine the source of vaginal bleeding, whether it was from the uterus or from the vagina. The speculum, in which a cotton tampon was inserted, was placed in the vagina and observed. If the cotton was blood stained they assumed it came from the uterus; if only the outer wall alone of the speculum was stained, the inference was that they were dealing with vaginal bleeding.[1]

That the ancient Greeks, 500 B.C., used the speculum is questionable. It can be assumed that they did since they used rectal specula, sounds and catheters. According to K. A. Ligeros,[2] Hippocrates used the speculum or "mitroscope," which was similar to the Cusco duckbill speculum of the 19th Century. Shapiro states that there is no proof that Hippocrates ever used a speculum; the ulcerations that Hippocrates described were noted by touch and not by visualization with a speculum.[3]

Galen[4] (A.D.130-200) made the first record of a speculum. In 1818, two specula were found in the excavations of Pompeii that must have been buried for 1800 years, since A.D. 79.[5] These were beautifully made bronze dilators; one contained three blades, the other four blades which diverged when a centrally located screw was turned. These specula were the type used in the time of Galen and Celsus (27 B.C.-A.D. 50), and very likely in the Middle Ages.

Soranus (A.D. 98-177) wrote an entire chapter on the speculum in his book on gynecology. A number of others, in the second cen-

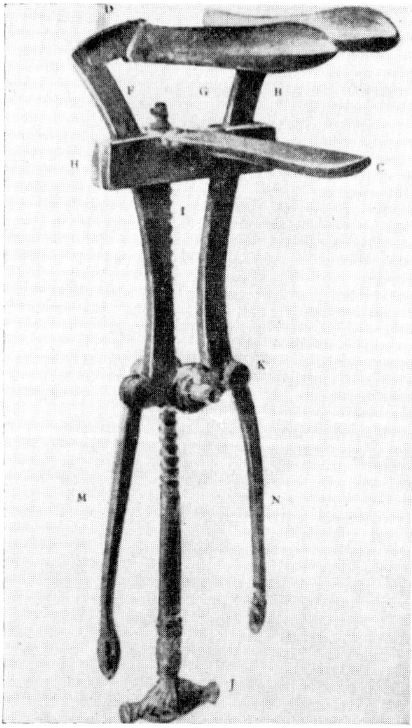

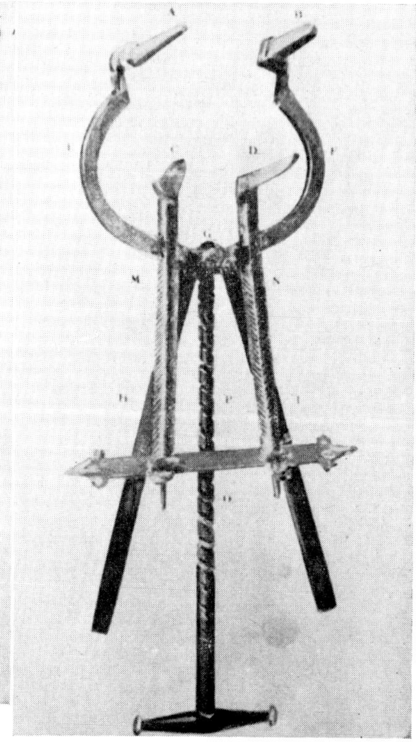

Fig. 176. Trivalved speculum from Pompeii. (Leonardo, R. A.: *History of Gynecology*. New York, Froben, 1944.)

Fig. 177. Quadrivalved speculum from Pompeii. (Leonardo, R. A.: *History of Gynecology*. New York, Froben, 1944.)

tury, were familiar with the speculum. They were Aretaeus, Archigenes, Aspasia, and Leonides (who practiced in Alexandria and was a contemporary of Soranus). Leonides wrote of its use, saying:

> When a deep fistula has perforated the sphincter, either one that has commenced in the anus or one that has begun higher up, it may have been stopped in the sphincter. After exploring, one dilates the anus, just as one dilates the vagina of a woman, with the anal dilator, and by this we mean to say the dioptra.

Aetius in the 6th Century and Paulus of Aegina in the 7th Century used the cylindrical type of vaginal speculum. Before using, the length of the vagina was measured; then the speculum was introduced. Sometimes a conical and other times a valvular type with

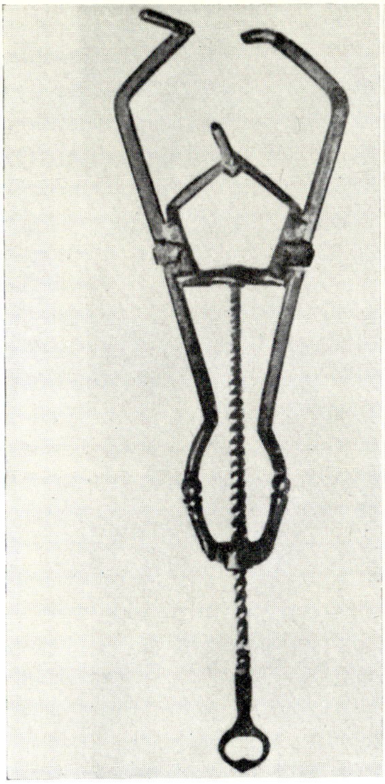

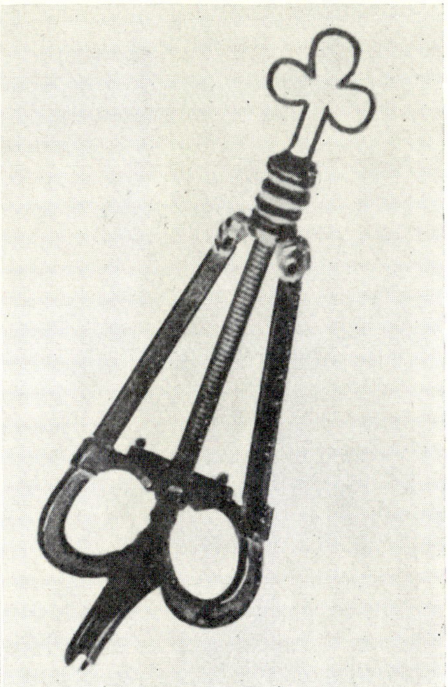

Fig. 178. Speculum of Fourteenth Century. (Leonardo, R. A.: *History of Gynecology*. New York, Froben, 1944.)

Fig. 179. Speculum of Fifteenth century. (Leonardo, R. A.: *History of Gynecology*. New York, Froben, 1944.)

single or several blades was inserted; these blades opened by turning a screw.

Albucasis[6] in 1085, described specula of ebony and boxwood, and also the screw type used by Aetius. Many centuries then passed with hardly a mention of the speculum.

Pierre Franco in 1586 described one similar to Paulus' of the 7th Century.

Paré (1510-1590) talked of the speculum when he discussed cancer, and so did Guillemeau. They used it to visualize the cervix.

Jacob Rueff in 1587 published *De Conceptu et Generatione Hominis*,[7] which contains the description of a three-bladed speculum used to dilate the vagina and to aid in delivery of the child by seizing the head with sharp hooks. Had he left out the cross bars on his instrument and flattened the blades and removed the hooks on it, he would have invented the obstetrical forceps and would have been able to extract a living instead of a dead child. The book does have a representation of an apertorium which is the first known illustration of a smooth-bladed forceps.

Astruc temporarily revived the speculum again in 1761, but it was not until Recamier's time in the early 19th Century that it again was reintroduced (1801 to 1818). At first it was a steel tube with polished walls.[8] He discovered that, in spite of his having enlarged the diameter of this tubal instrument, the extent of the visual field was equal only to the diameter of the speculum. So he modified it by making two half-cylinders which could be separated and thus increase the visual field. When Recamier enlarged his tubal speculum, users of it noticed that the patients were very uncomfortable from its size, so Dupuytren reduced its size, narrowed the external end and equipped it with a handle.

Actually, at that time, very little use of the speculum was made since the time of Hippocrates in the 4th Century B.C. until Osiander,[9] in 1801 to 1808, used a speculum in hysterectomy and vaginal amputation of the cervix in carcinoma. But it was Recamier, in 1818 who popularized it more than anyone else.

Ricord came along about this time and introduced a bivalve speculum.

To Sims, whose immense fame from vesico-vaginal fistula has already been discussed in the preceding section of this chapter, we are indebted for devising the "spoon speculum" which made it possible for him to operate with accurate visibility. He also developed a double-ended duckbill speculum,[10] and one with interchangeable blades.

Segales developed a popular trivalve speculum, and Charriére invented a quadrivalve instrument.

Sir William Fergusson of London modified Recamier's tubular speculum in 1870. It is this speculum that was modified by the addition of a water cooling device, and used later (not *too* long ago) as the "Percy" treatment of cancer of the cervix. This speculum consisted of a cylindrical tube of glass coated with mercury, covered by India rubber, and thoroughly varnished throughout. It was

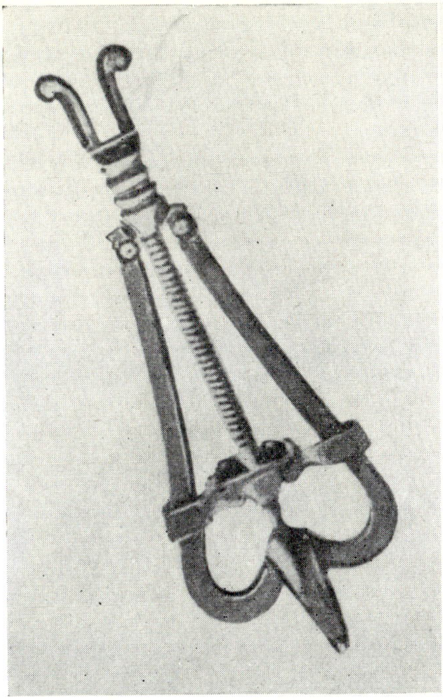

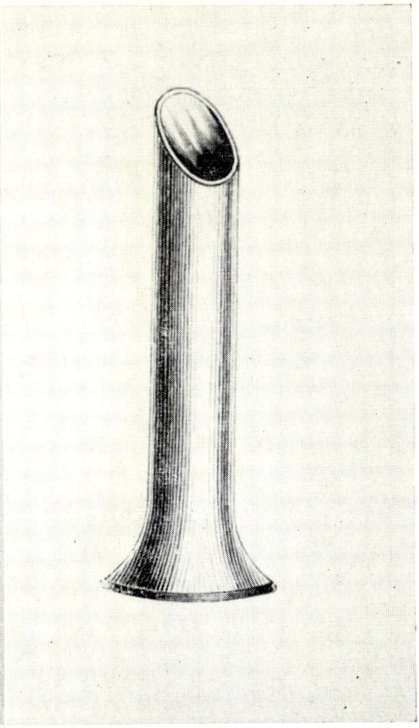

Fig. 180. Speculum of Sixteenth Century. (Leonardo, R. A.: *History of Gynecology* New York, Froben, 1944.)

Fig. 181. Fergusson's speculum. (Hirst, B. C.: *Text Book of Obstetrics*. Philadelphia, Saunders, 1918.)

considered the best, the most useful, and cleanest speculum in its day.

M. Cusco and Brewer invented a speculum like the one commonly used today. Many of the bivalve specula opened at the distal (inserting) end, so that the proximal end through which you look remained the same since they worked on hinges; this was a distinct disadvantage. This was obviated when Bozeman invented a bivalve speculum in which the blades remained parallel when opened. He also used a duckbill speculum similar to Sims'; in fact, there is some controversy about who was first in devising it. At any rate they came into being at approximately the same time.

Collins, Goodell and B. C. Hirst developed similar bivalve specula, that opened parallel. Hirst's speculum was made of wire, so that the lateral walls of the vagina were exposed to increase the area of visibility.

Thomas invented a telescopic vaginal speculum which consisted of two cylinders of metal, one sliding into the other, so that it could be made longer or shorter to accommodate to the length of the vagina.

Martin, in the latter part of the 19th Century, invented a bath speculum, which was a vaginal dilator introduced during the bath to allow inward bathing of the vagina. It never became popular.

In recent years there have been many improvements in the speculum; to mention only a few:

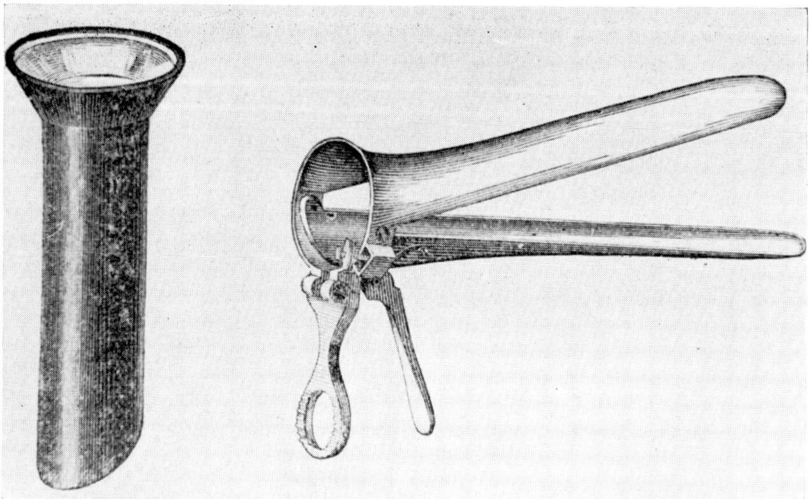

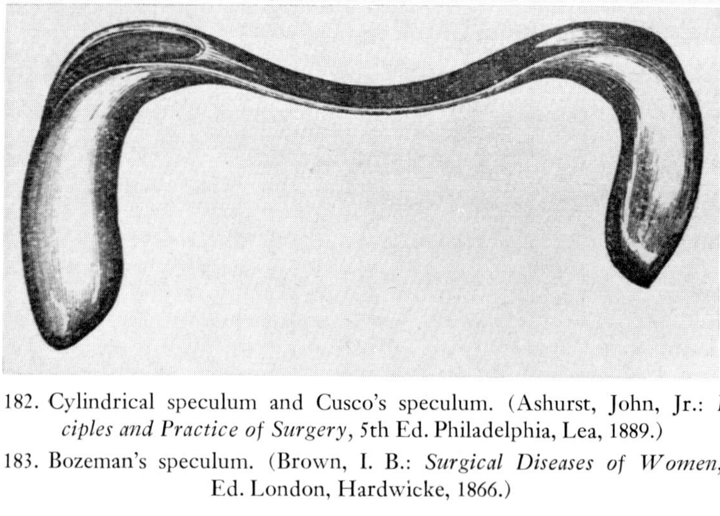

Fig. 182. Cylindrical speculum and Cusco's speculum. (Ashurst, John, Jr.: *Principles and Practice of Surgery*, 5th Ed. Philadelphia, Lea, 1889.)

Fig. 183. Bozeman's speculum. (Brown, I. B.: *Surgical Diseases of Women*, 3rd Ed. London, Hardwicke, 1866.)

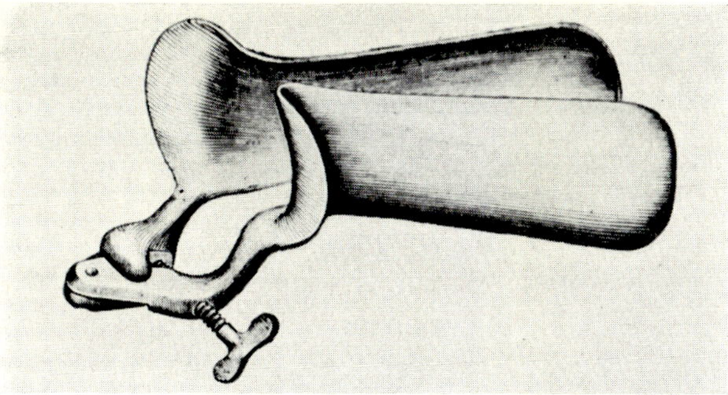

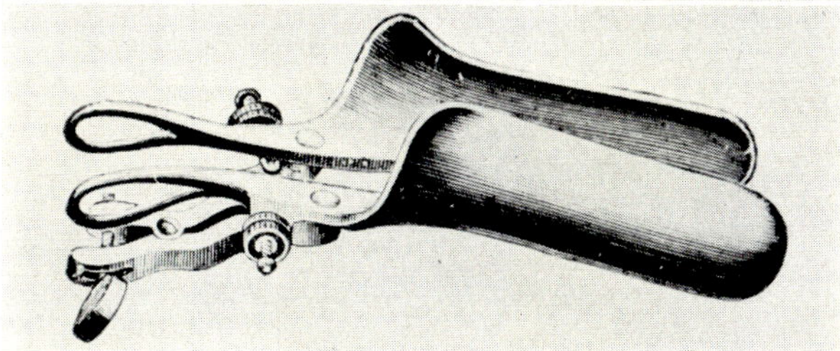

Fig. 184. Collin's speculum. (Hirst, B. C.: *Text Book of Obstetrics*. Philadelphia, Saunders, 1918.)

Fig. 185. Goodell's speculum. (Hirst, B. C.: *Text Book of Obstetrics*. Philadelphia, Saunders, 1918.)

Arthur W. Erskine,[11] in 1938, described an ingenious "expanding speculum for transvaginal Roentgen therapy." A special multibladed speculum is used; the blades are expanded by a wrench mechanism after it is inserted, the x-ray tube is attached, and x-rays directed to the upper vagina and cervix. In more recent years, still other improvements in this type of x-ray therapy speculum have been made.

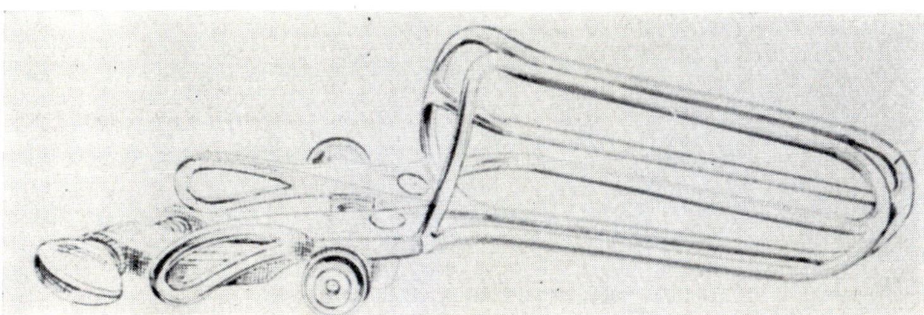

Fig. 186. Hirst's bivalve speculum. (Hirst, B. C.: *Text Book of Obstetrics*. Philadelphia, Saunders, 1918.)

Arthur Bowen[12] devised a cup to attach to a speculum for collecting tissue in curettage.

John Stallworthy[13] described in 1941 a modification of the Graves' speculum, in which illumination is obtained through a curvlite lower blade which lights up.

As late as 1889, Ashurst, in his book, describes the use of the speculum, in the following manner (this was the accepted method): "the speculum should always be introduced well warmed and oiled, under cover of the patient's garments or bed clothes, without any exposure of the person."

First Occurrences and Outstanding Events

A. Vesico-Vaginal Fistula

Vesico-vaginal fistula was found in mummified Queen Henhenit in 2050 B.C.

Avicenna, in A.D. 1037, was the first to recognize incontinence as the result of a fistula produced in labor.

van Roonhuyse, in 1663, was the first to give practical suggestions for its cure.

Sims, in 1849, was the first to do the operation for vesico-vaginal fistula successfully (published in 1852).

In 1845 Sims adopted the position that became known, for the first time, as the Sims' position.

First hospital for women was started by Sims in New York, in 1855. (Kennedy had started a similar hospital, the Rotunda, in 1835.)

First women's clinic was established in 1841, by Bedford in New York.

First scientific approach to vaginal repairs, including fascia, was by Emmet in 1870.

B. History of the Speculum

The Hebrews in 1300 B.C., as stated in the Talmud, were probably the first to use a speculum.

First specific record of a speculum was by Galen in the second century.

Recamier (circa 1801-1818) reintroduced the speculum after a long lapse of time.

The "spoon speculum" of Sims made it possible to operate with clear visibility for vesico-vaginal fistula. He later developed a double ended duckbill speculum, and one with interchangeable blades.

References

A. Fistula

1. Sims, J. M.: *The Story of My Life*. New York, Appleton, 1894.
2. Falk, H. C. and Tanger, M. L.: Vesico-vaginal Fistula; historical survey. *Obst. & Gynec., 3*:337-341, 1954.
3. De Lamballe, Jobert: *Traites des Fistules Vesico-uterines*. Paris, Baillière, 1852.
4. Mettauer, J. P.: Vesico-vaginal Fistula. *Boston M. and S. J., 22*:154, 1840.
5. Mahfouz Bey, N.: Urinary and recto-vaginal fistulae in women. *J. Obst. and Gynec., Brit. Emp., 36*:581-589, 1929.
6. Lower, W. E.: Vesico-vaginal fistula. *Ann. Surg., 92*:774-778, 1930.
7. van Roonhuyse, Hendrik: *Heelkonstige Aanmerkkingen*. Amsterdam, T. Jacobsz, 1663, pp. 135-57.
8. Fatio, Johannes: *Helvetisch, vernunstige Wehenmutter* (op. posthum.). Basel, J. R. Imhoff, 1752.
9. Wyeth, J. A.: *With Sabre and Scalpel*. New York, Harper, 1914.
10. Graham, Harvey: *Eternal Eve*. London, Heinemann, 1950, p. 448.
11. Emmett, T. A.: *A Memoir of Dr. James Marion Sims*. New York, Appleton, 1884.
12. Leonardo, R. A.: *History of Gynecology*. New York, Froben, 1944, p. 231.
13. Emmett, T. A.: A study of the etiology of perineal laceration, with a new method for its proper repair. *Tr. Am. Gynec. Soc., 8*:198-216, 1884.

B. Speculum

1. Thompson, C. J. S.: The Evolution and Development of Surgical Instruments. *Brit. J. Surg., 26*:232, 1938.
2. Ligeros, K. A.: *How Ancient Healing Governs Modern Therapeutics*. New York, G. P. Putman, 1937.
3. Schapiro, I. and Deneffe, V.: L'antiquité du speculum. *Chronique Méd., Par., 6*:553-558, 1901.
4. Leonard, C. H.: Ancient Gynecology. *Obst. Gazette, ancinn., 3*: 505, 1880.
5. Newnham, W. H. C.: On the Evolution of Gynecology. *Bristol Medico-Chirurgical J., 32*:257, 1914.
6. Thompson, C. J. S.: *The History and Evolution of Surgical Instruments*. New York, Schuman, 1942.

7. Rueffus, Jacobus: *De conceptu et generatione hominis.* Tiguri, C. Froschoverus, 1587, p. 24.
8. Recamier, Joseph: Invention du speculum plein et brise. *Bull. Acad. med., Paris, 8*:661-668, 1842.
9. Ricci, J. V.: *Genealogy of Gynecology*. Philadelphia, Blakiston, 1950, p. 350.
10. Thomas, T. G.: *Practical Treatise on the Diseases of Women*, 4th Ed. Philadelphia, Lea, 1878, p. 67.
11. Erskine, A. W.: Expanding speculum for transvaginal Roentgen therapy. *Am. J. Roentgenol., 5*:42, 1939.
12. Bowen, Arthur: Bowen speculum cup. *Am. J. Surg., 42*:435-436, 1938.
13. Stallworthy, John: Useful speculum. *Brit. M. J., 2*:696-697, 1941.

Chapter XVIII

OPERATIVE GYNECOLOGY AND OBSTETRICS

A. GYNECOLOGICAL OPERATIONS

So far, in the 19th Century, we have discussed the epoch making discoveries of anesthesia, bacteriology and pathology that formed the basis for the revolutionary advances of obstetrics and gynecology; operative procedures came into being in this century that would have been impossible without these discoveries. Many of the same operations are used today with improvements, of course, but are basically unchanged. We shall, therefore, describe them and at the same time give a historical résumé of the evolution of each one. We shall begin with vaginal hysterectomy; this is often concerned with plastic procedures, particularly procedentia for a diseased uterus. Then we will discuss abdominal hysterecomy which was concerned largely with fibroids and malignancy in the early history of this operation.

Vaginal Hysterectomy

The stimulus for the performance of this operation occurred when Osiander of Göttingen performed the first radical operation in Germany in 1801 for uterine cancer; he amputated the carcinomatous vaginal portion of the uterus.[1] From 1801 to 1808, he excised the portio for cancer eight times. It was not long after this before many men began to do vaginal hysterectomy. However, we should go back to the very first attempts at vaginal hysterectomy and note the sequence of events in the development of this operation which reached its pinnacle in the 19th Century.

The history of vaginal hysterectomy goes way back to Soranus of Ephesus, in the 2nd Century A.D., when he amputated a gangrenous inverted uterus.[2] As far back as the 5th Century B.C., the Hippocratic era, vague reference can be found to this operation. Berengario da Carpi of Italy, performed a vaginal hysterectomy in A.D. 1517, and again at a later date, using the technique of Soranus. In 1560, Andrea della Croce performed this operation. Early in the 17th Century, several midwives and a Dr. Schenck of Grabenberg, reported a series of twenty-six cases. In 1783 Marshall did vaginal hysterectomies, and from 1794 to 1799 Monteggia, in Italy, and Hunter, in Scotland, reported such cases. At this period of development we reach the contribution of Osiander, already mentioned.

It was through the contribution of Osiander in Germany that all subsequent vaginal hysterectomies were supposed to have followed. Some believe that it was Conrad Langenbeck, in 1813, who did the earliest vaginal hysterectomy for cancer. In France, Lauvariol was the first to perform this operation. Baudelocque performed twenty-three complete hysterectomies on inverted or prolapsed uteri between 1800 and 1816. The operations in the early part of this period were not actually vaginal hysterectomies, but only those executed about 1816. When necessary, he artificially prolapsed the uterus and then cut it away. This was the method of procedure used by Osiander of Göttingen also. In 1819, according to Mathieu,[3] Windsor treated a patient with a long standing uterine inversion by tying a silk ligature above the uterus and tightening it daily. After twelve days he successfully completed the amputation by cutting off the uterus distal to the ligature. In 1817, four years after Langenbeck's operation, Paletta in Italy performed the operation for uterine cancer; his technique was the same as that of Soranus, Avenzoar, Berengario and others of the early period. In 1822, Sauter (1766-1840) removed a carcinomatous uterus through the vagina; some authors consider this the first such case.

In 1829, the first authenticated case in the United States was done by John Collins Warren of Harvard, but the patient died on the fourth postoperative day. Others to perform vaginal hysterectomy were:

Herman and Werneberg of Pittsburgh, in 1832, for cancer.

Esselman of Nashville, in 1843, for an inverted fibroid uterus.

Henning, in 1878, removed the adnexa with the uterus. A similar procedure was done by Kiexter (or Kiester) in 1848, according to Richard A. Leonardo in his "History of Gynecology" published in 1944.

The operation was virtually abandoned because of the high mortality until Vincent Czerny (1842-1916) of Heidelberg systematized the operation in 1879, and thus brought it into practical and general use. Later the original work of Billroth, Wolfler, Mikulicz, Schroeder, Kocher, Teuffel, Martin, Harlden, Doyer, and Spencer Wells brought the operation up to date.[4]

Before discussing abdominal hysterectomy it becomes necessary to diverge a little. Whereas prolapse was the reason for vaginal hysterectomy in most instances (and quite a number of prolapses complicated by malignancy), abdominal hysterectomy involved the cure of fibroids mainly, and in a number of instances carcinoma. Along with hysterectomy for fibroids, the procedure of myomectomy appears. In the records we have one case of vaginal approach in myomectomy, but the abdominal approach was the more common route. Because abdominal hysterectomy was closely related to fibroids and carcinoma, we shall give a very brief account of the history of fibroids and of carcinoma before enumerating the historical evolution of the operations pertaining to those conditions.

Fibroids: William Hunter had written an excellent paper on "fleshy tubercles," his term for uterine fibroids, yet many surgeons still considered them malignant. During the time of Recamier and Lisfranc, physicians confused "interstitial hypertrophy" (fibroid tumors) with cancer, often being unable to distinguish clearly one from the other. Astruc mistakenly said, in 1776, that the scirrhous tumors were due to abortions. In ancient times, Hippocrates and others probably recognized malignant tumors. This difficult question was finally resolved by James Henry Bennet of London in 1845. In his book, *Inflammation of the Uterus*, he clearly distinguished between malignant and non-malignant uterine tumors, and he, more than anyone else, showed that fibroid growths are benign.[5]

The removal of fibroid tumors was attempted by the vaginal route and via the abdomen; both myomectomy and hysterectomy were performed.

Eugene Koeberle (1828-1915) of Strassburg performed a case of vaginal myomectomy in 1856.

Washington L. Atlee (1801-1878) was a graduate of Jefferson, and became Professor of Medical Chemistry at the University of Pennsylvania. He was one of the early ovariotomists in the United States, performing 246 such cases. He was threatened with arrest, when he first began to do ovariotomy, by his colleagues who were highly incensed at his attempt. He practiced in Lancaster, Pennsylvania, with his brother John, for many years.

Most surgeons were attempting to cure fibroids by hysterectomy and getting terrific mortalities. The feeling of the profession was echoed in the London *Medico-Chirurgical Review* as follows:

> We consider extirpation of the uterus, not previously protruded or inverted, one of the most cruel and unfeasable operations that ever was projected or executed by the head or hand of man.

Atlee approached the problem differently; he exposed the uterus through an abdominal incision but did not remcve the uterus; instead of hysterectomy, he enucleated the tumors only. So to him goes the honor of performing the first abdominal myomectomy in 1853.[6]

Hegar, much later, did the first abdominal myomectomy in Germany.

Abdominal Hysterectomy

Prior to the introduction of anesthesia and Listerism, gynecologists preferred the vaginal route to the abdominal approach because of less shock, better drainage and less peritonitis. When they began to do abdominal hysterectomies they chose total to subtotal for the same reasons that they preferred the vaginal procedure, and also because they feared the entrance of air through the cervical canal. Even after Listerism the outstanding physicians disapproved of the abdominal route; they made the unqualified statement that tumors in the muscle and even on the surface of the uterus were "out of our reach." James Y. Simpson, in 1863, considered it an utterly unjustifiable operation. In 1848, Charles D. Meigs said it was hopeless to attempt to do anything with fibroids that extended up into the abdomen.

Heath of Manchester, on November 21, 1843, did the first abdominal hysterectomy for fibroids; his pre-operative diagnosis was ovarian cyst. Charles Clay, in 1844, also of Manchester did the second abdominal case; it was a supravaginal hysterectomy and bilateral salpingo-oophorectomy. However, the patient died on the fifteenth day. In 1846, Bellinger did a hysterectomy. In 1853, Walter Burnham, of Lowell, Massachusetts operated a case; he had planned a myomectomy, but was forced to remove the uterus. He operated on fifteen cases (one was a sarcoma of the uterus which he did in 1853), but only three of his patients survived. In 1855, Kimball, also of Lowell, Massachusetts, did the first correctly diagnosed hysteromyomectomy. He was the first to drop the stump into the pelvis. Subsequently he performed four such operations with a mortality of 25 per cent. In 1863, eight years after Kimball's case, forty-two abdominal hysterectomies were reported with only nine survivals, five of them in the United States. Hegar and Kaltenbach showed a mortality of 72 per cent; in 1872 the procedure was condemned at Paris because of the high mortality, and for many years vaginal hysterectomy was done again.[7]

Another approach in the treatment of fibroids in the 19th Century that became quite popular, especially in America, was the therapy of electricity. In fact it assumed the proportions of a fad. It was begun in 1869, by Ciniselli of Cremona, who inspired Ephraim Cutter in 1874 to apply this form of therapy. Even earlier than this, a certain August Tripier described the treatment of fibroids by the electric current. After Cutter, Georges Apostoli (1847-1900) of France did important work in the treatment of uterine fibroids by electricity in 1883.

Malignancy

In the 19th Century the earliest hysterectomy was done for malignancy rather than for fibroids, by Langenbeck in 1813, per vaginum. Some years later the abdominal route was used. The sequence of performance of hysterectomy for carcinoma follows:

Vaginal

1813: Conrad Langenbeck of Germany was the first to perform hysterectomy for carcinoma. It was the first vaginal hysterectomy of the 19th Century for any reason.

1817: Paletta of Italy.

1822: Sauter.

1829: John Collins Warren, of Harvard.

1879: Czerny, who greatly improved the technique; its performance was much the same as it is today.

1898: Schauta, started the radical operation with removal of glands.

Abdominal

1853: Burnham of Massachusetts was the first to do an abdominal hysterectomy for malignancy, a sarcoma.

1878: Freund of Strassburg did the first hysterectomy for carcinoma by a highly improved technique; viz: packing off of the intestines and ligation of the vessels, closure of the broad ligaments by sutures, thorough peritoneal closure, and the patient's pelvis elevated during the operation, a position later popularized by Trendelenburg, and which now bears his name.

1898: Wertheim performed the first radical abdominal approach with the removal of glands.

When abdominal hysterectomy was condemned at Paris, because of its high mortality, vaginal hysterectomy was revived. But in 1878, when Freund did a hysterectomy through the abdomen for cancer by an improved technique, the abdominal approach began to be used again. His technique was a distinct advance over all previous methods. Improvements in technique by other men followed, so it was not too many years before abdominal hysterectomy returned to the forefront. The men who contributed most in its improvement were Reis, Werder, John G. Clark, Professor of Gynecology at the University of Pennsylvania, Howard A. Kelly, of Baltimore, and Wertheim. Clark's contribution was the catheterization of the ureters preoperatively and drainage of the pelvis through the vagina. Wertheim contributed to the technique of extended hysterectomy for carcinoma. Kelly showed a reduction in mortality to 5 per cent.

Other methods of therapy for uterine carcinoma occurred later in this century, and extended into the turn of the century. They were:

Amputation of Cervix

1652: Tulpius, at the suggestion of Paré.

1801: Frederick Benjamin Osiander, Germany, was the first to perform this operation for cervical carcinoma. He repeated it eight times.

The Percy Treatment

1870: Sir William Fergusson of London modified Recamier's tubular speculum by the addition of a water cooling device. This speculum was used in the treatment of carcinoma of the cervix and was known as the Percy Treatment.

X-ray and Radium

1895: X-rays were discovered by Roentgen

1898: Radium was discovered by the Curies.

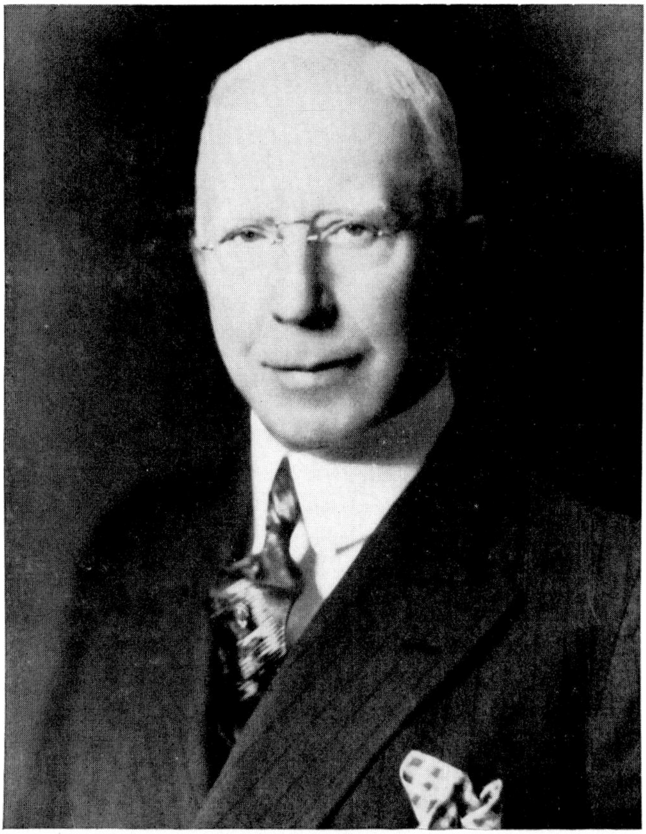

Fig. 187. George E. Pfahler.

1900: Pusey and Pfahler were the first to use x-rays for endometrial carcinoma.

1902: Transvaginal cone therapy was first described by Cauldwell.

1903: Abbe, of America, was the first to apply radium to cervical carcinoma.

Early 1900's: High voltage x-ray machines, cyclotron, betatron, 100,000 mev. atom smasher (used as a reactor mainly), radio-active isotopes, atom pile, and cobalt (cobalt replacing superhigh voltage x-ray machines).

Diagnostic Procedures

1842: Recamier introduced curettage.

1872: Simon reintroduced it in France, especially for cancer.

1927: Schiller devised a test for cancer of the cervix.

(?) Papaincolaou smears; dates back to the late 19th Century, becoming popular only in recent times.

The advances in therapy of carcinoma of the uterus were, without doubt, due partly to the increased knowledge of the subject of carcinoma, which makes a more intelligent approach possible. In the history of carcinoma we note that carcinoma was always more or less suspected since the Egyptian era. Pastes and the cautery were used in treating it. Galen wrote about tumors, he described malignant tumors and even classified them. The diagnosis was made by the presence of ulceration especially if foul discharges accompanied it. They knew the lesion was crab-like in growth. According to Galen, the cause was due to the action of "black bile." He gave a hopeless prognosis in these cases. It was Galen who wrote that different kinds of bile caused different diseases; he discussed and probably began the theory of "humors" as caused by certain type of bile.[8]

Contributions to the problem of malignancy versus benignity were made as follows:

17th Century: Beginning with Harvey, Malpighi, Sanctorius, Mayow, DeGraaf, Leeuwenhoek and Willis.

18th Century: In latter part of this century, Morgagni and Bichat contributed; and very late in this century Hunter differentiated cancer from benign lesions, but not too much attention was given to his views in this matter.

19th Century: Virchow's work stimulated most contributions in this field of malignancy versus benign. Shortly after contributions in Germany, Henry C. Coe, and Cullen cleared up this confusion in America. In England in 1845, the monumental work of Bennet definitely established the difference between fibroids and malignancy.

Histopathology of high caliber started in the early 19th Century, as evidence of this we have the contribution of Bayer in 1821, who reported the first ovum. Early in this century carcinoma was accurately described, but its epithelial origin was not definitely established.

1852: Robin of Paris was the first to show that carcinoma began in the epithelium and infiltrated the tissues, ulceration often resulting.

1865: Cornil of Paris also showed epithelial origin of carcinoma. Thiersch did the same on the skin.

1872: Waldeyer showed that all carcinoma came from epithelial tissue.

1858: Wagner of Leipsig described carcinoma faithfully, but did not realize its epithelial origin.

1878: Veit and Ruge made important contributions.

1888: Sir John Williams, with the above two, Veit and Ruge, all made important contributions to add to our knowledge of carcinoma.

Malignancy, as Treated Today: Present-day treatment of cancer begins with the education of patients for routine check-ups. Scheffy has shown that 28.3 per cent of all cancer patients benefited by no delay from the time of the first symptom to the time of the first treatment, and that doctors, alone or in combination with the patients, are responsible for 33 per cent of delayed therapy. All of this shows progress but not sufficient emphasis on the education of the doctors.

Surgical treatment, which we have already discussed, is usually combined with radiation. It is the latter form of treatment that we shall now discuss. The advances in radiation therapy consist in delivering larger and more accurately measured doses to tumor bearing areas. This means increased intensity, increased filtration to eliminate the caustic rays, divided doses to permit recovery of normal tissue, rotation of the portals of approach, interstitial application, intra-arterial approaches and the use of radioactive isotopes.

To increase the depth of rays, increase of voltage to 1,000 kv machines has been added. To increase intensity has led to the cyclotron and the betatron, which can deliver 300 mev. A new 100,000 mev. atom smasher is contemplated by the United States government, but, because of the expense involved for therapy, may be used mainly as reactors.

A radioactive isotope differs from its sisters only in that it emits radiation and has a different atomic weight, but chemically it is no different. In 1953 there were 850 known elements and their isotopes. Now there are more than 1400. Some are natural isotopes, others are artificial. The Curies produced the first artificial radioactivated isotope by bombarding aluminum with alpha particles from radium. Radium as a source is still sometimes used, but most isotopes today are made by the use of the cyclotron or the betatron, or by highly energized neutrons of the atomic pile.

The application of radioactive isotopes produced with the uranium chain reactors are divided for specific uses into those dependent on physical placement of radioactivity based on the use of gamma radiation, and those dependent on chemical placement which utilizes beta radiation. Physical placements use radioactivity from external sources, interstitial sources such as gamma ray sutures, needles or infiltrating colloids, and intracavitary sources such as gamma ray applicators or colloid infusions. The chemical placements may use colloid deposition such as radiated gold; selective absorption such as iodine for the thyroid gland. Gold-198 emits both beta and gamma rays, but it is the beta rays which are used for most of the therapy. Cobalt-60 emits a beta ray of low intensity which can be readily screened out thus offering pure gamma rays. Activated gold in colloidal form, while more easily handled, is less stable and of shorter life, so that cobalt is more economical. Colloids are used in body cavities such as the chest and abdomen, intravenously. This form (colloid) of therapy is used particularly for infusions and has little if any effect on the tumor masses. Cobalt can do anything that radium does. Many clinics are replacing expensive supervoltage x-ray machines with the less expensive cobalt pack.[9]

Today, radiation therapy is used in conjunction with other forms of treatment in addition to surgery. The additional agenda are, to mention a few, mustard of nitrogen and hormones and the indirect surgical procedures such as castration, adrenalectomy and hypophysectomy. The efficacy of all these new methods remains uncertain; the final outcome is still in the process of evaluation.

Ectopic Pregnancy

One of the major operative procedures that received energetic attention in the 19th Century was ectopic pregnancy. This condition had been known for many centuries; the help these patients received was practically nil. They were usually discovered at postmortem examination. The first recorded case of ectopic is that of Albucasis, 11th Century. His patient had an abdominal swelling that underwent suppuration and eventual drainage through the abdominal wall with passage of the fetal skeleton. As far back as the 18th Century some idea as to the possible etiology of this condition was being discussed; in 1752, Boehmer believed that in some way sterility was the cause. Henry Oldham, of the Guy Hospital, said, in 1845, that pelvic inflammatory disease caused it. In the 18th Century ectopic pregnancy was classified into its various types by Bianchi. By the 19th Century the symptomatology and the pathology had become fairly clear, as well as knowledge of the various types, but treatment was still out of the question.

As far back as the latter part of the 16th Century, the only recorded attempts at operation, were by Jacob Noierus in 1595, and by Felix Plater in 1598. The procedure consisted of making an abdominal incision and extracting the fetus, nothing more. There is no record of this procedure for the 17th century except for the first case of ovarian pregnancy with rupture which was reported, in 1682, by de Saint Maurice of Perigod; this case was abstracted by Smellie in 1877. A case was reported by Mauriceau in the 17th Century, but there is some question as to the authenticity of its being an ovarian pregnancy. The first authentic case of ovarian pregnancy was reported by Catherine von Tussechenbroek in 1899. The 18th Century contains records of three performances in the United

States: the first by Bard, of New York, in 1759; the second by Dr. William Baynham, of Virginia, in 1791; the third by Mr. M. C. Knight in 1795.[10]

In the 19th Century, some remarkable cases of vaginal section for extra-uterine pregnancy were performed in the United States. Yet, the situation in the early part of this period had not changed from that of previous years, when not too many surgeons were ready to open an abdomen. In 1816, John King, of South Carolina, performed the operation. The record states: "cut through the walls of the vagina and removed through the incision, by means of the forceps and abdominal pressure, a living child which had been carried the full term of gestation in the abdominal cavity outside the uterus. The life of the mother was also saved."[11]

While ectopic pregnancy was a hopeless condition before the advent of anesthesia and Listerism, a change began to take place when asepsis and anesthesia began to be practiced. And peculiarly enough, it began with a man who scoffed at Lister and his practices. He did practice asepsis, however, in a round-about way; he insisted on scrupulous cleanliness of instruments, wound and everything connected with the operation. This man was Lawson Tait. About this time the literature on ectopic was tremendous, and among the more influential early writers was John S. Parry, of Philadelphia,[12] and Gill Wylie of New York. In 1876, Parry reported a study of 500 cases with 336 deaths. He felt that the fetus caused the mother's death, so the line of therapy should be directed to the fetus, to kill it and prevent its further encroachment. Medical methods were employed, and Simpson used surgical means such as puncturing the mass (sac); this entire theory was soon abandoned. At best, the death rate was five in six cases operated; if not operated, only one in three died.

Lawson Tait (1845-1899) was graduated from Edinburgh and practiced in Birmingham. He was friend, pupil and assistant to Simpson. In 1883, he did the first operation for ruptured ectopic pregnancy.[13] In the beginning he did general surgery; later he confined his surgery to gynecology. He did thousands of abdominal sections with scarcely a death. Although he scoffed at the idea of Lister's antiseptic measures, Tait's insistence on scrupulous cleanliness in the preparation of his instruments and his practice of flushing out the abdominal cavity with warm or boiled water at the conclusion of a laparotomy, marks him as a pioneer in aseptic, as distinguished from antiseptic, surgery. And yet he was disdainful of Listerism. He was one of the greatest ovariotomists of the day. The routine repair of a rectocele by use of the flap-splitting technic was originally devised by Tait;[14] it is almost the same procedure that is used today. Besides ovariotomy, ectopic pregnancy, and cystocele repair, he was the first to do uterine fixation, salpingectomy, and bilateral oophorectomy for fibroids to shrink the fibroids instead of doing hysterectomy, a procedure for which the mortality rate was still too high. The first salpingectomy was performed for inflamed tubes. In 1883, he reported sixty-two cases without a fatality. It was not until 1892 that the profession accepted the procedure. According to his pupil, McKay, Lawson Tait added to the advancement of operative gynecology more than anyone who had preceded him.

Plastic Surgery and Prolapse

The history of vaginal plastic surgery goes back to Trotula, in the 11th Century, for it was she who sutured a complete tear of the perineum; the procedure she employed was almost the same as is used today. Paré did repairs of torn perinea in the 16th Century. Later Dieffenbach (1792-1847), a German surgeon and Roux, a Frenchman did repairs on a scientific basis.

It remained for Emmet, in the 19th Century, to demonstrate the value of the fascia and the necessity of uniting all the deeper structures in the performance of a plastic repair. Simon, Hegar and Tait went even further in the development of this procedure, particularly on the posterior wall. In 1856, Sims did a simple oval denudation and a repair of the anterior wall. In 1888, Sänger devised an operation of flap splitting and elevation of the bladder, a procedure introduced in 1887 by Hedra of Texas. Skene, in 1892, did important work on cystocele, tucking in the anterior wall of the vagina.

The history of cystocele is linked with prolapse because the ancients did not always clearly distinguish between the two. The Egyptians treated prolapse by medicaments, fumigations and mechanical as well as astringent effects. The Greeks did the same, i.e., Hippocrates and later Soranus;[15] however, they both spoke of surgical measures. They usually waited until the uterus became gangrenous and probably used the cautery. Many of the early physicians tried to cure prolapse by forming scar tissue, either by use of the cautery or a little later by denudation.

Romaine Gerard, in 1823, suggested surgical occlusion of the vagina for prolapse. In 1831 Heming had success with a procedure somewhat similar to the Le Forte operation. In 1892, Mackenrodt and Dührssen both reported vaginal fixation, an operation first done in America by Vineberg in 1894. Shucking suggested bringing out the uterus into the vagina and fixing it to the denuded canal. Freund, in 1895, was the first to do this; later Fritsch and Wertheim performed it. From this evolved the Watkins interposition operation in 1898. This became displaced by Mayo's vaginal hysterectomy. Then came the Manchester operation which was brought to America by Shaw in 1933; this was primarily an operation of support by shortening the parametrial tissues and not simply advancing the bladder.

Uterine Displacements

The 19th Century witnessed a flood of procedures for the correction of uterine displacements. In 1716, vanDeventer described retroflexio-version in pregnancy. He made an unsuccessful attempt at replacement of a retrodisplaced uterus by the use of fingers and knee-chest position; the uterus contained a four-month pregnancy. Before 1840, operations for the correction of retrodisplaced uteri were not permitted. Alquié,[16] in 1840, suggested to the French Academy of Medicine that the round ligaments could be shortened by drawing them through the inguinal canals, a procedure he had performed on cadavers only. The Academy held to the opinion that the operation was impracticable and commended him for not having tried it on a living woman. It was not attempted until 1864, by Deneffe, who failed to find the round ligaments. In 1843, Simpson described the value of the uterine sound in identifying uterine displacement. This may be the origin of the later ill-advised practice of placing a sound in the uterus to correct retrodisplacements which have not responded to manual treatment.

Amussat, in 1850, tried to produce adhesions in the vaginal vault posteriorly by the use of the cautery. Koeberle at Strasbourg in

1869, sutured the ovarian pedicles to the laparotomy wound in order to correct the uterine displacement. Lawson Tait, in 1880, fixed the uterus to the incision in the abdomen. Alexander of Liverpool in 1881, and Adams of Glasgow in 1882, successfully shortened the round ligaments; the procedure suggested by Alquie in 1840. Olshausen in 1885 or 1886, performed ventral fixation for retroversion or prolapse. This procedure was also done at the same time, though independently, by Howard A. Kelly. In 1888, Kelly and also Sänger did a fixation through the vagina. Later Kelly writes, "We don't need to do suspension operations."[17]

Mackenrodt in 1892, Winter in 1893, Justner in 1894, and Vineberg, Bode and Wertheim all used the anterior vaginal section for shortening the round ligaments. Then came the Gilliam suspension in 1900, Webster in 1901, and Baldy in 1902. The Montgomery suspension came in 1906.

Pessaries

Pessaries go back to ancient times, and were used as late as the Arabian period, after which their use declined somewhat until the 16th Century.

The year 1854 marked a fresh epoch in the evolution of gynecology; then it was that the great war of uterine displacements and pessary manufacturers began. Hodge in America, who in 1866, invented the horse-shoe pessary and other models. Velpeau, in France, and Graily Hewitt, in England, stood forth as champions of the immense importance of malposition of the uterus in the causation of pelvic disease. Today we know that very considerable changes in the position of the uterus are perfectly compatible with the enjoyment of excellent health.

Sounds

The Egyptians used sounds for medication and probing; Wierus, in 1657, used a sound for exploration, comparable to our modern sounds, and Lair, in 1828, discussed the use of the uterine sound in diagnosis. His suggestions passed unnoticed until Recamier's use in 1842. One year later, in 1843, sound was introduced into use simultaneously by Simpson, Huguier and Kiwisch, each of whom claimed credit for its discovery.

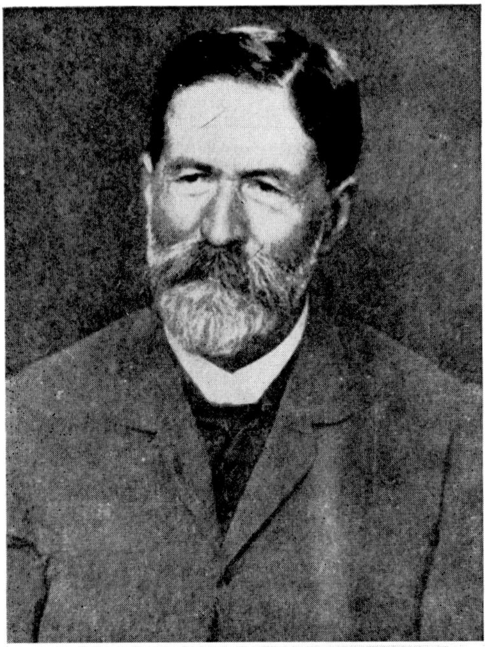

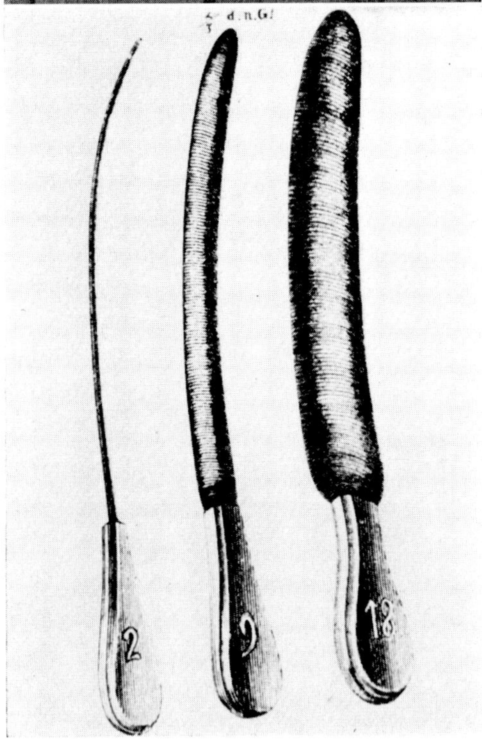

Fig. 188. Alfred Hegar. (*Obstetrics and Gynecology, 6*:No. 6, p. 679, Dec. 1955. New York, Hoeber.)

Fig. 189. Hegar's original dilators. (*Obstetrics and Gynecology, 6*:No. 6, p. 681, Dec. 1955. New York, Hoeber.)

Dilators

During the Arabian period, dilators of the cervix were used in the form of sponge tents. In 1831, Schnackenberg tried to produce cervical dilatation by using a bladder attached to a syringe. A much more successful method was devised by MacIntosh of Edinburgh, who used graduated sounds; it was used for the treatment of dysmenorrhea in 1832. In 1851, an efficient apparatus, the colpuerynter was invented for this same operation by Carl Brown. In 1872, Thomas suggested and used cervical dilatation by the use of sounds of hard rubber; he used twelve different sizes. Each sound was left in place for fifteen minutes, a very slow procedure which was tedious, painful and the results uncertain. Today when we speak of dilators, we associate them with the name of Hegar.

Alfred Hegar (1820-1914) was born in Darmstadt, Germany. The Hegar dilator[18] is used today in some clinics for doing "time dilatation" in dysmenorrhea. Hegar distinguished himself not only for his dilators, but he is known for the early sign of pregnancy, the Hegar sign, which is attributed to his assistant C. Reinl by some authors. Other contributions were repair of urinary fistulae, perineorrhaphy, and myomectomy (he was the first German to do this operation). In the treatment of fibroids he did ovariectomy to shrink the tumors; he did his first bilateral oophorectomy of normal ovaries to create an artificial menopause in 1872. His contribution of dilators also has been questioned; some attributed them to Peaslee of Dartmouth College in 1870. In both instances, the Hegar sign and the dilators, we find the publications were made by Hegar and that is the reason their discovery is credited to him.

Curette

Recamier (1774-1852), who reintroduced the vaginal speculum and uterine sound and was one of the first to perform posterior colpotomy, also developed the use of the curette in 1842. It was pronounced unscientific and barbarous by Chassaignac, Scanzoni and others. It was used little, and, eventually, not at all. Simon reintroduced it in France, in 1872, in treating malignant tumors. Doléris, Hegar, Kaltenback and Olshausen used it for endometritis. It has been modified in recent years and made safer. A form of curette was used in ancient times for performing abortions. In fact as far back as prehistoric times, crudely made instruments, apparently suitable for performing a uterine dilatation and curettage, have been discovered by archaeologists.[19]

B. CESAREAN SECTION

The first innovations of major importance in the operation of cesarean section did not occur until the latter 19th Century. A brief history of the operation will acquaint us with the difficult and slow progress that had been encountered since its discovery.

As far back as mythological times, one can find references to this operation. In ancient European folklore one finds innumerable references to it. But in the writings of the Egyptians, Greeks and Romans, it is never mentioned as performed on the living mother; however, it was known to the ancient Jews. In the Talmud we find references to the cutting open of the abdomen and to babies delivered through the flanks of women which clearly suggest the abdominal cesarean operation. Maimonides, commenting on the "Nidda" is quoted as saying that a woman who cannot bear a child in the natural way, shall be opened in the side and, in this way, delivered of her offspring.

In the sequence of events in the development of this operation we see that, in the beginning, the cesarean operation was performed only upon the dead mother to provide a separate burial for the child, that it later was done upon the dying mother where the child showed signs of life, and finally, upon the living mother in the effort to save both baby and mother.

Rösslin and Guillemeau in the 16th Century, mention the operation on the dying or dead mother with a live baby, but there is no record to show that they saved any babies. In the 17th Century, Mauriceau endorsed the procedure. Schwarz, who collected the records of 346,941 births from 1836 to 1848, states that of 107 cesarean operations in this group not a single baby that was removed from a dead mother was saved. However, there are scattered instances recorded where babies were saved.

In making the incision in such cases, certain precautions were assumed because of the ever-present possibility of the supposedly dead mother being alive and only in a state of collapse. In the 15th Century, Alexander Benedictus suggested the lateral abdominal incision on the dead mother to avoid injuring the liver. Buelin, Baudelocque, Guillemeau and others entered into the discussion of how and where the incision should be made. The median incision was adopted in France and Germany in the middle of the 18th Century. It was contended that a median incision would occasion less loss of blood and less protrusion of bowel.

It was not until the early part of the 16th Century that we find the first authentic account of the operation on the living mother. This operation, plus the reintroduction of version by Paré a short time later, helped to develop the science of obstetrics. Francis Rousset in 1581, is credited with being the first of the French writers to advocate cesarean section on the living woman. He cited a case that had been operated six times, but died at the seventh cesarean because her surgeon had previously died. Paré, in commenting on this said that he thought it marvelous that this were possible, but he could not comprehend its possibility. The attendant dangers of such an operation were too great for him to give his sanction for its performance. He said:

> In order to give issuance to the child it would be necessary to make a large wound in the epigastric muscles, and likewise to the matrix where, its being imbued with a great quantity of blood, making there so great a division, there would be a very large hemorrhage from which death would result. Besides having consolidated the place the scar would not allow the matrix to afterwards dilate in order to carry a child. There are still other accidents which could occur, and the worst the sudden death of the mother, and I would never advise doing such work where there is so great a danger with not a single hope.[1]

Not only did Rousset never perform the operation, but he never saw it done. So the only credit due Rousset is that he was the first to suggest the operation.

The first account of the operation, according to some authorities, but nevertheless disputed by others, was an account by Marcellus Donatus in the Middle Ages. The operator was Christopher Bain of Italy, in 1540, and, though the mother lived, the baby was dead when extracted.

The most authentic account of this operation was made by Caspar Bauhin in 1588, in which he states that Jacob Nufer, a swine spayer

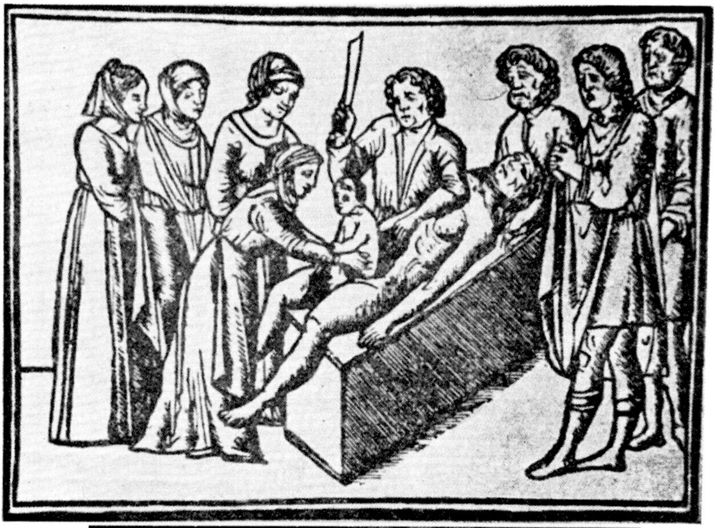

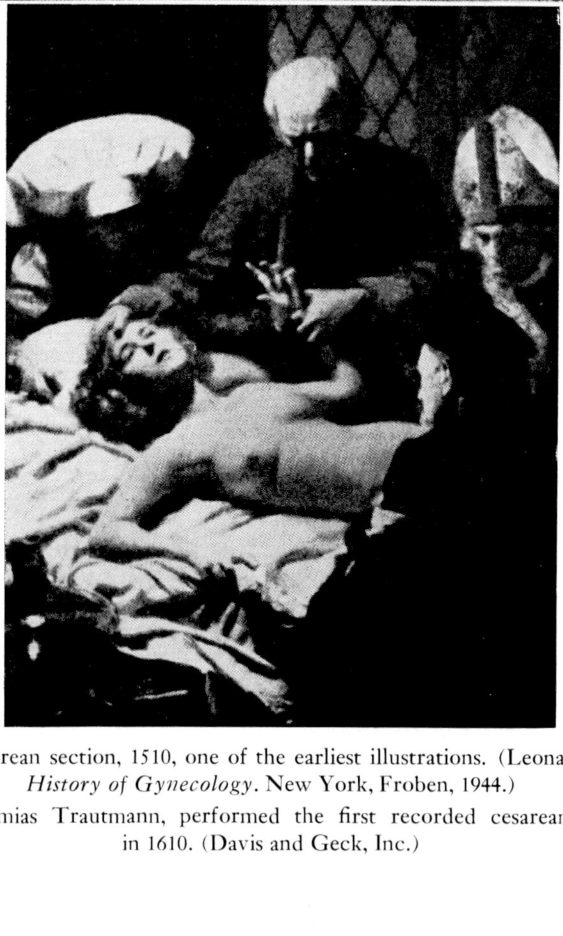

Fig. 190. Cesarean section, 1510, one of the earliest illustrations. (Leonardo, R. A.: *History of Gynecology*. New York, Froben, 1944.)

Fig. 191. Jeremias Trautmann, performed the first recorded cesarean operation in 1610. (Davis and Geck, Inc.)

at Sigerhausen, Switzerland, opened the abdomen and uterus of his wife in A.D. 1500. It was her first labor, long and painful and not progressing. Several stonecutters and thirteen midwives were in attendance but none could help her. Nufer obtained permission from the civil authorities to do a cesarean operation. All the midwives were invited, but only two were sufficiently hardy to remain as assistants. The baby was extracted from the abdomen through a neat incision, which was sutured and healed well. Later Nufer's wife gave birth to twins, and gave birth four times more. The baby lived to be seventy-seven years old. This cesarean operation has gone down in history as the first authenticated cesarean.[2]

On April 21, 1610, the first such operation reported in detail and by good authority was by a surgeon named Trautmann of Wittenberg. The report was made by Daniel Sennert.[3]

From the 16th to the early 19th Century, there was much opposition to the operation. Paré condemned it and would not even watch it. Osborn preferred craniotomy on the living child to cesarean section. Manning in the 18th Century would only perform cesarean on the dead. In the 19th Century, Baudelocque was called an assassin for advocating cesarean operations in extreme contractions of the pelvis. Such opinions were no doubt the result of the high mortality. Baudelocque had forty-two deaths in seventy-three operations; Velpeau in 1831 had a mortality of at least one out of two cases. In the same year J. Burns and S. Cooper reported not a single recovery in Great Britain. Dr. Denman stated that all patients died who were operated. Mortality figures of 73, 90, 83, and 79 per cent were reported by other men. However some prominent men favored the operation. Smellie justified its performance though he himself never did it. Scipione Mercurio did much to popularize it in Italy in the 16th Century. Even Denman, who said they all died, said it was proper to do the operation under certain circumstances. In 1827, the first successful cesarean section was performed in the United States by John L. Richmond (1785-1855), of Newton, Ohio. This was an operation done on a Negro woman with a pocket knife and the kitchen table; the patient recovered fully in twenty-four days.[4] (See First Occurrences and Outstanding Events under B. Cesarean)

The first half of the 19th Century saw no solution to this prob-

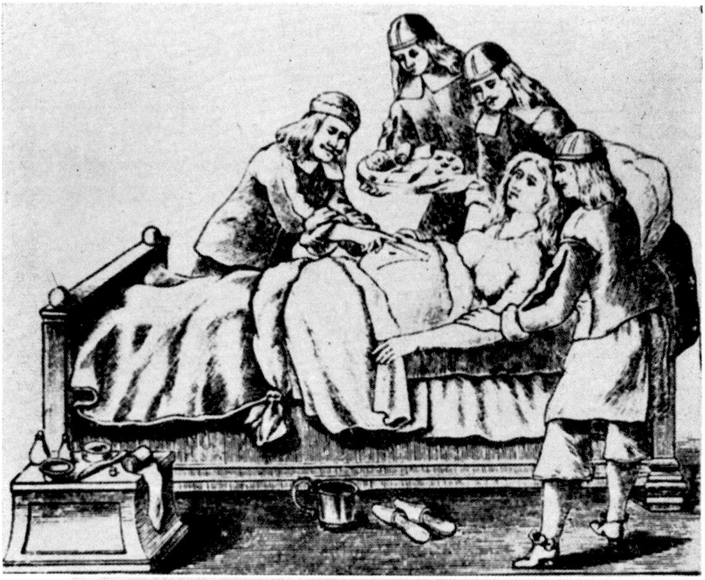

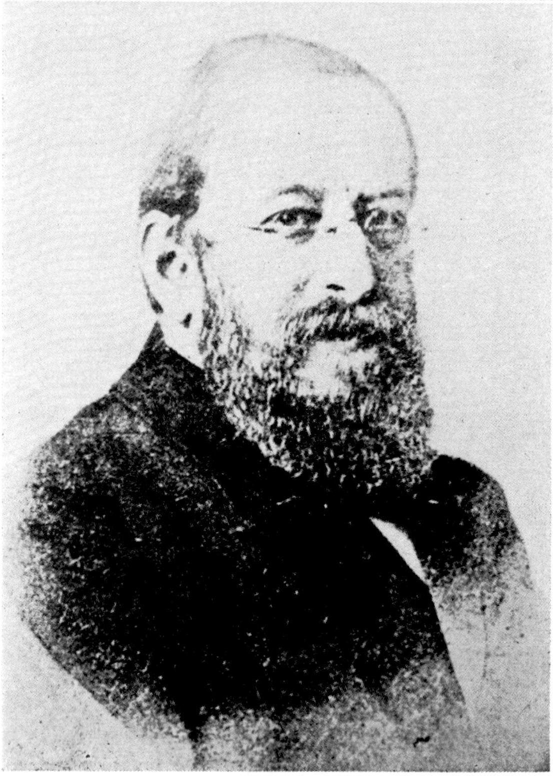

Fig. 192. Cesarean operation during the early Seventeenth Century. (Reproduced from the *Armamentarium Chirurgicum* of Scultetus, 1595-1645.)

Fig. 193. Max Sänger. (Findley, Palmer: *Priests of Lucina*. Boston, Little, 1939.)

lem. Vicious debates on cesarean versus craniotomy continued, particularly in Britain and the United States, for the mortality was still 75 per cent. Barnes and Hicks favored mutilation operations while Greenhalgh, Hodge, and Dewees favored cesarean.

In 1876, the first innovation of major importance was the Porro operation (amputation of the body of the uterus). Six years later, in 1882, it became unnecessary to sacrifice the uterus because Ferdinand Adolph Kehrer and Sänger developed a technique to close the uterine incision by sutures. An effort to suture a ruptured uterus had previously been made by Lebas in 1769. Improvements in surgical technique and a better understanding of the indications and contraindications followed, and today we have not only a perfected technique of the classical cesarean but also other procedures which prevent exposure of the peritoneal cavity to the hazards of contamination. Alfred Dührssen in 1896 introduced vaginal cesarean section. Alexander J. C. Skene, of the United States, performed the first extraperitoneal cesarean section successfully in 1876. However, it was earnestly introduced by Frank of Cologne in 1907. With the contributions of Latzko, Sellheim, Justner and others the extraperitoneal cesarean section became well established.

So far as the records show, the cesarean operation was not performed on the living woman in the time of Julius Caesar. This fact should effectually dispose of the popular belief that the name of the operation was derived from the alleged manner of birth of Julius Caesar. It is the consensus that the name was derived from the "lex regia," in the time of Caesar, in which it was ordered that an abdominal section must be performed on all dead and dying women, when in the advanced stage of pregnancy, to save the child for the state. Later, the "lex regia" became known as the "lex cesaria" and from this law the name cesarean was derived.

First Occurrences and Outstanding Events

A. Operations

Osiander did the first vaginal hysterectomy (really a cervical amputation) for carcinoma, in comparatively modern times, in 1801.

First recorded vaginal hysterectomy was by Soranus in the 2nd Century A.D.

Langenbeck, in 1813, did the first actual vaginal hysterectomy for cancer.

John C. Warren did the first authentic vaginal hysterectomy in the U.S., in 1829.

James H. Bennet of London, in 1845, was the first to differentiate fibroids from malignancy.

Washington L. Atlee, in 1853, performed the first abdominal myomectomy.

Heath, in 1843, did the first abdominal hysterectomy for fibroids.

Kimball, in 1855, did the first abdominal hysterectomy for fibroids, correctly diagnosed.

Burnham, in 1853, did the first hysterectomy, abdominal, for malignancy (sarcoma).

Wertheim, in 1898, did the first radical hysterectomy with gland removal.

Tulpius, in 1652, was the first to amputate the cervix.

X-rays were discovered by Roentgen in 1895.

Radium was discovered by the Curies in 1898.

Pusey and Pfahler were the first to use x-rays for endometrial carcinoma, in 1900.

Abbe, in America, was the first to use radium for cervical cancer in 1903.

Galen was the first to clinically distinguish cancer.

Bayer, in 1821, reported the first human ovum seen.

Robin of Paris, in 1852, was the first to show that cancer originated in the epithelium.

First recorded case of ectopic pregnancy by Albucasis in the 11th Century A.D.

First attempt at operation for ectopic pregnancy in 1595 by Jacob Noierus.

First case of ovarian pregnancy with rupture in 1682 operated by de Saint Maurice.

First case of ovarian pregnancy reported was by Catherine von Tusschenbroek in 1899.

First case of ovarian pregnancy operated was by John Bard, of New York, in 1759.

Also listed as first operation for ruptured ectopic (besides attempt of Noierus in 1595) was that by Tait in 1883.

Tait was the first to do uterine fixation, salpingectomy and bilateral oophorectomy for fibroids.

Trotula, in the 11th Century, did the first plastic.

Emmett was the first to show necessity of fascial repair in plastic operations.

Ancients used medication and cautery (to form scar) for prolapse.

Heming in 1831 did a procedure like the LeForte for prolapse.

Mackenrodt and Dührssen did fixation for prolapse in 1892.

Watkins, in 1898, interposed the uterus for prolapse.

Mayo did vaginal hysterectomy for prolapse.

Shaw, in 1933, was the first to introduce to America, the Donald, Fothergill or Manchester operation for prolapse.

Alquié, in 1840, suggested operation (shortening of round ligaments) for retroflexion. He did not perform it, however.

Deneffe, in 1864, performed the operation suggested by Alquié, with a death.

First pessaries go back to Arabian era.

Hodge in 1866, invented the horseshoe pessary in the U.S.

First sounds were by Wierus in 1657.

First dilators also go back to Arabian era.

First graduated sound by MacIntosh, of Edinburgh, in 1832.

Recamier, in 1842, developed the curette.

B. Cesarean

First cesarean was recorded by the ancient Hebrews, in the Talmud.

First cesarean with living mother and baby by Nufer in A.D. 1500.

First detailed account of cesarean by Trautmann in 1610.

John L. Richmond in 1827, performed the first successful cesarean in the United States.

Ephraim McDowell is sometimes mentioned as the first American to perform a successful cesarean.

Jesse Bennett, shortly after 1801, did the first successful cesarean in the United States (on his wife), according to a report by John Hull of England.

First major innovation in cesarean operation by Porro in 1876.

Kehrer and Sänger, in 1882, were the first to close wound of uterus with sutures. (Similar effort was made by Lebas in 1769.)

A. Dührssen did the first vaginal cesarean in 1896.

Skene, in 1876, did the first successful Extraperitoneal cesarean.

References

A. Operations

1. Ricci, J. V.: *Genealogy of Gynecology*. Philadelphia, Blakiston, 1950, p. 350.

2. Leonardo, R. A.: *History of Gynecology*. New York, Froben, 1944, p. 313.
3. Mathieu, A.: History of Hysterectomy. *West. J. Surg., Obst. and Gynec., 42*:No. 1, p. 2, Jan. 1934.
4. Leonardo, R. A.: *History of Gynecology*. New York, Froben, 1944, pp. 311, 316.
5. Bennet, J. H.: *A Practical Treatise on Inflammation, Ulceration and Induration of the Neck of the Uterus*. London, Churchill, 1845.
6. Atlee, W. L.: *The Surgical Treatment of Certain Fibrous Tumors of the Uterus*. Philadelphia, Collins, 1853.
7. Leonardo, R. A.: *History of Gynecology*. New York, Froben, 1944, pp. 316-320.
8. Mettler, Cecilia and Mettler, F. A.: *History of Medicine*. Toronto, Blakiston, 1947, chapt. V.
9. Smith, F. R.: An etiologic aspect of cancer. *Obst. & Gynec., 13*: 119-127, 1959.
10. Ricci, J. V.: *Genealogy of Gynecology*. Philadelphia, Blakiston, 1950, p. 398.
11. King, John: *Analysis of the Subject of Extra-uterine Foetation, and of the Retroversion of the Gravid Uterus*. Norwich, Wright, 1818, pp. 9-12.
12. Parry, J. S.: *Extra-uterine Pregnancy*. Philadelphia, Lea, 1876.
13. Leonardo, R. A.: *History of Gynecology*. New York, Froben, 1944, p. 334.
14. Tait, R. L.: On the method of flap-splitting in certain plastic operations. *Brit. Gynec. J., 3*:367-76, 1887-8; 7:195-214, 1891-92.
15. Rawls, R. M.: Cystocele, *Am. J. Obst., Vol. 78*:328-329. Sept. 1918.
16. Leonardo, R. A.: *History of Gynecology*. New York, Froben, 1944, p. 338.
17. Kelly, H. A.: Reminiscences in Development of Gynecology. *Connecticut State M. J., 1*:463, Nov. 1937.
18. Speert, Harold: Gynecologic Eponyms, Alfred Hegar: Hegar's sign and dilators. *Obst. & Gynec., 6*:No. 6, pp. 679-683, Dec. 1955.
19. D'Angelo, G. J.: Dilatation and Curettage, a development covering 3000 years. *Obst. & Gynec.*, 2:No. 3, pp. 322-324, Sept. 1953.

B. Cesarean

1. Findley, Palmer: *Priests of Lucina*. Boston, Little, 1939.
2. Thorek, Max: *Modern Surgical Technic*, Vol. III. Philadelphia, Lippincott, 1938, p. 1738.

3. Sennert, Daniel: De Mulierum and Infantium Morbis, in *Practicae Medicinae*. Frankfurt and Wittenberg, T. Mevii, 1649, IV, 2, pp. 439-442.
4. Leonardo, R. A.: *History of Gynecology*. New York, Froben, 1944.

Chapter XIX

PRACTICE AND TEACHING METHODS

ALTHOUGH THE 19th Century ushered in the period of greatest advance, we should not be misled and assume that medicine at this time was anything like it is today; the methods used in the practice of our specialty and the teachings of this period were still comparatively crude. The text books and illustrations are interesting; many of the books were beautifully illustrated with engravings by good artists, others, like G. Spratt's[1] book, *Midwifery*, of 1850, are graphically illustrated by superimposed dissected plates, some of which are in color. Each plate has a number of superimposed drawings that can be lifted and turned over by a hinge effect to disclose the underlying drawing, with as many as a half dozen superimpositions. It is indeed an old form of illustration found in common usage in the 19th Century. This type of illustration, with dissected plates, dates back to the 16th Century, yet Spratt, in his preface, proudly proclaims them to be an innovation in medical illustration.

One of the earliest books to be so illustrated was by Georg Bartisch of Frankfurt in 1584; the plates are hand colored and detailed. Another book similarly illustrated was by Gasparo Aselli of Milan in 1627; the book is *De Lactibus sine Lacteis venis*. Although not printed in superimposed plates to represent anatomic relations as were Spratt and Bartisch's books, this book of Aselli's is considered the earliest anatomic illustration in color printing; it describes the lacteal vessels which he discovered. Four colors are utilized—black, dark red, light red and white (the color of the paper)—to show the

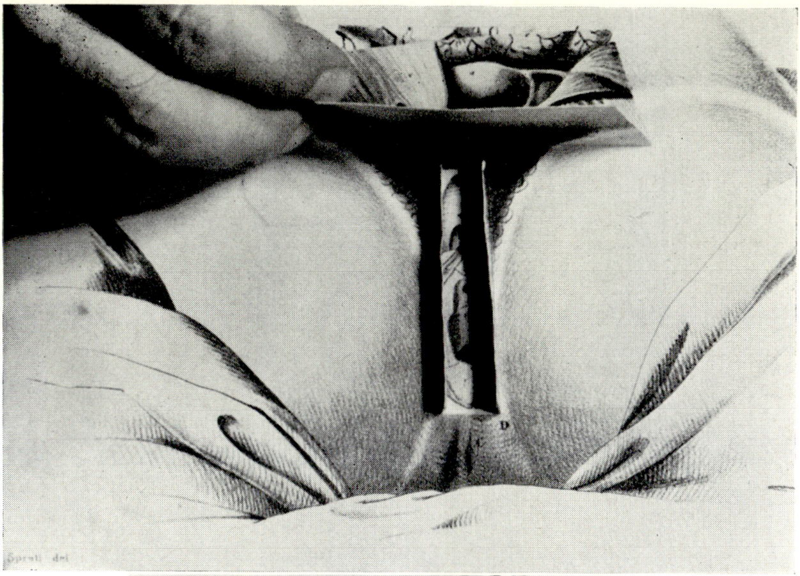

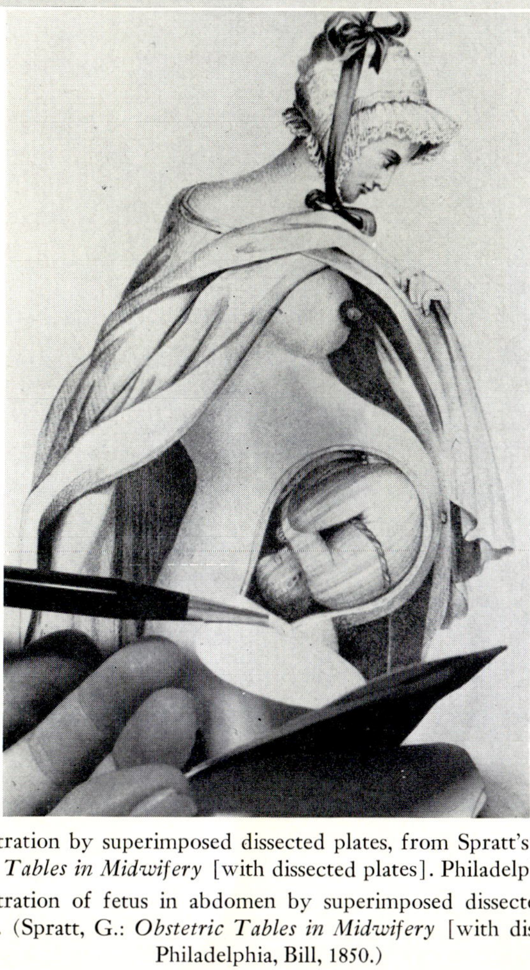

Fig. 194. Illustration by superimposed dissected plates, from Spratt's book. (Spratt, G.: *Obstetric Tables in Midwifery* [with dissected plates]. Philadelphia, Bill, 1850.)

Fig. 195. Illustration of fetus in abdomen by superimposed dissected plates from Spratt's book. (Spratt, G.: *Obstetric Tables in Midwifery* [with dissected plates]. Philadelphia, Bill, 1850.)

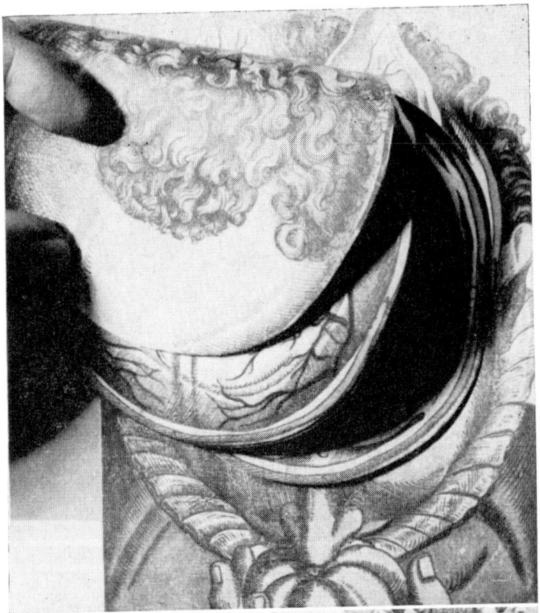

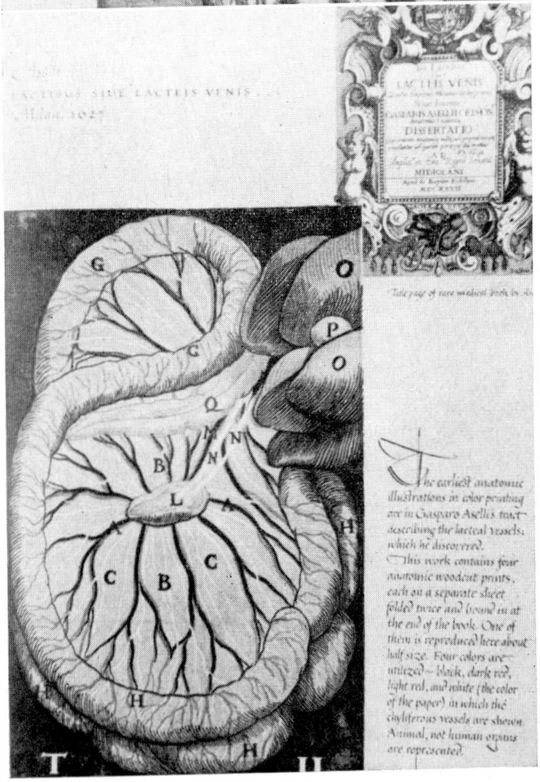

Fig. 196. One of the earliest medical illustrations by superimposed dissected plates, by Georg Bartisch of Frankfurt, in 1584. (Dunham, J. S., ed.: *What's New*, No. 180, [The History of Medical Division, of the armed forces medical library]. Chicago, Abbott Laboratories, 1953, p. 9.)

Fig. 197. Earliest medical illustration in color by Gasparo Aselli of Milan, in 1627. (Dunham, J. S., ed.: *What's New*, No. 180, [The History of Medical Division, the armed forces medical library]. Chicago, Abbott Laboratories, 1953, p. 11.)

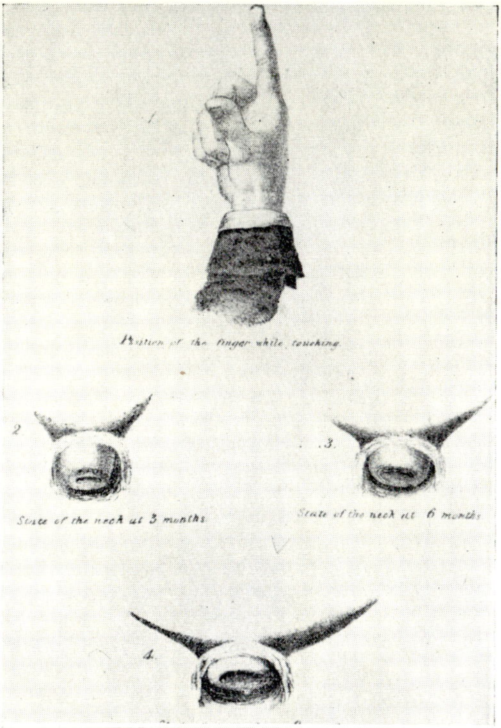

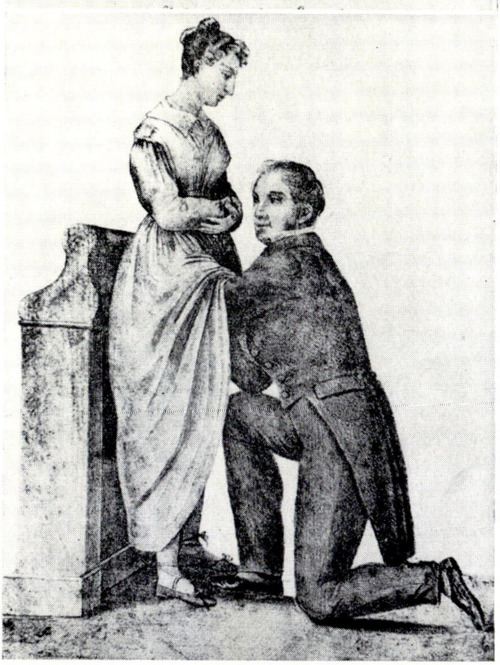

Fig. 198. Finger palpation (touching) of cervix in pregnancy. (Doane, Sidney: *Maygrier's Midwifery*, 6th Ed. [transl. by] New York [Clinton Hall], Redfield, 1833.)

Fig. 199. Touching the female erect. (Doane, Sidney: *Maygrier's Midwifery*, 6th Ed. [transl. by]. New York [Clinton Hall], Redfield, 1833.)

chyliferous vessels. Animal and not human organs were represented.[2]

Examination of female patients had not yet attained the level comparable to the standards of today. Examinations were still made under covers, as was catheterization, and any other manipulations that did not require the outright inspection of the external genitalia. An interesting dissertation on examination of patients, particularly in pregnancy is given in a book by Sidney A. Doane in 1833. He says:

> "Of touching": Among the modes of determining the existence of pregnancy, "touching" is the most essential, as it unites all the conditions requisite to establish the sensible and positive signs of pregnancy. Considered in this respect, touching may be defined as a manual operation, the object of which is to ascertain the changes in the situation, the figure and the consistence of different parts of the uterus, not only during pregnancy, but also during and after parturition. In order that this operation may be successful, the index finger of one hand must be introduced into the vagina to discover the state of the neck, the opposite hand being applied to the abdomen, to judge how much the uterus is developed, and from combining these two modes of investigation, to form an opinion of the existence of pregnancy, and then to determine the period of gestation.
>
> "Of touching the female standing": This mode is advantageous in every respect. The parts of the female are in their natural position, and the accoucheur cannot be mistaken. The mode of proceeding is as follows: the female stands erect; her back, supported by some vertical plane, should remain motionless during the operation; her legs are separated, and the pelvis carried forward; the hands hang down, or are gently crossed on the abdomen; and the whole form should be perfectly at ease. The accoucheur then oils the index finger of one hand, introduces it by the posterior commissure within the vagina, passes it up to the neck of the uterus, which is generally situated to the right and backward; by examining carefully, he determines its extent and size, its degree of resistance and flaccidity; if the os tincae be open, the end of the finger is carefully introduced, to judge how much it is shortened, and thus to determine the period of pregnancy; the neck not being able to yield thus and to lose its extent and resistance without contributing to the dilatation of the uterus, and thus

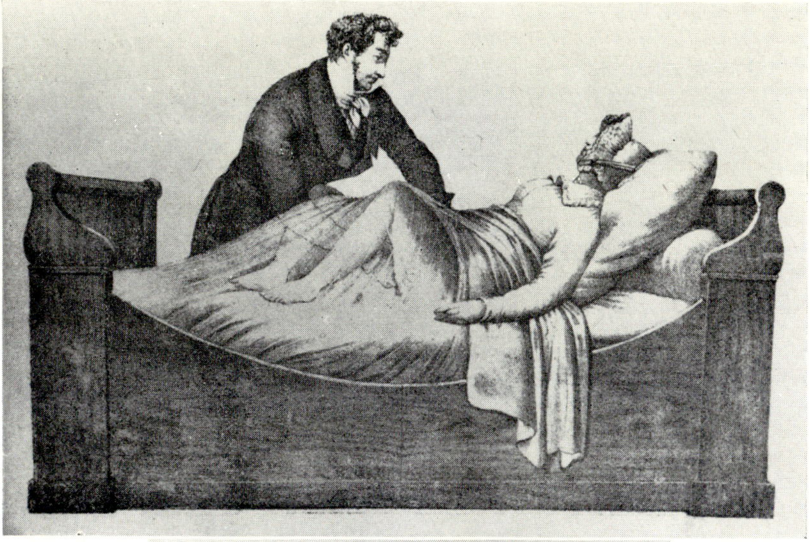

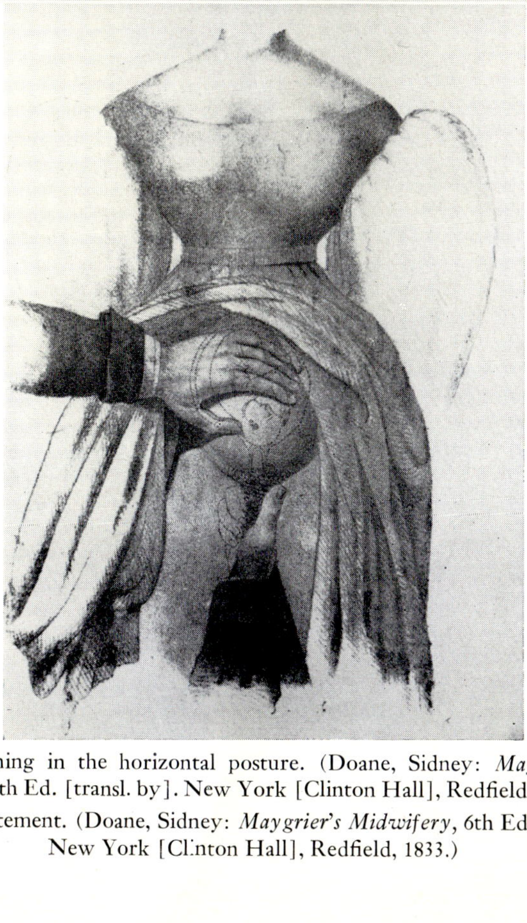

Fig. 200. Touching in the horizontal posture. (Doane, Sidney: *Maygrier's Midwifery*, 6th Ed. [transl. by]. New York [Clinton Hall], Redfield, 1833.)

Fig. 201. Ballottement. (Doane, Sidney: *Maygrier's Midwifery*, 6th Ed. [transl. by]. New York [Clinton Hall], Redfield, 1833.)

concurring in its enlargement. While the accoucheur thus passes the index finger within the vagina, he must place the palm of the opposite hand on the abdomen, to judge of the changes in the figure and size of the uterus, produced by the progress and development of pregnancy; he must also determine the height to which the uterus has risen, by pressing slightly on that part of the abdomen to which its base corresponds.

"Of touching the female reclining": The mode of touching while the female is reclining differs a little from that just mentioned and must be practiced whenever the preceding mode would not afford the same results. It is most advantageous during the first three or four months of pregnancy. During labor both methods can be employed with the same success; but after parturition and during the period of lying-in, the female to be touched must always be in a horizontal posture, and consequently lying down. In order to practice it successfully, the head of the female should be gently flexed on the chest, the legs upon the thighs, which are slightly separated. The accoucheur should stand on the right side of the female, if he is touching with his right hand, and vice-versa, if the left hand be used; the index finger is introduced into the vagina, as before, and the other hand is placed upon the abdomen.

"Ballottement": To ascertain the presence of the child in the uterus, we proceed in the following manner; we easily see a depression between the neck and the adjacent part of the bladder, to the base of which the lower part of the uterus corresponds; the head of the fetus is generally situated near this point, after the fourth month of pregnancy; here also the accoucheur must place the extremity of his finger, while the opposite hand is applied to that part of the abdomen where the base of the uterus is situated; then by an alternate action, sometimes by the hand placed on the abdomen, sometimes by the finger in the vagina, he raises and depresses the child. This is called ballottement. Ballottement can rarely be performed before the fourth month of pregnancy; before this time the head of the child is too small, and the quantity of the waters of amnios proportionately great, to perceive it through the parietes of the uterus. Ballottement is most easily performed from the fourth to the seventh month, as the head is then more elastic. Further, this phenomenon so wonderful in its effects, not only demonstrates the certainty of pregnancy but also that the child is living; since a dead fetus never responds as

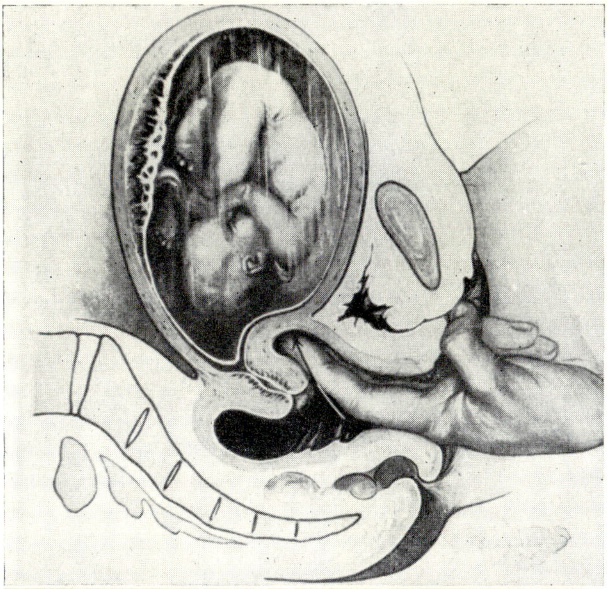

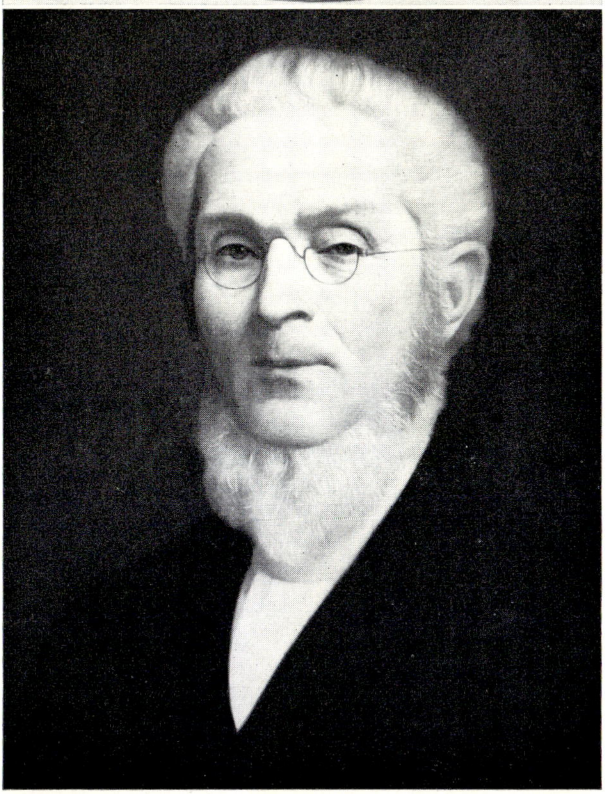

Fig. 202. Ballottement, head returning to finger. (DeLee, J. B.: *Principles and Practice of Obstetrics*, 5th Ed. Philadelphia, Saunders, 1929.)

Fig. 203. Dr. Joseph Warrington. (Pennsylvania Hospital, Woman's Building, Philadelphia.)

> promptly and lightly to the motions impressed upon it. After the seventh month, the head of the child becomes heavier, the water diminishes so that ballottement is almost impossible. In fact this is stronger proof of pregnancy, as the child's head then occupies most of the superior strait, in which it seems already engaged, and the finger easily passes over its whole surface.[3]

DR. JOSEPH WARRINGTON (1808-1888) was born in Westfield, New Jersey, graduated from the University of Pennsylvania in 1828, practiced at 229 Vine Street, Franklin Square, and died in Moorestown, New Jersey. In 1828, Dr. Warrington conceived the idea of establishing a course in instruction on nursing care of maternity cases, and by 1832, he had organized one of the best known of the older charitable institutions in the city, "The Philadelphia Lying-in Charity for Attending Indigent Women in Their Own Homes." The course to the nurses consisted of systematic lectures in addition to bedside instruction in the homes of patients. Their original quarters were at Eighth and Race Streets; in 1888, they went to Eleventh and Cherry Streets, where they remained until 1929, when the Pennsylvania Lying-in Hospital took over the training, including doctors.

In 1842, Dr. Joseph Warrington published a small book on obstetrics.[4] It is a compendium written in question and answer form, and was intended as a review for students who were contemplating taking an examination in obstetrics. A few of the questions and answers, in order to acquaint us with a method of teaching in the mid-19th Century, are hereby enumerated:

1. *Q.* Is the external examination sufficient to enable the accoucheur always to diagnosticate pregnancy?
   A. No, it is liable to fail from a variety of circumstances.
2. *Q.* What other resource is there?
   A. Examination per vaginum.
3. *Q.* What is this process called in professional language?
   A. The touch.
4. *Q.* What is the relative importance of this operation to the accoucheur in pregnancy and diseases of the uterus?
   A. By some high authority it is regarded as important to the accoucheur, as the lever to the mechanic, and the compass to the mariner.

5. *Q.* What conduct should the accoucheur observe when about to make this kind of examination?

   A. That which has regard to the sense of delicacy, on the part of the female.

6. *Q.* To whom should he make the proposition for an examination?

   A. To a third person, as a nurse, the husband, or some matronly female.

7. *Q.* How should he dispose of himself, while such a proposition is communicated to the patient?

   A. He should retire into another room until the decision is made.

8. *Q.* What arrangements should be made in order to conduct the examination most satisfactorily?

   A. The room should be darkened, and the patient lightly dressed, and placed in the suitable position.

9. *Q.* Should the physician insist upon having a third person present?

   A. He should always do so if it be at all practicable.

10. *Q.* What is the rule for carrying the hand under the coverings?

    A. The clothes should be properly raised at their lower edges, by the left hand, and then the right hand with the index finger lubricated, passed cautiously up under the clothes without uncovering the patient.

11. *Q.* Suppose your patient to be standing, how should she be arranged?

    A. She should be allowed to rest her hips against something firm, and then recline forward as if to lean upon the examiner.

12. *Q.* How should the examiner be situated?

    A. Either upon a low seat, or resting upon one knee, in front of the patient.

13. *Q.* To what portion of the genital fissure should the finger be carried?

    A. Always to the posterior commissure, avoiding contact with the mons veneris if possible.

Catheterization, among other manipulations in examining or treating a patient, was performed without uncovering the patient.

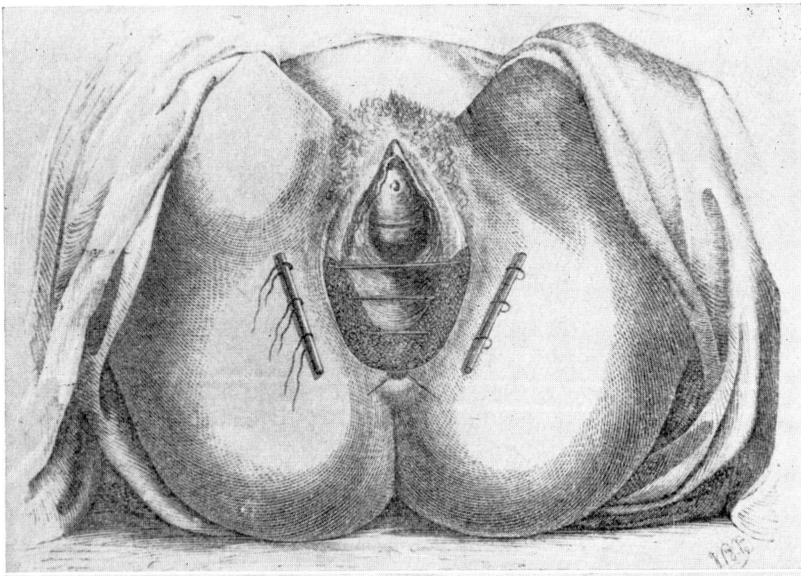

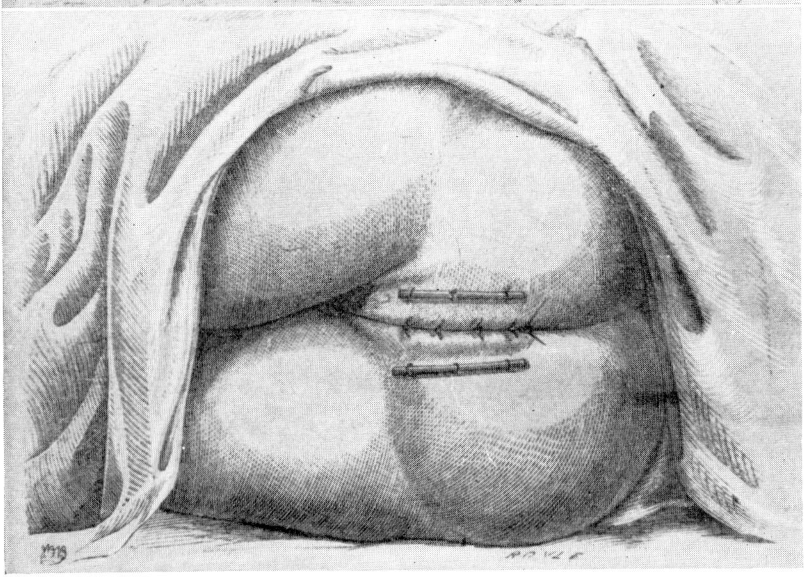

Fig 204. Operation on perineum. Quill sutures, untied. (Brown, I. B.: *Surgical Diseases of Women*, 3rd Ed. London, Hardwicke, 1866.)

Fig. 205. Operation on perineum. Quill sutures, tied. (Brown, I. B.: *Surgical Diseases of Women*, 3rd Ed. London, Hardwicke, 1866.)

Occasionally the catheter was mistakenly pushed either into the vagina or the rectum, thus contaminating the bladder when it was finally catheterized.

As for the operating techniques of this period, the methods in vogue are well described in I. Baker Brown's text book of 1854,[5] published in London. The question of sepsis was being hotly debated, but nothing definite was yet decided despite the impending discoveries of Holmes, Pasteur, and Virchow. Surgeons were beginning to be more scrupulous in their cleansing of wounds (as taught by Lister); they tried (as was preached by Symes) silver wire and numerous other materials and techniques to prevent infection. A method for suturing in vaginal plastics is described in Brown's book and may be of interest:

> The sutures are double, to allow them to enclose the quills or (as used) the pieces of elastic catheter, cane or bougie, around which they loop on one side, and are tied over on their free ends on the other. For the quill sutures I prefer stout twine, well waxed, to silk, as I believe it to be less irritating, and productive of less suppuration. Insertion of interrupted sutures, "The Quill Sutures" being firmly secured, the sides of the "fissure" become approximated, the divided surfaces in apposition. To bring together the outer margins, along the line of the skin, it is advisable to pass three or four interrupted sutures, and these answer best when metallic, consisting either of iron or silver wire, or copper silvered. These sutures are removed in eight to ten days. Just twisting wire has been used, and also lead shot. The lead shot is, as the name describes, pellets of lead with a hole to thread the suture through. When the shot is pushed up to the tissues at the desired spot (where you would make a knot), you compress the lead shot with a compressing instrument and it holds. (This technique has been used in a few instances as recently as ten years ago.)

This book by I. Baker Brown is considered to be the first purely surgical work on gynecology to be published.

By the end of the 19th Century, surgery compared almost favorably with that of today, still it was a dogged and cumbersome type of performance because the 20th Century innovations of antibiotics, transfusions and early ambulation were as yet unknown. I think

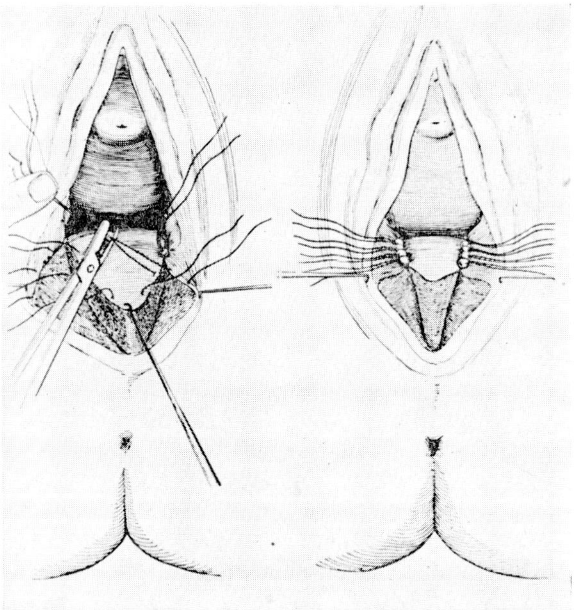

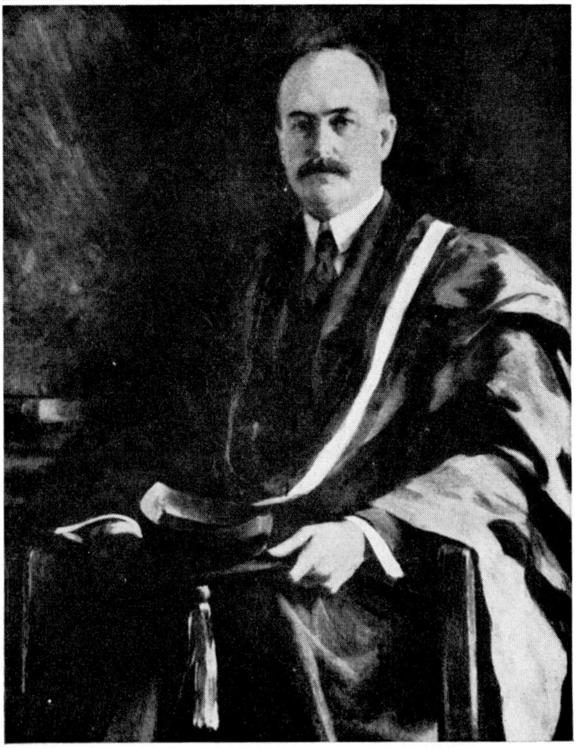

Fig. 206. Operation on perineum. Sutures secured with perforated shot. (Penrose, C. B.: *Disease of Women*. Philadelphia, Saunders, 1897.)

Fig. 207. Charles B. Penrose. (Addison, Agnes: *University of Pennsylvania Medical School, Portraits*. Philadelphia, University Press, 1940.)

the procedures that best exemplify this is the treatment of "inversion." In C. B. Penrose's book "*Diseases of Women*,"[6] printed just before the turn of the century, 1897, an interesting account of the treatment of chronic inversion of the uterus is given:

> The woman should be kept in bed for a few days before the operation (the procedure of replacement). Saline laxatives should be administered. The parts should be prepared by vaginal injections of hot water in large quantity, administered three times a day. A large bag (Barnes) should be placed in the vagina for

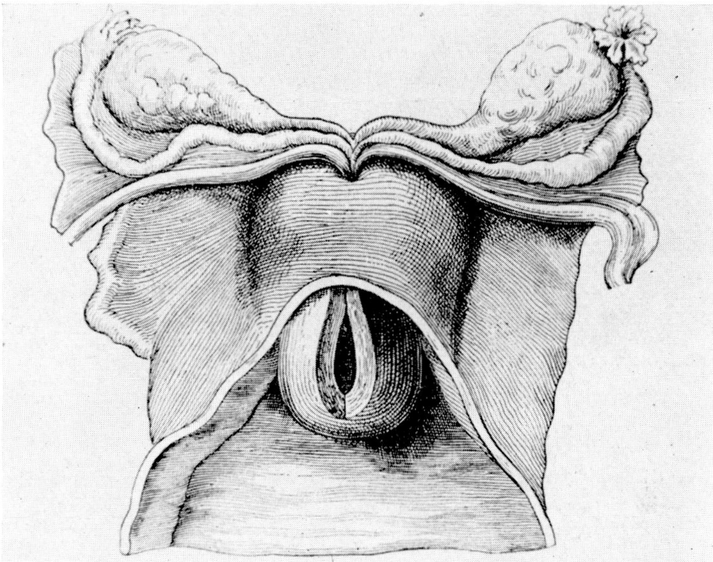

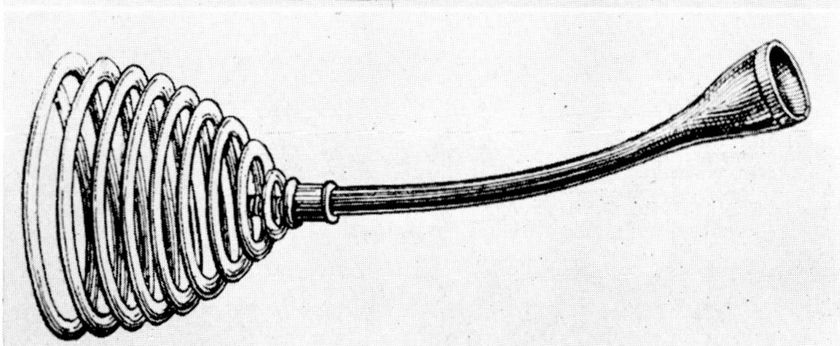

Fig. 208. Complete inversion of the uterus. (Skene, A. J. C.: *Diseases of Women*. New York, Appleton, 1889.)

Fig. 209. White's repositor for inversion of the uterus. (Penrose, C. B.: *Diseases of Women*. Philadelphia, Saunders, 1897.)

two or three days before the operation, in order to distend the genital tract sufficiently to admit the hand. In some cases the pressure of such bag, applied for from one to eleven days, has itself effected reduction. At the time of operation an anesthetic should be administered and the woman should be placed in the lithotomy position. The bladder should be emptied.

Penrose continues by quoting Emmet:

> "My hand was passed into the vagina, and, with the fingers and thumb encircling the portion of the body close to the site of inversion, the fundus was allowed to rest in the palm of the hand. This portion of the body was firmly grasped, pushed upward, and the fingers were then immediately separated to their utmost; at the same time the other hand was employed over the abdomen in the attempt to roll out the parts forming the ring, by sliding the abdominal parietes over its edge. This maneuver was repeated and continued. At length, as the diameter of the uterine cervix and os was increased by lateral dilatation with the outspread fingers, the long diameter of the body of the uterus became shortened, and the degree of inversion proportionally lessened. After the body had advanced well within the cervix, steady upward pressure upon the fundus was applied by the tips of all the fingers brought together.

Penrose's book further states that reduction may be aided by the use of White's repositor. This instrument consists of an India rubber cup set on a curved iron staff which has at its other end a stout spiral spring. The cup is placed against the inverted fundus, and the spring against the body of the operator, who is thus enabled to maintain continuous pressure during the manipulations of his fingers.

Reduction of chronic inversion by manual methods is a long and exhausting process, requiring sometimes three or four hours for its accomplishment. It is advisable to have several assistants for mutual relief. It may be necessary to desist, and to repeat the operation when the condition of the patient permits it. In case reduction can be but partially accomplished, or when, from any cause, the attempt at reduction has to be temporarily abandoned, the result of the work done may be preserved by a method of Emmet's of freshening the edges of the cervix and bringing them into apposition by suture. This procedure not only prevents the complete inversion from

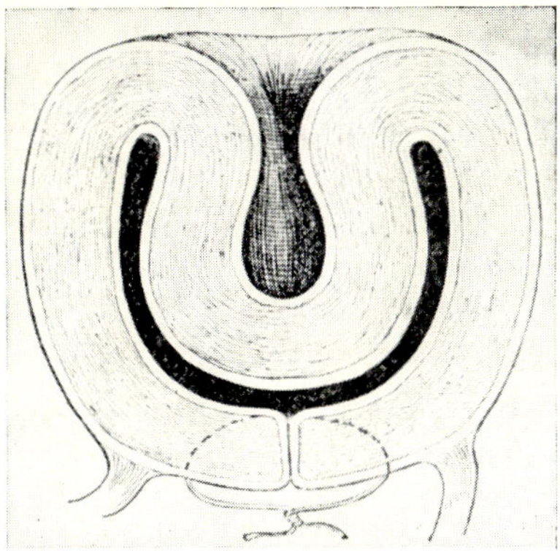

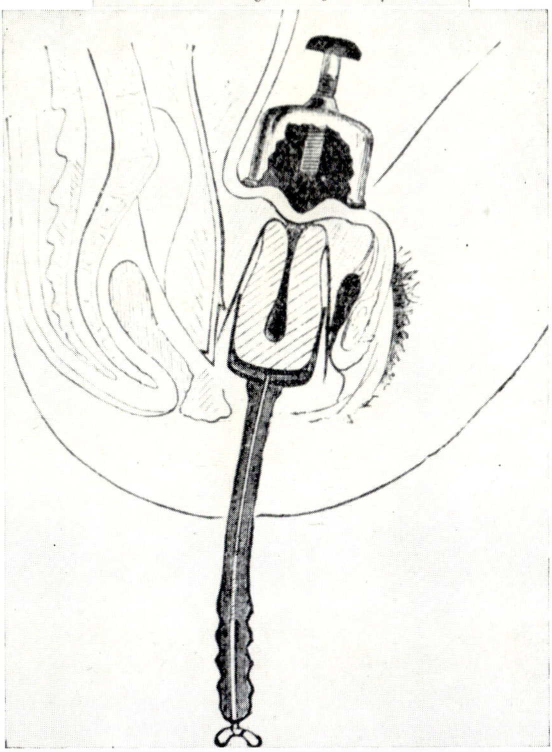

Fig. 210. Emmet's method of retaining partially reduced inversion. (Penrose, C. B.: *Diseases of Women*. Philadelphia, Saunders, 1897.)

Fig. 211. Byrne's method of reduction. (Skene, A. J. C.: *Diseases of Women*. New York, Appleton, 1889.)

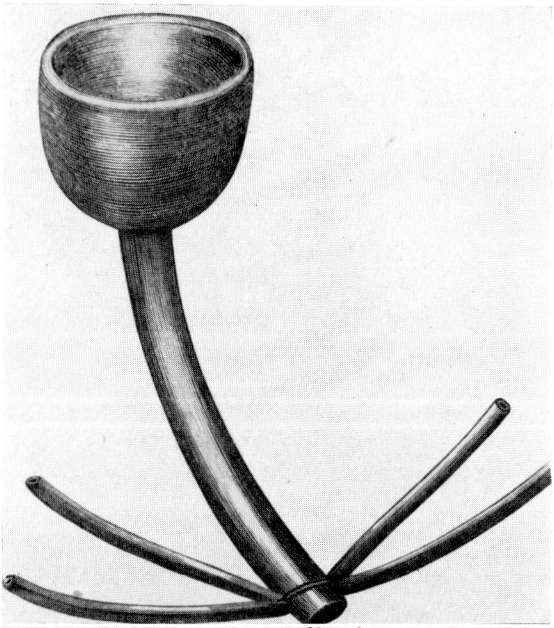

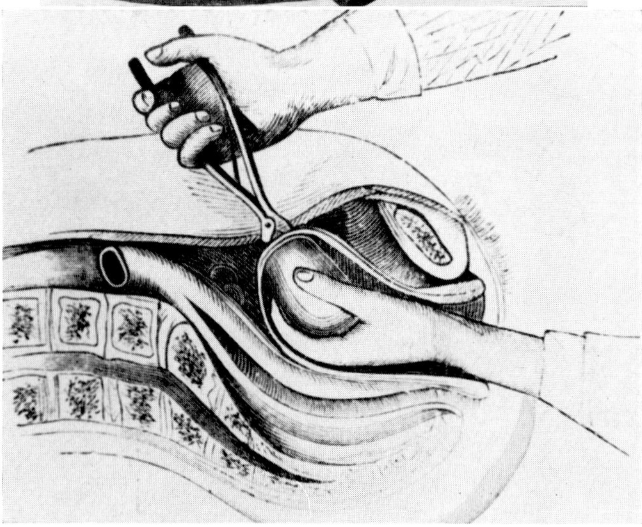

Fig. 212. Cup pessary to produce gradual pressure. (Skene, A. J. C.: *Diseases of Women.* New York, Appleton, 1889.)

Fig. 213. Replacement of uterus by dilatation through the abdomen. (Skene, A. J. C.: *Diseases of Women.* New York, Appleton, 1889.)

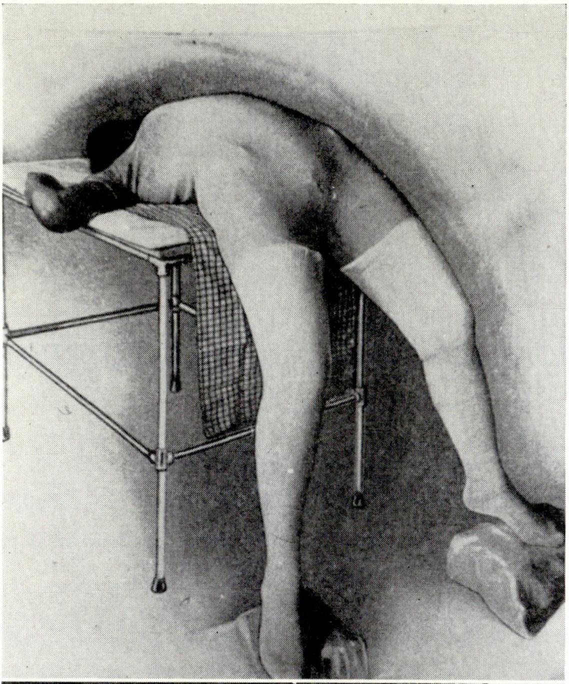

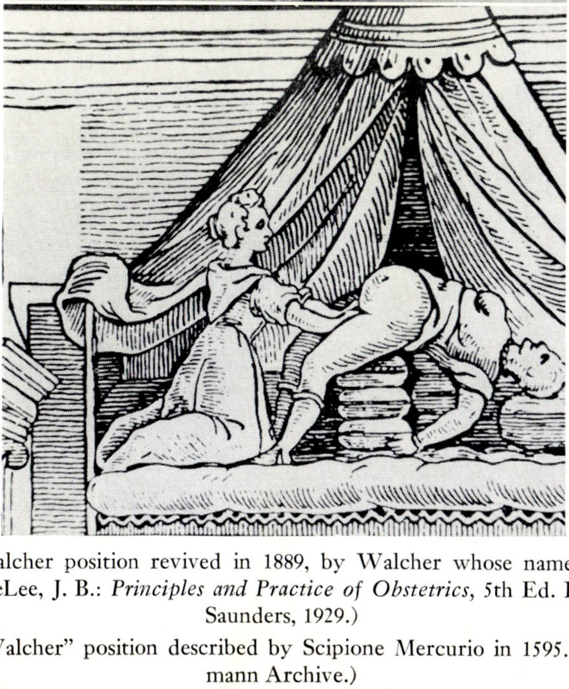

Fig. 214. Walcher position revived in 1889, by Walcher whose name is still appended. (DeLee, J. B.: *Principles and Practice of Obstetrics,* 5th Ed. Philadelphia, Saunders, 1929.)

Fig. 215. "Walcher" position described by Scipione Mercurio in 1595. (The Bettmann Archive.)

returning, but the traction produced by stretching the cervix over the fundus itself favors reduction.

Other methods of taxis used for chronic inversion are described in Skene's book[7] of 1889, such as John Byrne's (Brooklyn) method of reduction, which was considered the most useful by Skene. When chronic inversion is not reduceable by taxis, then gradual reduction by continuous pressure is used. This is effected by a cup and stem held in place by a perineal band of rubber or elastic fastened to a bandage around the pelvis. This is usually worn for two days, then changed and replaced if necessary.

When the above methods fail, Thomas' method is employed. This is accomplished through an incision of the abdomen, dilatation with a steel instrument made like a glove stretcher over the cervical ring, intra-abdominally, and reposition of the inverted uterus, by one of the methods mentioned, by the other hand in the vagina. This is not offered as a method of treating inversion of the uterus, but as a substitute for amputation.

If, after careful trial of conservative methods, reduction of an inverted uterus is found to be impossible, the physician may be compelled to perform hysterectomy.

It is of interest that in the latter 19th Century certain techniques relative to the position of the patient on the table were developed or revived. There is the "Walcher position" which Walcher revived in 1889. It was first described and published in 1595 by Scipione Mercurio's midwifery hand book in Venice and Padua, he called it the "hanging leg position."[8] Later, in 1738, Melli gave it prominence. This position was used to facilitate delivery because it lengthened the true conjugate from six to twelve millimeters, especially in flat pelves. Today it is seldom used, probably because it becomes quite painful to the patient after about thirty minutes. A curious fact stated by DeLee of Chicago[9] regarding this situation is that he has had better results by the use of the exaggerated lithotomy position, which is contraindicated because it contracts the inlet. Dr. DeLee states that in the exaggerated lithotomy position, the thighs force the uterus up, correcting the pendulous belly so common with contracted pelvis; the uterus and child are straightened out, the former being thus allowed to act with more directness,

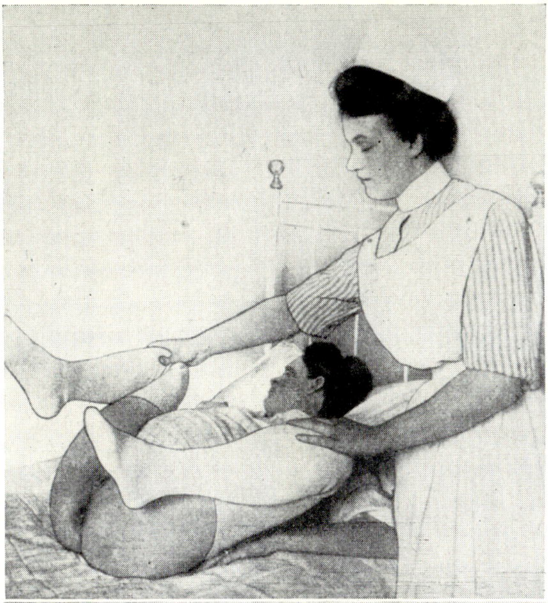

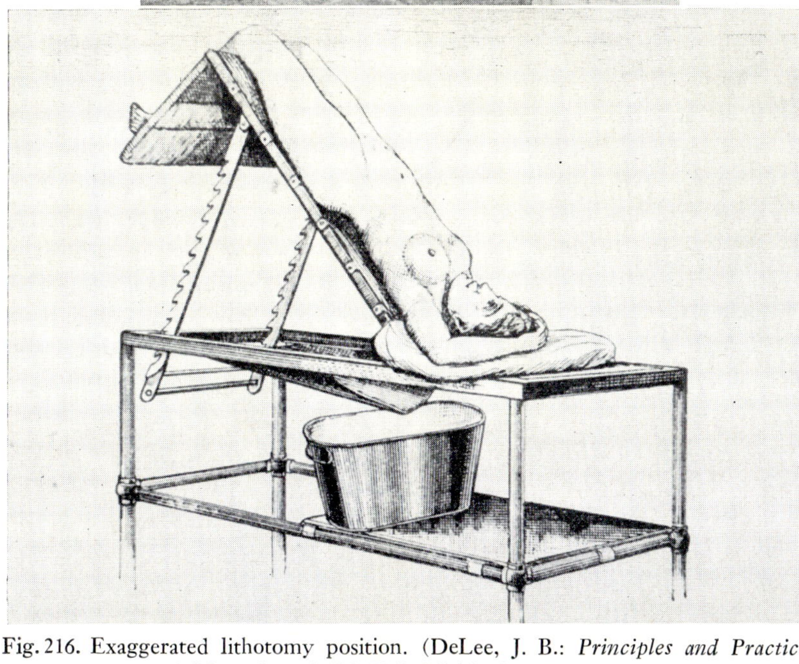

Fig. 216. Exaggerated lithotomy position. (DeLee, J. B.: *Principles and Practice of Obstetrics*, 5th Ed. Philadelphia, Saunders, 1929.)

Fig. 217. Trendelenburg position. (Penrose, C. B.: *Diseases of Women*. Philadelphia, Saunders, 1897.)

and the latter being brought into better position over the inlet. It is also possible that an occasional parietal bone or ear presentation is corrected. The patient can be kept in this position for several hours as against a half hour in the Walcher position.

Another technique that was revived in the 19th Century was the inclined operating table, with the patient's head lower than the pelvis, the position well known to the Salernitans. It is the Trendelenburg position, reintroduced by F. Trendelenburg in 1881. Even today it is used in many operations.

FEMALE UROLOGY: ITS CONTRIBUTORS AND CONTRIBUTIONS OF THE 19TH CENTURY

FRIEDRICH TRENDELENBURG (1844-1925) of Berlin, applied the "Trendelenburg" position first at a vesico-vaginal fistula operation and at a lithotomy. From his successes with it in these cases he was led to an intensive study of urinary-tract surgery, to which he contributed many ideas.

ALEXANDER J. C. SKENE (1838-1900), of Brooklyn, was born in Scotland, graduated from Long Island College in 1863, and was the first to discover certain glands in the female urethra, beneath the mucous membrane, the physiology of which he did not know.

HOWARD A. KELLY (1858-1943) developed the bimanual examination in gynecology which was used systematically during the 19th Century. He said:

> Our ancestors used simple finger touch or digitation. They felt the cervix and that was about all. Then they would insert, often with difficulty, a not too efficient vaginal speculum and in spite of poor exposure and visibility, they would have to make their diagnosis.[10]

Kelly stated that an abnormal ureter can be felt more easily, but even a normal one is palpable. He conceived the idea of putting the patient in the knee chest posture and, using a small diameter open cylindrical speculum, he endeavored to inspect the interior of the urinary bladder with light reflected from a mirror on his forehead. The whole bladder distended atmospherically, so that he was able to see very well.

> From that moment, the entire category of bladder diseases and the upper urinary tracts in women became the perquisite of gy-

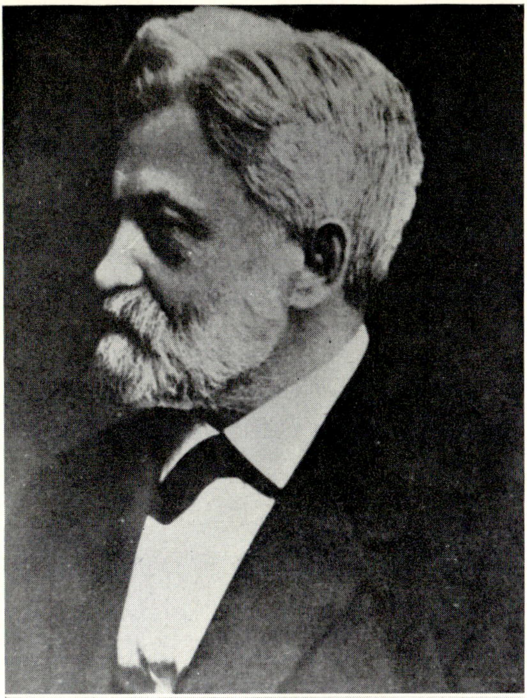

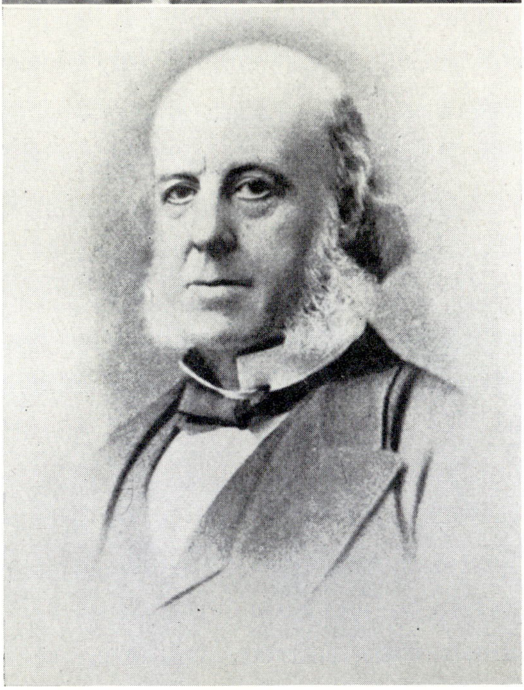

Fig. 218. Carl S. F. Credé. (Findley, Palmer: *Priests of Lucina*. Boston, Little, 1939.)
Fig. 219. John Braxton Hicks. (The American Gynecological Society.)

necologists through the revelations of a direct visual exploration, instrumental touch contacts, and an ability to remove bits of tissue in the urethra and bladder, including as stated, ureters, renal pelves, and kidneys.[11]

Three men,[12] Credé, Hicks and Duncan, were teachers of great caliber; they made lasting contributions to obstetrics in the mid-19th Century. A brief word for each follows:

Carl Siegmund Franz Credé (1819-1892) was born in Leipsig. His two outstanding contributions are the external expression of the placenta and the prophylactic management of ophthalmia neonatorum. Attempts to assist nature in the delivery of the afterbirth had been made from prehistoric times. Women had been tormented with sneezing powders, emetics, pommeling of the abdomen, traction on the cord, and thrusting the oiled hand into the uterus. Credé used gentle friction and external pressure. Evidence of this method goes back to ancient times and even to primitive peoples. The same procedure was employed by Mauriceau in the 17th Century, Johnson and White in the 18th Century, and Baudelocque, Osiander and Bard in the 19th Century. Credé never did claim priority to this procedure; he cited Plenck as the originator.

John Braxton Hicks (1825-1897) was born in Rye, Sussex. He was an honorary fellow of the Philadelphia and Boston Obstetrical Societies, and the American Gynecological Society. His contributions were many, but two stand out. They are: (a) combined external and internal version; instead of inserting entire hand, he used one or two fingers only; and (b) on the condition of the uterus in obstructed labor, etc. He advised watchful waiting, a tonic uterus made delivery impossible, an atonic uterus invited hemorrhage, therefore, wait and it would adjust itself. He observed that the uterine contractions in labor differed only in their intensity from the rhythmical contractions experienced throughout pregnancy.

James Mathews Duncan (1826-1886) was born in Aberdeen. He was assistant to Simpson and helped him in the discovery of chloroform in obstetrics. He aspired to the chair of midwifery in the University of Edinburgh, but he was bitterly disappointed. His contributions were the anatomy of the cervix in pregnancy and after labor, he explained placenta previa and hemorrhage from it.

It was his thesis on puerperal mortality that gave him his greatest distinction.

The following contributions are mentioned at this time because they are more or less isolated facts that did not previously fit into any properly correlated place; nevertheless, they are 19th Century contributions and shall therefore be enumerated now.

The first American article on a purely gynecological subject was published in 1806. It was "The History of a Hemorrhage from a Rupture on the Inside of the Left Labium Pudendi" by Nathaniel W. Appleton of Boston, published in the *Transactions of the Medical Society of Massachusetts.*

Primary carcinoma of the fallopian tube was reported for the first time by Orthmann in 1888. Since then over 300 cases have been found in the literature.[13]

Hydatidiform mole had been studied inconclusively over the past centuries. Its etiology was clinched in the 19th Century by Virchow, although Malpighi and Marchand and Vallisnieri had said that mole was diseased chorionic villi. Hippocrates and Aetius of Amida and other ancient writers mentioned and described mole. The first clinical accurate notation of mole was made by Nikolaas Tulpius (1593-1674). He is the surgeon depicted in Rembrandt's *Anatomy Lesson.* Mauriceau in 1664 removed a mole by finger manipulations. Paul Portal in 1685 described it quite accurately. Ruysch in 1691 ascribed mole to disease of the ovum. Madam Boivin of Paris said in 1827 that the cysts were echinococcic.[14]

Chorio-epithelioma was reported for the first time by Sänger in 1899.

Fetal heart sounds were authentically heard for the first time in 1822. The stethoscope that was discovered by Laennec in 1819 was instrumental in the discovery of fetal heart sounds by Kergaradec a pupil of his. He used the stethoscope to hear the splashing sounds that a baby must make in moving around *in utero.* Instead he picked up its heart beat. This is the first time that this phenomenon was noted; it was published in his *Memoire sur l'Auscultation Applique a l'Etude de la Grossesse.*[15]

Eclampsia was a problem that had been known for a couple of centuries; its solution began by the work of John Charles Weaver

Lever who was born in 1811 at Plumstead. He was the first to recognize the presence of albumin in cases of eclampsia and that it was always associated with pregnancy, and was relieved on delivery of the victim. Further work in this field was done by Alexandre Henri Pilliet, a French pathologist who was born in 1858 and died thirty-seven years later. He showed that eclampsia was associated with changes in the liver.

Pelvimetry was another important contribution of this century; it was the result of the work of Gustav Adolf Michaelis, who was born in Hamburg in 1798. He published a book *Das enge Becken* in 1851 in which he recorded thousands of pelvic measurements and found that any pelvis that measured less than 8.75 cm. at the true conjugate should be regarded as an abnormally contracted pelvis. He stressed the importance of pelvimetry and showed that it could be used as an indication for cesarean section. This was a continuation of the work done by Deventer, Smellie and Baudelocque.

Menstruation continued to be poorly understood until the latter part of the 19th Century. The association between menstruation and the reproductive processes was a matter for speculation only. There had been some pretty good guesses, however, about the migration of the ovum through the tubes and about probable changes in the mucosa of the uterus preparing for its reception. In 1839, the first suggestion that ovulation controlled menstruation was made by Augustin Nicolas Gendrin. In 1843, Girdwood demonstrated that the ovary controlled menstruation. It had been believed that intercourse acted as a trigger releasing the ova; but, in 1844, von Bischoff showed that Graafian follicles rupture periodically without reference to intercourse.

In 1863, a theory on menstruation that was rather generally accepted was set forth by Pflüger. He believed that pressure was set up in the follicle by some reflex irritation, and this, in turn, sent impulses through the ovarian nerves to the cord which was returned to cause pelvic congestion which led to menstruation. Johnstone was of the opinion that menstruation was a result of the upright position of man. But the concept that comes closest to the modern idea of menstruation is that women menstruate because they do not conceive; Powers, Sigismund and His were the exponents of this

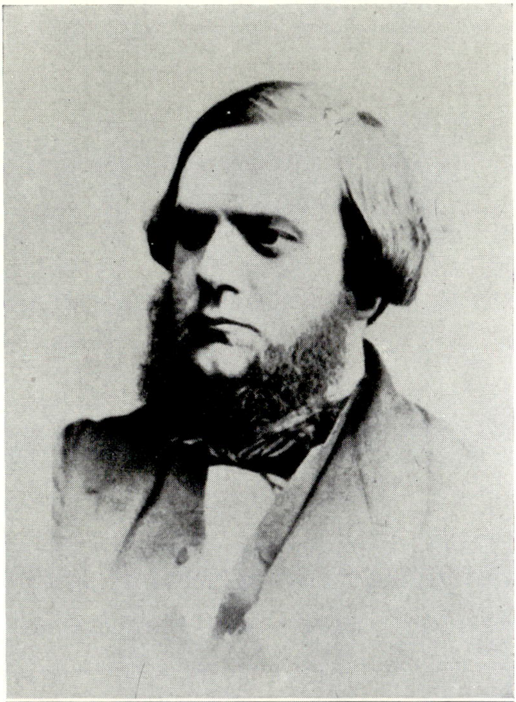

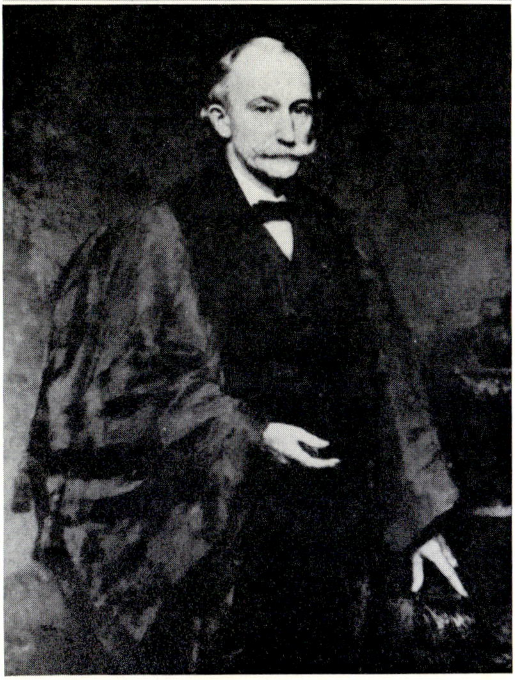

Fig. 220. James Matthews Duncan. (The American Gynecological Society.)

Fig. 221. Richard A. F. Penrose. (Addison, Agnes: *University of Pennsylvania Medical School, Portraits*. Philadelphia, University Press, 1940.)

concept. Mary Putnam Jacobi, Stephenson and Raciborski sponsored still another concept, "the menstrual wave"; i.e., that the menstrual flow instead of being a pelvic phenomenon only, is really a local manifestation of a profound rhythmic change affecting the entire organism (Novak).

Changes within the uterus have been controversial for a long time. In 1873, Kundrat and Engelmann, and, in 1885, Leopold corroborated his findings, and asserted that widening of the glands, dilatation of blood vessels and infiltration with round cells, took place in the endometrium just prior to menstruation. Williams, in 1876, concluded that the uterine mucosa is entirely cast off during menstruation; these were unreliable deductions because the studies were made upon autopsies. In 1882, Moricke arrived at an opposite conclusion from curettings at known stages of the menstrual cycle; that no tissue is lost at menstruation. The best work of this period was done in 1896 by Westphalen, both from curettings and freshly excised uteri. He described cyclic changes in the mucosa:

> Beginning about ten days before the period, and characterized by gland hypertrophy, secretory activity and hyperemia. With menstruation comes a loss of tissue, followed by a period of regeneration, not completed, he believed, until the fourteenth or fifteenth day.

Gebhard envisaged a similar cycle, but considered that there was no characteristic or extensive loss of the endometrium. It was not until the early part of the next century, the 20th, that the cycle of changes in the endometrium was definitely established. (Menstruation, its further progress, is continued in next chapter.)

As late as 1900 and even for a few years afterwards, medical students were graduated without ever having seen an actual delivery, much less doing a delivery or even assisting in one. There were no obstetrical clinics as yet. The best example of obstetrical teaching that bordered on the practical was exemplified by RICHARD A. F. PENROSE (1827-1908), who was Professor of Diseases of Women and Children at the University of Pennsylvania. Besides being instrumental in opening the wards at the Philadelphia Hospital for instruction of students, he was a brilliant didactic teacher. With his mannikin, "Mrs. O'Flaherty," he gave a dramatic presentation of childbirth. This was the nearest approach to an actual delivery that students were permitted to witness.[16]

The status of obstetrics and gynecology at the end of the 19th Century can best be appreciated by the following anecdote told by W. R. Nicholson, who was Vice-Dean of Obstetrics and Gynecology in the Graduate School of Medicine of the University of Pennsylvania for many years:

> In the very early years of the Philadelphia Obstetrical Society, its members did not accept new concepts as readily as they do today [according to Dr. Nicholson]; they were eager and fractious and if they were divided in opinions on gynecological matters they did not hesitate to make their views known. Not only did they argue vociferously and at length, but on a number of occasions, members of the Society actually came to blows. Gynecology was a comparatively new specialty and the Philadelphia Obstetrical Society was even more recent. Many gynecological opinions had not been clearly crystallized as yet so that bitter differences were common. The general surgeon with the feeling that this young, new specialty was infringing on a field of medicine that belonged to him, felt justified in his ridicule and abuse of the gynecologist since the behavior of the gynecologists themselves was anything but commendable. At a meeting of the Society, a prominent gynecologist presented a paper in which he discussed pus tubes. At the end of his discussion he was severely criticized, and was practically called a liar; as far as many of the men present at the meeting were concerned there was no such entity as a pus tube. After much heated discussion, the author of the paper stated that at the very next meeting he would present indubitable evidence of pus tubes. So at the next meeting, Doctor X requested the floor and when granted he walked up to the speaker's platform carrying a bucket. He said, "gentlemen, in order to prove to you without a shadow of doubt that there is such a thing as a pus tube, I have collected a number of them; in fact I have a bucket full, which I shall gladly pass around for examination." In spite of his evidence which soon infiltrated the entire audience, voices of protest and doubt nevertheless arose. Arguments started and not many moments passed before many of these loud and personal "discussions" ended in fisticuffs. The pus tubes were used as weapons in the melee and the meeting had to be adjourned.

The 19th Century was the greatest that medicine has ever seen. In the beginning of this period gynecology was that branch of medicine in which obstetricians were called upon to perform certain surgical procedures that occurred in women incident to child-bearing, so that therapy was mostly medical and conservative. At the close of the century gynecology had increased in scope to become a major specialty.

Ovariotomy was the first surgical feat and this was before anesthesia; vesico-vaginal fistula operations followed, then by the middle of the century hysterectomy and other operations were devised; these advances in gynecological surgery were contingent not only upon the discovery of anesthesia, but probably more from the development of bacteriology and pathology, so that the control of infection (Listerism) was the crux of these advances.

While gynecology came into its own, obstetrics improved only in so far as management to prevent infection (puerperal fever) was concerned, and this applies to obstetrical operative procedures also, such as cesarean section.

By the end of the century, the field of endocrinology had attained importance; many of its mysteries were beginning to unravel.

First Occurrences and Outstanding Events

Earliest medical illustrations with superimposed plates was by Bartisch of Frankfurt in 1584.

Earliest anatomic illustrations in color by Gasparo Aselli of Milan in 1627.

I. Baker Brown's Book, the first purely gynecological surgery text book was published in 1854.

Walcher position, revived by Walcher in 1889, was first practiced by Scipione Mercurio in 1595.

Trendelenburg position revived by Trendelenburg in 1881 was first used by the Salernitans.

Skene was the discoverer of the urethral glands named after him.

H. A. Kelly developed the bimanual examination in gynecology; also the Kelly air cystoscope.

Credé contributed the prophylactic management of ophthalmia neonatorum, and the Credé method of pracental extraction by external manual friction. An old method, however; Credé cites Plenck as the originator.

Hicks devised external internal version.

Duncan assisted Simpson in the discovery of chloroform, used in labor.

First American article on purely gynecological subject matter was by Nathaniel W. Appleton in 1806.

Orthmann, in 1888, was first to report primary cancer of Fallopian tube.

Etiology of hydatidiform mole was clinched by Virchow in the 19th Century.

Chorio-epithelioma was reported for the first time by Sänger in 1899.

Fetal heart sounds first heard by Kergaradec in 1882.

John C. W. Lever was the first to recognize albumin in cases of eclampsia.

Alexandre Henri Pilliet was the first to show that eclampsia was associated with changes in the liver.

Girdwood in 1843 showed that the ovary controlled menstruation.

Gendrin in 1839 suggested that ovulation controlled menstruation.

Kundrat and Engelmann showed that there was widening of the glands, dilatation of blood bessels and infiltration of round cells in the endometrium just prior to menstruation.

Best work in menstruation in 19th Century (1896) was done by Westphalen who noted shedding of the mucosa.

References

1. Spratt, G.: *Obstetric Tables in Midwifery* (with dissected plates), 1st Am. Ed. (from 4th London Ed.) Philadelphia, Bill, 1850.
2. Dunham, J. S., ed.: *What's New*, No. 180 (The History of Medical Division, of the armed forces medical library). Chicago, Abbott Laboratories, 1953, pp. 9-12.
3. Doane, Sidney: *Maygrier's Midwifery*, 6th Ed. (transl.). New York, Redfield, 1833.
4. Warrington, Joseph: *Obstetric Catechism.* Philadelphia, Crolius, 1842.
5. Brown, I. B.: *Surgical Diseases of Women*, 3rd Ed. London, Hardwicke, 1866.
6. Penrose, C. B.: *Diseases of Women.* Philadelphia, Saunders, 1897.
7. Skene, A. J. C.: *Diseases of Women.* New York, Appleton, 1889.
8. Mercurio, G. S.: *La commare o riccoglitrice.* Venetia, Ciotti, 1601.
9. DeLee, J. B.: *Principles and Practice of Obstetrics*, 5th Ed. Philadelphia, Saunders, 1929.
10. Kelly, H. A.: *Medical Gynecology*. New York, Appleton, 1908.

11. Kelly, H. A.: Reminiscences in the Development of Gynecology. *J. Connecticut M. Soc., 1*:459, 1936.
12. Findley, Palmer, *Priests of Lucina*. Boston, Little, 1939.
13. Leonardo, R. A.: *History of Gynecology*, New York, Froben, 1944, p. 350.
14. Ricci, J. V.: *Genealogy of Gynecology*. Philadelphia, Blakiston, 1950, p. 298.
15. Le Jumeau de Kergaradec, J. A.: *Mémoire sur l'auscultation appliqué a l'étude de la grossesse*. Paris, Màquignon-Marvis, 1822.
16. Addison, Agnes: *Portraits in the University of Pennsylvania*. Philadelphia, Univ. of Pennsylvania Press, 1940.

Chapter XX

CONTEMPORARY OBSTETRICS AND GYNECOLOGY (1900-1950)

IN THE FIRST HALF OF THE 20th Century, x-ray and radium, blood transfusions and parenteral therapy, endocrines and antibiotics have been the chief contributions to medicine. These discoveries were not necessarily revolutionary; they have not basically and materially changed the practice of medicine, but they have added vastly to our armamentarium against disease.

Modern medicine was made possible by two outstanding events that occurred in the last part of the 19th Century; they are anesthesia and bacteriology.

Anesthesia

The 20th Century advances in anesthesia contain numerous refinements. Its inception and development in the 19th Century has been discussed in the preceding pages. During the latter 19th Century, chloroform was used most of the time, but by the end of this period it was shown that ether was just as effective and much safer, so it displaced chloroform. Today we have inhalation anesthesia, which is usually gas-ether, cyclopropane and trilene; the intratracheal route which is very recent; intravenous anesthesia for pentathol; spinal and caudal routes; rectal anesthesia of ether; and, of course, local anesthesia. Extremely complex machines have been developed to such an extent that the anesthetists have become highly specialized, and in cooperation with the surgeon have practically taken over the procedures almost completely. It has removed a heavy responsibility from the surgeon, who can now give his undivided attention to the surgical problem undertaken. While it is in this century that these methods of anesthetization have been developed, interest and experiments in this facet of medicine go back to previous centuries.

In preliminary attempts at various forms of anesthesia, we can go as far back as 1633, when the first attempt at rectal anesthesia was made by John Gerarde, who published his *Herball* in London, in which he praised the qualities of the garden poppy. Said Gerarde:

> The leaves, Knops, and seed stamped with vinegar, woman's milke and saffron . . . and put in the fundament as a clyster causeth sleepe.[1]

In 1847, the rectal technique was tried again by using ether and water by the Frenchman Marc Dupuy and the Russian Nikolai I. Pirogoff. The biggest advance in this type of anesthesia came in 1913, when James T. Gwathmey developed an oil ether colonic absorption technique. By 1930, Gwathmey reported on 20,000 cases using it in labor and with good success.

Intravenous anesthesia was first attempted 300 years ago, when a Mr. Robert Boyle, at the instigation of Dr. Christopher Wren, first injected opium in the circulation of dogs in 1656, using the discovery of Harvey's circulation as the basis for this idea. Later, in 1833, Hales, an American, and Charles Pravaz added to our knowledge of intravenous methods of therapy. Following this we note attempts at subcutaneous injections for anesthetic purposes; it was begun by Francis Rynd in 1845, and carried further by Alexander Wood of Edinburgh. The first actual intravenous anesthesia in man was performed in 1874 by Pierre Cyprien Ore, of Bordeaux, in which a testicle was removed entirely without pain; choral hydrate was the drug used. Many others attempted this technique, but because of the high mortality that resulted, it was abandoned. It was revived, in 1909, by Ludwig Burkhardt of Wurzburg, who used a solution of 5 per cent ether. In 1911, "hedonal" was used and although not in general use by civilian practitioners, it was used extensively by the military personnel during the first world war. In 1912, paraldehyde was used and, in 1923, the barbiturates replaced all other drugs for this purpose.

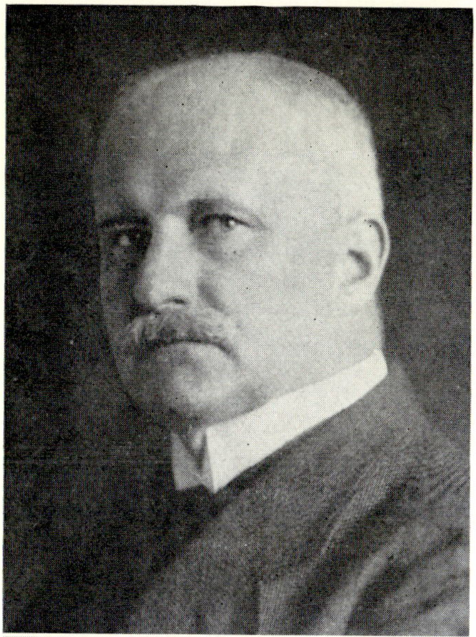

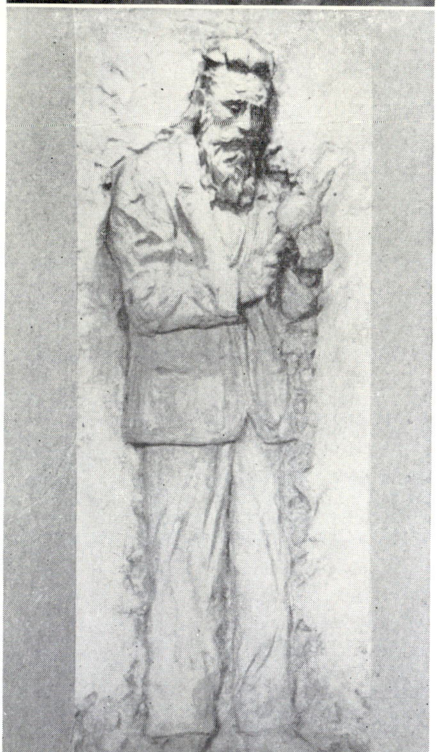

Fig. 222. August Bier, was the first to attempt spinal anesthesia in 1899. (Culver Service.)

Fig. 223. William Roentgen. (*MD Medical News* Magazine, June, 1958. New York, MD Publications, Inc. [Photo by Jas. Coyne, sculptor Doris Appel.])

Cocaine, which is used largely in local anesthesia and in spinal anesthesia has an interesting history. Cocaine, from which its derivatives are used, was isolated in 1859, by Niemann. In 1884, Carl Holler first used it locally, in the eye, as a topical application; then Reclus, in Paris in 1866, used it by the infiltration technique. William S. Halstead in 1884 dissected an entire axilla with this drug.

J. Leonard Corning suggested the practicability of spinal anesthesia in 1885. In 1899, August Bier allowed his assistant Hildebrandt to give him a spinal anesthetic of a strong cocaine solution; this was the first time this type of anesthetic was attempted on a human. He was paralyzed for three months but finally recovered fully. The form of cocaine derivative has been steadily improved, so that, by the time of the Second World War, this form of anesthesia was used almost as often as inhalation anesthesia. It has been greatly used in obstetrics, in some clinics almost exclusively; results show that fewer stillbirths and less neonatal deaths occurred than with inhalation anesthesia.

A drug much used in anesthesia is curare, which was evolved by Claude Bernard, in 1865, although it had been noted, in 1800, by Von Humboldt as the alkaloid poison used in the arrows of aborigines. It was first used as a muscle relaxant in anesthesia by Griffith and Johnson of Canada in 1944. It is more practical in gynecology than obstetrics because of its relaxing qualities.

Twilight sleep came at the turn of the century. In 1902, came the first use of morphine and scopalamine in obstetrics. Barbiturates are used as basic drugs before general anesthesia is given. Intravenous anesthesia for obstetrics can be said to be in the experimental stage as yet, because of possible ill effects on the baby.

In 1939, trichlorethylene was introduced in Great Britain, by a Mr. Chalmers. This drug, "trilene," is being used now in deliveries. It is prepared in inhalators so that the patient herself can control its administration between pains.

Caudal anesthesia, which was described in 1901, by Sicard and Catheline, was first used, in 1942, by Edwards and Hingson for producing analgesia in obstetrics.

Simpson's development of the use of chloroform in maternity

cases was contingent on the fad of hypnotism that prevailed at that time and which he found unsatisfactory; he replaced mesmerism with chloroform. Today there is a revival of "mesmerism" in a sense, by such methods as those of Dick Read, who first presented this subject in 1933.

Radiology

Another facet of medicine that began at the end of the 19th Century became highly developed in the first half of the 20th Century was x-ray and radium.[2]

Wilhelm Conrad von Roentgen (1845-1923) was born at Lennep in the Ruhr. He studied at the Polytechnic School in Zurich. He was professor of physics at the University of Wurzburg. He did extensive research on gases, and, by 1888, had built quite a reputation with a contribution on the electrical effects of moving dielectrics. In 1895, he confined his research exclusively to the cathode ray, and evacuated vessels through which high tension electric charges were passed. Geissler, Leonard and Crookes tubes were used by him in his experiments. During one of his experiments his wife was holding a piece of specially prepared paper for him while he made a test with his tube, and they were both amazed when they saw the shadow of Mrs. Roentgen's bones of the hand. This was in 1895, when he read his famous "Preliminary Communication on a New Kind of Rays." He called them x-rays, and they became known as Roentgen rays later. After much publicity letters poured in from all over the world; they were envious, abusive or fearful at this discovery of "death rays." The x-ray craze spread rapidly, commercial houses began to manufacture machines and reaped a financial harvest; Roentgen, on the other hand, was barely able to buy tubes for further experimentation. The danger of x-rays was not generally realized at this time, but it was not long before medico-legal situations began to arise, and proper precautions were instituted. Among the numerous honors conferred upon him was the first Nobel prize in 1901. By the time he died, in 1923, many improvements had been made by other scientists, such as the high voltage machines in use today. Until now, nothing in medicine offered so much in the way of diagnosis and therapy as did this discovery.

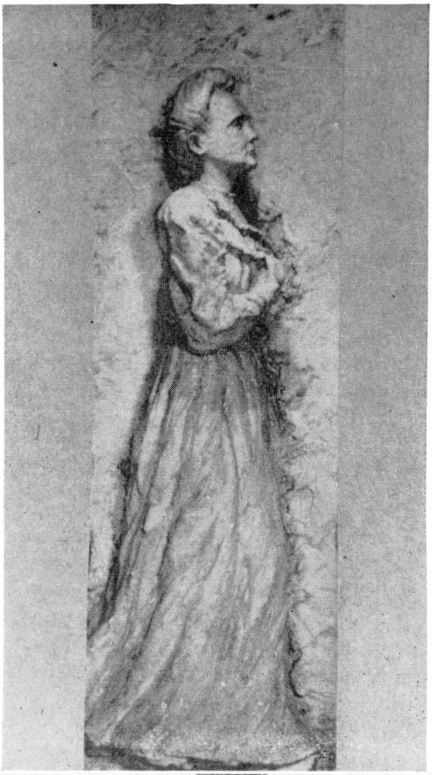

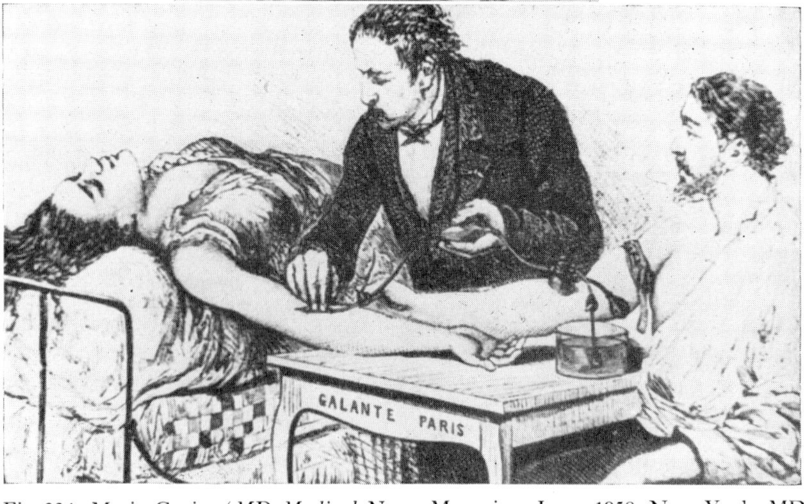

Fig. 224. Marie Curie. (*MD Medical News* Magazine, June, 1958. New York, MD Publications, Inc. [Photo by Jas. Coyne, sculptor Doris Appel.])

Fig. 225. Postpartum blood transfusion, circa 1850. (The Bettmann Archive.)

MARIE CURIE (1867-1934), née Sklodowska (Marie displacing the name Manya) was born in Warsaw, where she taught mathematics and languages. She moved to Paris, studied physics and mathematics for which she was awarded a master's degree.

She went to work in Pierre Curie's laboratory and, in 1895, they were married. Dr. Pierre Curie also had a master's degree; his father and grandfather were physicians. The study of fluorescent substances was in vogue, and one of the interested scientists was Henri Becquerel. The substance he was studying was a rare metal discovered by Klaproth; it was uranium and had been recovered from pitchblende. Becquerel made experiments with photographic plates as did Roentgen, and found that the effect was the same with rays from the metal as from the x-rays. Marie Curie was chosen to do the research with this new found radiating metal. She examined many other metals and found that thorium had the same properties, a property that she personally named "radioactivity." Pierre and Marie worked on this problem together. They separated the metal with the properties of radiation from pitchblende, and obtained polonium and radium as the active elements; this was in 1898.

Between them, Marie and Pierre wrote thirty-two papers within a period of five years, from 1899 to 1904. She ultimately showed that radium was two million times more active than uranium, that three different types of rays emanated from them, and that this radiation penetrated almost everything in its vicinity. What Marie Curie termed the "cataclysm of atomic transformation" was a continuing natural process; uranium was converted into radium, radium particles expelled atoms of helium with enormous force and were themselves broken down into polonium and other radioactive elements. These destroyed themselves in measurable or calculable periods of time which never varied. The physiological effects were noted by scientists who studied these effects, Pierre Curie and Becquerel exposed their arms to these radiations and noted that they became burned, severely in the case of Becquerel. The Curies and Becquerel received many honors.

Pierre Curie, who was born in 1859, was killed in 1906, when he was run down by a runaway horse and carriage. Marie Curie was awarded the Nobel prize in 1911. She travelled extensively, teaching and receiving highest honors in many countries. She died in 1934, from aplastic anemia.

The roentgen ray quickly passed through the stage where one delineated coins in a purse, or looked at the skeletons of mice as a matter of interest. It began to be utilized early as a means of diagnosing fractures of the long bones, and was destined to become an important instrument for the advancement of pelvimetry, but the more complicated uses such as visceral studies came later. In time it was used for the diagnosis of pelvic tumors, patency of the tubes, and uterograms.

The progress of radiation was phenomenal, and attempts to treat carcinoma were made. The first to apply x-ray treatment to cancer of the uterus were Pusey and George Pfahler. The latter was Chairman of the department of Radiology at the Graduate School of Medicine of the University of Pennsylvania. In 1903, Abbe[3] was the first to use radium for cervical cancer in America. With the technical improvements in filters and instruments and methods, radium displaced x-ray in many of the therapy cases. In 1904, Danlos made the first reports on the use of radium in cervical cancer. Wickham and DeGrais, in 1906, were among the early men to apply radium to cervical cancer; then came Cheron and Rubers, in 1909, and Duval, in 1911.[4] Now the cyclotron, betatron, atom smasher, isotopes and cobalt are used.

While anesthesia was being more highly developed and radiation was being invented and investigated, surgery was already well developed. although operations then considered very major would be termed as minor procedures today. In general surgery the operator often had to be content with incision or mere drainage rather than indulge in the removal of a diseased organ; for instance, cholecystotostomy was the rule, and practically no cholecystectomies were done. Gastroenterostomy was just beginning to emerge as a very formidable procedure in the management of gastric ulcer; radical gastric resection was practically unknown. It must be remembered that anesthesia still consisted of the use of ether, some chloroform and occasional nitrous oxide. As yet there was no parenteral therapy, no blood transfusions of any consequence, no endocrines and no antibiotics. Neurosurgery was in an embryonal state, chest and especially heart surgery had not yet appeared. In the treatment of shock the Murphy drip was used, and hyperdermoclysis was just coming into use.[5]

It was not very long before these practices became obsolete. Progress in transfusions, endocrinology, increased knowledge of sterility, development of pregnancy tests, discovery and perfection of the "wonder drugs" (sulfa and penicillin), improved clinical pathology, and better hospitals and teaching facilities brought the practice of obstetrics and gynecology to the present day level.

We shall discuss each one of these factors briefly.[6]

Transfusions

Transfusions were done by dissecting the median basilic veins of the recipient and donor, anastomosing them and stopping only when it was thought enough blood had gone to the recipient. Later came the syringe method, and improvements gradually brought us to our present methods.

The improvements came very slowly; the common occurrence of blood transfusion reactions was responsible for the lack of interest in transfusions. It was Braxton Hicks who gave transfusions a shot in the arm when he hit upon the idea of inserting sodium phosphate in the blood to prevent clotting. But reactions continued, and it was not until the turn of the century that transfusions became comparatively safe. It was Landsteiner who showed, in 1900, that there were different blood groups, and that the proper ones could be used with each other without reaction. The sodium phosphate that Braxton Hicks had used at the end of the 19th Century was displaced by the use of citrate in 1914. Then came the blood banks. Incidentally, Landsteiner was given the Nobel prize in 1930. He had discovered by 1928, that instead of four groups there were thirty-six. Further developments occurred, just prior to 1940, when Alexander S. Wiener discovered the Rh factor. Besides helping in transfusions by practically removing all hazards of reaction except for the occasional sub-group, it saved many infant lives by exchange transfusions.

Endocrinology

The endocrine factor in gynecology has become one of the big and important divisions of gynecology. The menstrual cycle was practically understood by the end of the 19th Century. However it remained for the early part of this century (19th) to definitely establish the cycle of changes in the endometrium. This was done by

Hitschmann and Adler,[7] in 1908, who studied uteri removed at various stages of the menstrual cycle. During the previous century there was much controversy as to whether or not there was much loss of tissue during menstruation. This question was convincingly settled in 1915 by Schroeder,[8] who showed that not only was there tissue loss, but that extensive amounts were extruded.

By the end of the 19th Century, the fact that the ovaries controlled woman's reproductive life was generally accepted. As late as 1895, Morris had grafted ovarian tissue in castrated women and restored ovarian function more or less. Then, in 1903, Fraenkel[9] showed that corpus luteum had endocrine activity, which developed in pregnancy and regressed if there was no pregnancy, with recurrence of period. Our modern concepts of menstruation go back to 1923, when Allen and Doisy showed that uterine bleeding followed a fall in the estrogen level in the blood. Then pituitary hormone was found (first by Oliver and Schafer in 1895), which later was pinned down to the posterior pituitary gland by Blair Bell in 1909. Further Palmer and Mocquot showed, in 1940, that the body temperature elevated on ovulation. Liquor of the Graafian follicle was first demonstrated by Stockard and Papanicolaou[10] in 1917. The endocrine field has been one of the most ardently pursued subjects in modern times; libraries of literature have accumulated.

Sterility

Because of better understanding of the physiology of the female organs, and the development of endocrinology together with the progress of all the other scientific subjects in medicine, sterility has become better understood and remedied. Chemical and clinical tests such as the Hühner and the Rubin test have resulted in a systematic attack of this problem that was never possible before the 20th Century. This same knowledge has helped to perfect tests for pregnancy.[11]

Pregnancy Tests

The first laboratory diagnosis of pregnancy was attempted by Voge in the form of a flocculation test and was published in 1926. Two years later, in 1928, Ascheim-Zondek test was devised. In 1930, Hogben devised a test on frogs, results of which were obtained in twelve hours. In 1931 came the Friedman test. In 1943,

Kupperman used immature female rats and could tell the presence of pregnancy in two hours. Many modifications of these tests have been made, the chief aim being the time factor. Some of the tests can now be performed in matters of minutes for a result. However, most of these are still unreliable. It is interesting to examine the history of pregnancy tests, for attempts to diagnose pregnancy by many methods goes back to 1350 B.C. Such tests are recorded on the Berlin Medical Papyrus. One of these tests not only decided if the woman were pregnant, but also determined the sex. In this remarkable test (remarkable because Henriksen has applied this test to fifty cases with a 75 per cent positive and an 85 per cent correct negative result), wheat and spelt were watered daily with the woman's urine. If both grew, she was pregnant; if the wheat grew she would have a boy; if the spelt grew the child would be a girl; if neither grew, she was sterile.

The Egyptians anticipated our present knowledge that urine contained hormones 33,000 years ago. About 400 B.C., Hippocrates suggested that a woman be given hydromel (honey and water) to drink upon going to sleep; if she was seized with tormina (abdominal distention) she was with child, if not, she was not pregnant. The urine in pregnancy, according to Magnus, 13th Century, would float milk, and on the authority of Rueff, 16th Century, would cover an iron needle with black spots. Savonarola, in the 16th Century, stated that from the commencement of gestation to the sixth month, the urine is lemon colored with cloudiness in its surface and a deposit in the center resembling carded wool. Solingen, in the 17th Century, claimed that wine mixed with urine would assume the appearance of water in which beans had been stewed. All these tests from Hippocrates down have not been corroborated by Henriksen, as was the test from the Berlin Papyrus.[12]

Sulfa and Penicillin

Important improvements in therapy that followed the discoveries and progress of bacteriology began in 1935 when Domagk demonstrated the effectiveness of a dye "prontosil" in its action against the streptococci. Soon thousands of improved sulphonamide compounds were evolved. Then penicillin came on the market. It was discovered by Fleming in 1929. It revolutionized the treatment of infections. Today, with the multitudinous antibiotics available for nearly all diseases, mortality and morbidity have been reduced beyond imagination.

Clinical Pathology

The advances due to clinical pathology and microscopy are manifest in untold numbers of newly discovered tumors and clarifications of misunderstood tumors. Up to 1920, Pfannenstiel's classification of ovarian tumors, in 1898, was the accepted standard. Its errors, especially in the field of solid ovarian tumors, were corrected by Robert Meyer in 1915. He described the granulosa cell tumors and later the arrhenoblastoma and the dysgerminoma, and Brenner cell tumors. By 1923, he was able to show elaboration of hormones, in the masculinizing and the feminizing growths. Their malignant or non-malignant potentials were learned. In 1912, histological classifications of the different grades of malignancy were begun by Kermaumer and Schottlaender[13] in Vienna; this work was done on the cervix.

In recent years much has been learned about endometriosis. Cullen and Von Recklinghausen first described this condition. In 1921, Sampson first demonstrated the frequency, importance and significance of endometriosis.[14]

Although much had been learned in the field of pelvic inflammation, such as Noeggerath's clinical reports on gonorrhea, Neisser's discovery of the organism, and Tait's surgical procedure of salpingectomy, patients were still dying too often. Incision and drainage instead of 'ectomy were instituted to avoid this, but to no avail. In 1932, fever therapy was used by Warren and Wilson, without too much success.

Schools and Hospitals

Scientific medicine began in the middle of the 19th Century, yet as late as 1890 conditions were so bad that they fostered fake medical schools, and as many as 161 such schools existed. It was the condition of medicine that prompted Oliver Wendell Holmes to assert, "if most medicine were thrown into the ocean it would be better for mankind but worse for the fishes."

Abraham Flexner made a survey of medical schools for the Carnegie Foundation in 1910, and characterized medical schools in the United States, as "shiftless, heterogeneous and multifarious." There were almost 500 schools in Canada and the United States 100 years ago. In 1910 they were reduced to 166. Today there are only 67, but these are reputable, a distinction that could not be applied before. Going back to the turn of the century, hospital internship was not required. Hospitals rarely extended internship more than twelve or eighteen months for those who participated. In lying-in hospitals internships rarely exceeded four to eight months, usually taken after a rotating internship in a general hospital. Except for complicated cases, few women went to the hospital for delivery fifty years ago. As late as 1935, 37 per cent of all babies were born in hospitals; in 1948, the figure is 86 per cent. In 1910, 40 per cent of the birth certificates were signed by midwives, and, in 1948, the figure was 5.3 per cent.

Medical teaching and hospital standards have risen tremendously in recent years, and central regulating agencies of the medical profession itself form the nucleus of these organizations. Better medical teaching, improved hospital care and better patient care is the result. However, a certain amount of regimentation has resulted, with a tinge of socialization in the offing. To offset this situation, medical insurance groups have been organized with the assistance and direction of physicians themselves. This has become nationwide in its scope, so that for the present the autonomy of the medical profession remains intact.

Progress in obstetrics has paralleled the improvements in gynecology. We shall discuss briefly only the more important conditions.

Toxemia

Around 1900, it was unusual to discover toxemia early in a patient, mainly because women reported late in pregnancy, or did not register at all. As late as 1917, blood pressure was seldom used; the first signs of toxemia noted were often the late signs, such as convulsions. Since eclampsia occurred only in pregnancy, it was argued that the prime therapeutic indication was to empty the uterus, and as soon as possible. As late as 1915, the mortality in many large hospitals was 38 per cent. Their aim was directed toward the pregnancy. However, a few obstetricians began to aim their therapy at the disease instead. E. Gustave Zincke gave veratrum viride with results far better than those of the radical school. His lower mortality was probably due as much to his non-interference with the pregnancy as to the effects of the drugs he used, for the eclamptic patient withstood shock poorly. In 1909, Stroganoff introduced a new idea in the therapy, and after its adoption the death rate fell perceptibly. William and Edgar, in 1910, called attention to the specific liver pathology, a central lobular necrosis. Cause of toxemia is still not known, but early diagnosis and more sensible treatment have reduced the risk of this dread disease.

Puerperal Sepsis

Although almost fifty years had passed since Semmelweis pointed out the cause of infection and its prevention, too many women succumbed to puerperal sepsis at the turn of the century. In 1914, in the United States, 4,664 women died of puerperal sepsis. To this number may be added many more who survived only to become pelvic cripples. In the conduct of labor, vaginal examinations were done exclusively and rubber gloves had only recently been introduced. Once developed, puerperal sepsis ran its course too often to a fatal termination, uninfluenced by nursing care or by attempts at local therapy, such as uterine curettement, hysterectomy, or the ligation of the pelvic venous trunks. The employment of intrauterine douches of alcohol, bichloride of mercury, and carbolic acid were abandoned after the reports of deaths from the absorption of the toxic substances used. There was no specific treatment available for blood stream infection. Trial was made of intravenous administration of antiseptic agents as Collargol, a silver salt, mercury, and even salvarsan was later tried. It was soon discovered that substances in sufficient strength to be bactericidal were inimical to the host. The discovery of antistreptococcic serum by Marmorek, and later of bacterial vaccines by Sir Almroth Wright, gave rise to a hope of cure only to be dispelled after thorough trial and it was not until thirty-five years later that chemotherapy in the form of sulfonamide compounds contributed something of real value. Still later Fleming gave us the first antibiotic, penicillin, which has been followed by many similar molds with their remarkable lifesaving action. Phlebitis and consequent embolism do not inspire the fear they once did because of the anticoagulants, like heparin and dicumarol, early ligation and early ambulation.

Placenta Praevia

Placenta praevia, fifty years ago, was managed by tamponade of the cervix and vagina for control of the bleeding, and upon removal of the pack, dilatation of the cervix was completed manually, version and extraction done. Tight packing was such an important consideration that Dr. Penrose, who was professor of Obstetrics at the University of Pennsylvania around the turn of the century, demonstrated the method of packing in one of his lectures by using a silk high hat which he seemed to pack interminably until the sides were about to burst: "That, gentlemen," he would say, "is the way you should pack the vagina." Even manual dilatation without preliminary packing was practiced by some, yet they apparently knew the danger of this procedure, as indicated in their writing. Hot styptic douches were employed in the effort to control bleeding. Before the seventh month, bed rest and applications of cold to the lower abdomen were used in an effort to carry the fetus to viability. Hydrostatic bags were occasionally used.

The two most rational procedures used up to forty years ago were Braxton Hicks version, which, although it meant a high fetal mortality, was far safer for the mother than manual dilatation, and the second was rupture of the membranes in the marginal previa. This latter is still good obstetrical practice. With the preceding management the mortality was anywhere from 10 to 40 per cent. For many years all cases of placenta previa were terminated the moment a diagnosis was made in order to guard the patient against a sudden hemorrhage which usually meant the loss of the baby in 70 per cent of the cases. Today a more conservative attitude is maintained; the patient is hospitalized, closely observed and prepared for any eventuality, such as the need of blood and cesarean operation. In this approach, not only has the patient mortality been reduced to less than 1 per cent, but the fetal mortality has been lowered to 20 per cent. Until 1912, it was considered objectionable to do a cesarean section for bleeding, especially in low implanted placenta. In 1931, Arthur H. Bill collected 2117 cases from the literature treated in the old way and got a mortality of 9.68 per cent. In 268 cases treated by cesarean the mortality was 1.78 per cent.

The etiology of premature separation of the placenta or abruptio was thought to be associated with trauma almost invariably. Toxemia as a cause was not usually considered. Early treatment comprised rupture of the membranes with or without a cervical pack and uterine stimulants. After cesarean became popular it was used widely in abruptio, but it had been discovered that the more conservative earlier treatment gives better results except in the patient with a long undilated cervix.

An additional factor in the improvement noted today in bleeding cases in pregnancy is the very recently discovered condition of "afibrinogenemia" in which the absence of fibrin prevents the blood from clotting. This condition occurs quite suddenly, particularly in prematurity and in cases of missed abortion. Cases suspected can have a blood test for fibrin within minutes, specially arranged sets for testing are maintained and always immediately available in the maternity, and the fibrin is always held in readiness for use.

Cesarean

In the beginning of this century, dystocia, especially when due to cephalopelvic disproportion, was often first recognized in the second stage of labor, and high forceps and craniotomy were not uncommon. Extensive lacerations, infections, and dead babies or babies with irreparable cerebral damage were the result. Cesarean section was not often done then, because it was contraindicated by actual or potential infection after repeated vaginal examinations and ruptured membranes, and many times after repeated attempts at delivery by forceps. Blood transfusion in cesarean is just as important as the necessary asepsis and anesthesia. With hemorrhage, pain and asepsis under complete control, cesarean has lost the terror with which it was regarded not too long ago. In a way, cesarean section almost belongs to this century, for it was only eighteen years before, in 1882, when Sänger first sutured the uterine incision. After this the death rate was markedly lessened; the mortality in Germany before Sänger's performance was 67 per cent; today it is 0.9 per cent.

Infant Mortality

Infant mortality has decreased appreciably since the early years of this period. In every well managed maternity, the nursery is staffed with pediatricians whose job it is to care for all delivered babies immediately, in fact, in questionable deliveries the pediatrician, or the pediatric resdent at least, is present at the delivery and looks after the baby from the moment it is delivered. Rh-negative babies where the biliruben rises above a certain amount, are given exchange transfusions regardless of clinical symptoms. This one procedure alone has prevented numerous cases of kernicterus. The condition of blindness in infants, retrolental fibroplasia, was found to be the result of excessive and prolonged oxygen given to newborns, the malformations which result from virus infections such as the German measles, and countless other contributions by pediatricians. This information has reduced infant morbidity and mortality tremendously.

Maternal Welfare

Preventive medicine in obstetrics is a comparatively recent addition to the many contributions to its progress. The effort to return a woman after childbirth to a state of health equal to that which she enjoyed before pregnancy, with a normal healthy child, is now known as material welfare. Dr. John William Ballantyne, born in Scotland, studied at the University of Edinburgh and was among the early obstetricians to encourage antenatal care. In the United States, the first attempts to establish adequate prenatal care were in Boston in 1912, under the guidance of Robert de Normandie. Results of preventive medicine have been short of astounding.

At the turn of the century in gynecology and obstetrics, surgical therapy was the foremost line of attack. The operations of gynecology were manifold and every woman presenting the slightest evidence of pelvic illness was immediately subjected to some form of operation. From the time that gynecology began and was recognized as a specialty in its own right, it has advanced very little in technique. Refinements have taken place, but no new major procedures. Today there is a tendency to more conservatism, partly because we have learned that many of our surgical approaches have not yielded the results expected. In some instances this policy has been pursued until very recently. After Sampson's demonstration of the frequency and significance of endometriosis in 1921, complete cure was thought possible only by total castration;[15] today we know that partial operation is just as efficacious in obtaining a cure. Conservatism has been made possible, in many instances, because of help from x-rays and radium, antibiotics and endocrines.

The evisceration operations for malignancy might be considered basically new. The Wertheim operation was very popular and just as radical as it is today except that lymph node dissection was not always done and the death rate was much higher. The Wertheim operation today is used for the early stages of malignancy, and radiation is used for the later stages; in the early part of the century, when it was done with such a tremendous mortality, Bonney of England was one of the foremost exponents of this procedure which he did regardless of stage or gland involvement.

When hysterectomy was done it was usually the subtotal variety, unless malignancy were present when total hysterectomy was performed. In 1945 the author wrote a paper on total hysterectomy in all cases, and without vaginal cleansing. This raised quite a furor. Nevertheless, at about this time gynecologists began to do total operations even though the patient may not have had preoperative preparation for a total procedure. Today subtotal operations are done only occasionally.

In the treatment of cancer cases by radiation it was eventually learned that the procedure was not as innocuous as first believed, and this applied to cases of malignancy with secondary infection. Some observers have found a mortality rate of 1 to 2 per cent in these cases; this is so with radium but not x-rays. With the use of transfusion and antibiotics, the mortality rate has steadily declined. In 1931, cases treated by radium for cervical carcinoma had a relative five year cure of 26 per cent, and Stage One cases alone showed a five year survival of 55 per cent. By 1948 the rates improved to 38 per cent, and for Stage One to 76 per cent. Improvement in these figures is continuing. This is attributed to the propaganda of early treatment and the general application of Papanicolaou smears. Examination of vaginal and cervical smears has been used in the United States more than any other country; in 1950, a professor of gynecology from one of the English schools, while visiting the United

States, was invited to attend a seminar at which cancer and the Papanicolaou smear were being discussed. He was greatly surprised that we never began the treatment of these cases (cancer) without a biopsy first. At his hospital in England, they rarely depended on biopsies or smears, they relied on their clinical judgment almost entirely. They had nothing comparable to the diagnostic clinics in the United States.

The influential gynecologists today have advised radiation for cervical cancer as the treatment of choice to be used by the average gynecologist. For clinics appropriately set up and with the staff properly trained, the surgical and radiation approach is advisable. Such clinics may be found in all the important medical centers. Among those with which the author is familiar is the one at the Pennsylvania Hospital, under the directorship of Dr. Robert A. Kimbrough, who is also Chairman of Obstetrics and Gynecology at the Graduate School of Medicine at the University of Pennsylvania and Professor of Gynecology at the university undergraduate school, with both of which the Pennsylvania Hospital is affiliated. The procedure of lymphnodectomy with uterine application of radium is the approach which Dr. Kimbrough has instituted at the Pennsylvania Hospital, implemented by a team chosen and well trained for this procedure. Although this work is in the experimental stage, it seems that the results will justify this approach. Evisceration operations in the more advanced cases are also practiced at this institution.

Although the tendency is to be more conservative, we are still too surgically minded. However, today we are beginning to stress prevention of gynecological disease; obstetrics has made greater advances in prophylaxis than gynecology, and prenatal care is the chief reason for this progress.

In the first half of the 20th Century, the greatest advances in gynecology and obstetrics are concomitant with the progress of medicine generally and in all its other specialties. This progress is the result of basic discoveries and their improvements.

The percentage of deaths from disease and infected wounds in the various wars is a good index to the progress of medicine: in the Crimean War, about 1800, 27 per cent died; in the Civil War, 1860, 6.5 per cent died; in the First World War, 1918, 1.9 per cent died;

in the Second World War, 1940, 0.1 per cent died. The factors responsible for the lessening of morbidity and mortality in these wars apply also to obstetrics and gynecology.

The discovery of anesthesia, development of asepsis, advances in gross and microscopic pathology, improved hospitals and educational facilities which resulted in the development of clinical and laboratory research, x-ray and radium, antibiotics, and endocrines were fundamentally responsible for the extraordinary progress of gynecology and obstetrics.

First Occurrences and Outstanding Events

Anesthesia became so refined and highly developed in the 20th Century that it has become a specialty in its own right.

Twilight sleep, the first use of morphine and scopalamine in obstetrics, started in 1902.

Trilene was first used in Great Britain in 1939 for obstetrical cases.

Roentgen discovered x-rays in 1895.

Curies discovered radium in 1898.

Landsteiner, in 1900 for the first time, showed different blood groups; this knowledge permitted blood transfusions to be performed without reactions.

Alex. S. Wiener, after 1930, discovered the Rh factor.

About 1945, total hysterectomy replaced the subtotal operation.

Hitschmann and Adler, in 1908, established various cycles of menstruation.

Schroeder, in 1915, established shedding of endometrium.

Fraenkel, in 1903, showed that corpus luteum had endocrine activity.

Doisey and Allen, in 1923, established our modern concept of menstruation (that uterine bleeding followed fall of estrogen level).

Blair Bell, in 1909, showed pituitary hormone came from the posterior pituitary gland.

Palmer and Mocquot, in 1940, showed body temperature elevation on ovulation.

Stockard and Papanicolaou, in 1917, were the first to demonstrate liquor of Graafian follicles.

Voge, in 1926, attempted the first laboratory diagnosis of pregnancy.

Domagk, in 1935, demonstrated the effectiveness of a dye; it was prontosil, and the beginning of the sulfas.

Fleming, in 1929, discovered penicillin.

Robert Meyer, in 1915, described hormonal ovarian tumors, and, in 1923, he described newer ones.

Sampson, in 1921, gave us complete understanding of endometriosis.

Today, early 20th Century, we have high voltage x-ray machines, the cyclotron and betatron, 100,000-volt atom smasher (used as reactor mainly), radioactive isotopes, atomic pile, and cobalt (cobalt replacing super high voltage x-ray machines).

Robert de Normandie, in 1912, established adequate prenatal care (clinics) in Boston.

References

1. Graham, Harvey: *Eternal Eve.* London, Heinemann, 1950, *p.* 612.
2. Graham, Harvey: *Eternal Eve.* London, Heinemann, 1950.
3. Fraser, J. R.: Progress in gynecology in the last twenty years. *Surg., Gynec. & Obst.*, Internat. Abst. Surg., *40*:452, June 1925.
4. *Ibid.*
5. Ricci, J. V.: *Genealogy of Gynecology*, foreword by Schuman, Edward. Philadelphia, Blakiston, 1950.
6. Graham, Harvey: *Eternal Eve.* London, Heinemann, 1950.
7. Hitschmann, F. and Adler, L.: Der Bau der Uterusschleimhaut des Geschlechtsreifen Weibes. Mit Besonderer Berucksichtigung der Menstruation. *Monatsschr. Geburtsh. u. Gynak.*, *27*:1, 1908.
8. Schroeder, R.: Anatomische Studien zur Normalen und Pathologischen Physiologie des Menstruationszyklus. *Arch. Gynaek.*, *104*:27, 1915.
9. Fraenkel, L.: Die Function des Corpus Luteum. *Arch. Gynaek.*, *68*: 438, 1903.
10. Stockard, C. R. and Papanicolaou, G. N.: The existence of a typical oestrous cycle in the guinea pig, with a study of its histological and physiological changes. *Am. J. Anat.*, *40*:159, 1917.
11. Rubin, I. C.: Forty years of progress in treatment of female sterility. *Am. J. Obst. & Gynec.*, *68*:324-333, 1954.
12. Graham, Harvey: *Eternal Eve.* London, Heinemann, 1950.
13. Schottlaender, J. and Kermaumer, F. *Zur Kenntniss des Uteruskarzinoma.* Berlin, Karger, 1912.
14. Sampson, J. A.: Perforating Hemorrhagic (chocolate) Cysts of the Ovary. Their importance and especially their relation to pelvic adenomas of the endometrial type. *Arch. Surg.*, *3*:245, 1921.
15. Fraser, J. R.: Progress in Gynecology in the Last Twenty Years. *Surg., Gynec. & Obst.*, Internat. Abst. Surg., *40*:452, June 1925.

NAME INDEX

SUBJECT INDEX